MRI: A Teaching File Approach

MRI: A Teaching File Approach

JOHN H. BISESE, M.D.
Georgia Baptist Medical Center
Atlanta Magnetic Imaging
(A Division of Health Images, Inc.)
Atlanta, Georgia

McGRAW-HILL BOOK COMPANY

New York St Louis San Francisco Colorado Springs Oklahoma City Auckland
Bogotá Caracas Hamburg Lisbon London Madrid Mexico Milan Montreal
New Delhi Panama Paris San Juan São Paulo Singapore Sydney Tokyo
Toronto

MRI: A TEACHING FILE APPROACH

Copyright © 1988 by McGraw-Hill, Inc. All rights reserved. Printed in the United States of America. Except as permitted under the United States copyright Act of 1976, no part of this publication may be reproduced or distributed in any form or by any means, or stored in a data base or retrieval system, without the prior written permission of the publisher.

1234567890 HAL HAL 89210987

ISBN 0-07-005403-7

This book was set in Palatino Bold by Compset.
The editors were Raymond Moloney and Julia White;
The production supervisor was Elaine Gardenier.
The cover was designed by Edward R. Schultheis;
Arcata Graphics/Halliday was the printer and binder.

Library of Congress Cataloging-in-Publication Data

MRI, a teaching file approach.

    Includes bibliographies and index.
    1. Magnetic resonance imaging—Atlases. I. Bisese,
John H. [DNLM: 1. Nuclear Magnetic Resonance—
diagnostic use—atlases. 2. Pathology—atlases.
WN 17 M939]
RC78.7.N83M75 1988   616.07'57   87-25998
ISBN 0-07-005403-7

CONTENTS

ORBITS/PITUITARY

CERVICAL

LUMBAR

ORTHOPEDIC

CHEST

ABDOMEN

PREFACE

In the summer of 1985, we began interpreting MR studies performed at a privately owned magnet based in the northern part of metropolitan Atlanta. This was the first clinically operational magnet in the area and offered us a unique opportunity to gain early extensive clinical experience with MRI. Within a year, we also began to interpret studies performed on a magnet based in downtown Atlanta. As our experience grew, the number of interesting cases accumulated rapidly. At the time this Atlas was begun, there were no works which attempted to chronicle or archive the interesting teaching cases. The MRI books published at that time were heavily biased toward physics and instrumentation and gave only brief attention to pathology.

The emphasis in this book will be on the MR appearance of the pathology: i.e., "What does it look like?" A second issue addressed here is the wide range of applications in the near future. Although the largest percentage of our day-to-day clinical experience is involved with the evaluation of the head and spine, a significant subset of orthopedic, abdominal, and pelvic cases has developed. The cases presented reflect a private clinical setting, both in a dedicated outpatient facility as well as in a large teaching hospital.

The variety of pathology described in this book is all the more remarkable as these cases were encountered as routine clinical problems, in a community, rather than an academic setting. By concentrating on those disease processes most likely to be encountered in the community at large, this Atlas is an attempt to provide a convenient and practical reference source for MR imaging.

MRI: A Teaching File Approach

1: Craniopharyngioma (.6T)

EXAM: MRI of the calvarium.

CLINICAL INFORMATION: Rule out tumor in 36-year-old female.

TECHNIQUE: Coronal and sagittal T1- and T2-weighted images were acquired.

FINDINGS: There is a large mass arising from the sella into the supersellar region and extending into and compressing the third ventricle. This also shows a secondary high-intensity signal focus, appearing to be cystic, which extends both to the right into the parahippocampal sulci and downward along the clivus. There are several large areas of signal void, probably representing calcification. Large mass with cyst in the areas of calcification is most consistent with a craniopharyngioma.

IMPRESSION: Craniopharyngioma.

DISCUSSION: The craniopharyngioma is a common tumor of the first two decades of life and constitutes approximately 16 percent of solid tumors seen in children. Our sample case is a 36-year-old, slightly older than the normal range. The second peak of patients seen occurs after the age of 50. The tumors rise from the remnants of Rathke's pouch. Calcification is more common in the younger patients. At surgery, a fluid resembling "crank-case oil" is removed from the cystic component of the tumor. The cystic portion of the tumor has a high cholesterol content, which appears as a region of high signal on the T1-weighted images.

REFERENCES: Pusey et al.: *AJR* **149**:383, August, 1987. *Neuroradiology,* Ramsey, p. 90, 2nd ed., 1985.

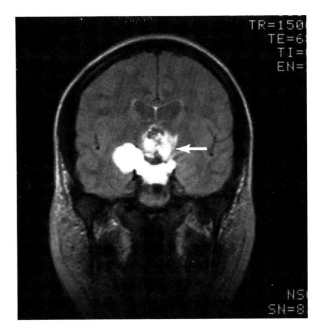

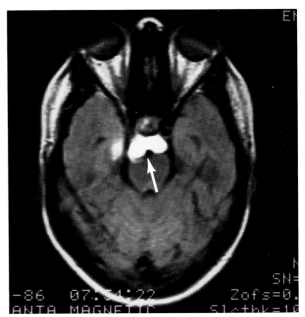

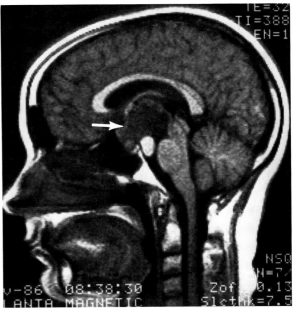

2: Metastases   (.6T)

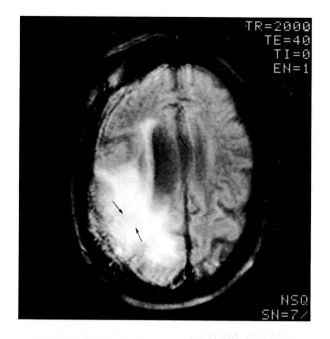

EXAM: MRI of the calvarium.

CLINICAL INFORMATION: 57-year-old with blurred vision, headaches, and clinical question of metastases.

TECHNIQUE: Coronal and axial T1- and T2-weighted images were obtained (2000/31,62).

FINDINGS: As with the CT, a large area of predominantly white matter and increased signal, representing edema, is seen in the right parietal lobe. There is, however, on MR, a suggestion within the central portion of the edema of a less intense area felt to represent a metastatic deposit.

IMPRESSION: Metastases.

DISCUSSION: The contrast seen on the MR images is secondary to the differences in the T2 relaxation rates. At times, however, the surrounding edema and the T2 characteristics of the metastatic lesions blend. This causes the metastatic focus to become invisible. We are unable at present to use an intravenous contrast agent, which is still in its experimental trials; however, with the anticipated appearance of intravenous gadolinium-DTPA on the market, a higher sensitivity to and differentiation of the metastases from edema is anticipated. However, in our experience, we have detected some metastases when CT was equivocal even with intravenous contrast. The ability to obtain images in the coronal and axial dimension with T1- and T2-weighting affords numerous views of an area which may be nonspecifically abnormal on CT.

REFERENCE: Claussen et al.: *AJNR* **6**:669, September/October, 1985.

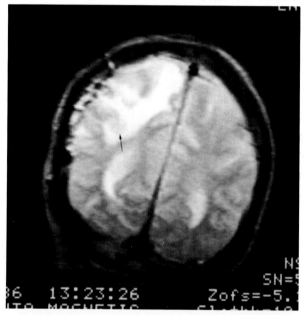

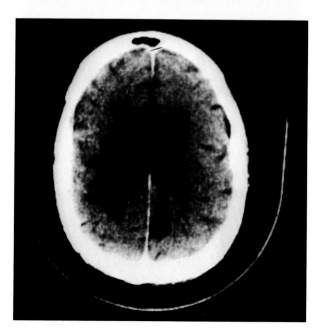

3: Low-Grade Glioma Versus Mesial Temporal Sclerosis   (.6T)

EXAM: MRI of the calvarium.

CLINICAL INFORMATION: 39-year-old with diagnosis of epilepsy since 1978. Recent CT demonstrated an abnormality. MR is to confirm this diagnosis.

TECHNIQUE: Coronal and axial T1- and T2-weighted images were acquired (2000/50,100).

FINDINGS: There is focal enlargement and increase in signal intensity in the right uncus with mild mass effect upon the right supersellar cistern.

IMPRESSION: Findings consistent with an intraaxial mass, such as a low-grade glioma, or possibly a focal area of mesial temporal sclerosis.

DISCUSSION: MR offers several advantages in the evaluation of temporal and middle fossa lesions in the workup of patients with seizure disorders. The most striking is the absence of artifacts normally encountered with CT because of the large amount of surrounding bone in the temporal region. Although, in our particular case, the artifacts do not degrade the diagnostic quality of the CT, there were artifacts on cuts lower to this. In addition, the ability to evaluate these areas in the coronal plane gives a better overall sense of the size of the lesion.

FOLLOW-UP: Low-grade astrocytoma by biopsy. Patient remains seizure-free on medication since these exams and workup.

REFERENCE: Brant-Zawadzki et al.: *Radiology* **150**:435, 1984.

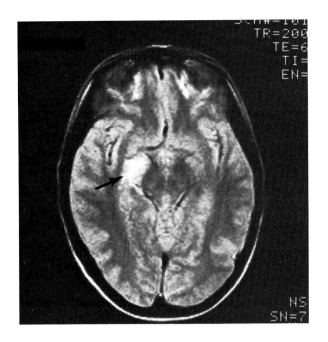

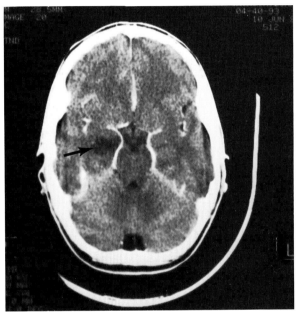

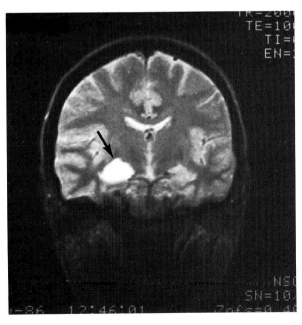

4: Glioblastoma Multiforme (.6T)

EXAM: MRI of the calvarium.

CLINICAL INFORMATION: 52-year-old female with dizziness for approximately 1 year.

TECHNIQUE: Axial and coronal spin density and T2-weighted images were obtained (2000/40,80).

FINDINGS: Soft tissue mass is identifed in and extending through the corpus callosum. There is increased signal on both the spin density and T2-weighted images, and the signal characteristics are heterogeneous, suggesting that internal portions of this tumor may represent calcifications. There is extensive anterior growth of the tumor invading the lateral ventricles. The posterior portions of the tumor are seen to extend into the occipital region, particularly on the right. The large size and aggressive features, as well as crossing of a midline structure, suggest this is a glioblastoma multiforme.

IMPRESSION: Glioblastoma Multiforme.

DISCUSSION: It is estimated that up to 15.5 percent of hemispheric tumors may be missed by CT, as pointed out by the authors of this reference article. We agree with them that MR should be their primary screening modality. In tumors as large as this, the diagnosis would be confidently made on either CT or MR. Of note in this case are the areas of decreased signal, representing calcification within the tumor. Also, our second reference, a paper presented at the 1987 ASNR meeting in New York, points out that features, already known to the CT investigator, of the gliomas may be graded. The features of corpus callosum involvement, larger amounts of edema, and hemorrhage from multiple cavities all indicate a tendency toward a higher-grade glioma or malignancy. All of these features are seen here, which strongly suggests that this is a Grade IV or a glioblastoma multiforme.

REFERENCES: Lee et al.: *AJNR* **6**:871, November/December, 1985.

Drayer et al.: Paper 96 presented at the meeting of the American Society of Neuroradiology, 1987.

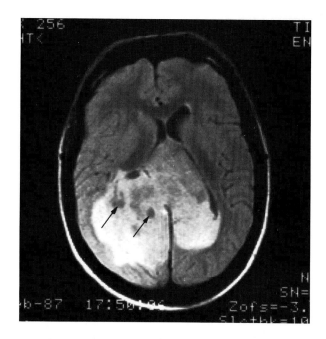

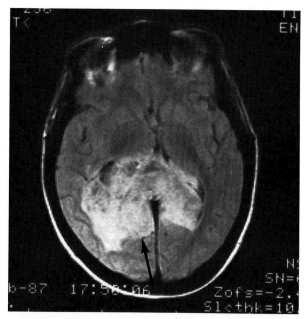

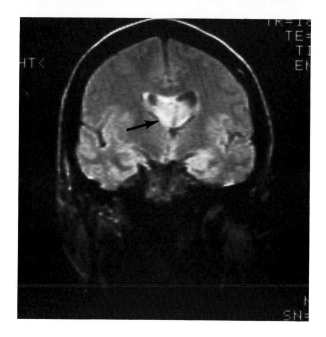

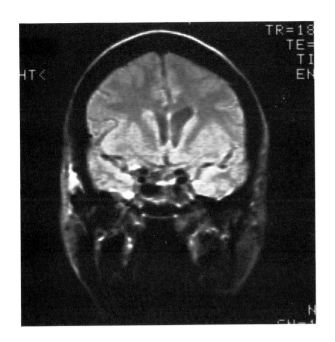

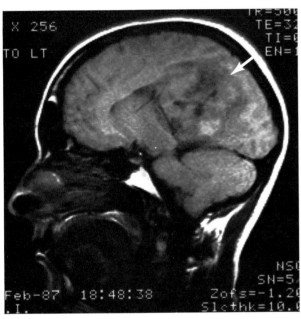

5: Colloid Cyst (.6T)

EXAM: MRI of the calvarium.

CLINICAL INFORMATION: 39-year-old male with headaches, nausea, and hydrocephalus. Rule out a colloid cyst in the third ventricle.

TECHNIQUE: Sagittal, axial, and coronal T1- and T2-weighting were acquired through the calvarium (2000/40,80).

FINDINGS: A rounded cyst-type lesion in the third ventricle with increased signal intensity on both the spin density and T2-weighted images is identified on all three planes. The margins are quite discrete. The lateral ventricles are enlarged with homogeneous increased signal seen surrounding the ventricles. A shunt device is identified with the tip in satisfactory position (not shown).

DISCUSSION: Fairly characteristic appearance of this somewhat rare benign lesion is well-documented on CT and now well-documented with MR. The high signal seen is attributed to the epithelia-secreting tissue of the cyst. Authors of our reference article have published a case in which there is a central low signal which they felt to represent high concentrations of sodium, calcium, iron, copper, and magnesium.

REFERENCE: Scotti et al.: *AJNR* **8**:370, March/April, 1987.

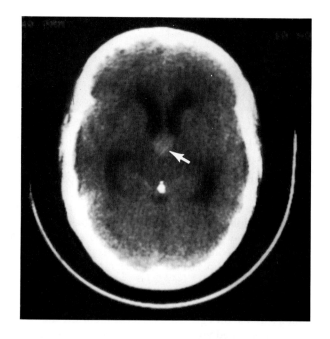

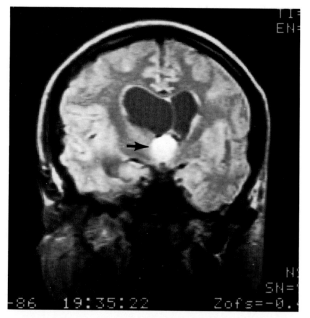

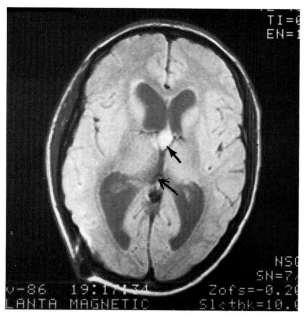

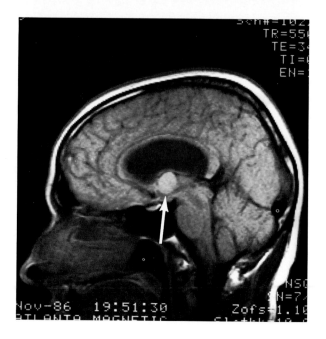

6: Metastases   (1.5T)

EXAM: MRI of the calvarium.

CLINICAL INFORMATION: 47-year-old female with known non-CSF primary malignancy now evaluated for possible CVA.

TECHNIQUE: Coronal and axial T1- and T2-weighting were acquired through the calvarium (2000/35,70; 1500/20,40).

FINDINGS: A well-circumscribed lesion is seen in the left parietal region with surrounding edema. When compared to a CT scan 5 months earlier, there is now marked increased signal in the white matter of the parietal region, extending down into the temporal region and into the occipital lobes. There has also been a dramatic increase in the size of what appears to be a solitary lesion. Mass effect is seen. When compared with the earlier CT scan, there has been an increase in size of a solitary malignant mass as well as increase in the amount of edema seen.

DISCUSSION: MRI is very sensitive in detection of edematous change and shows greater appreciation for the total extent of edema associated with a tumor. In this particular case, a tumor can be well-separated from the surrounding edema, and the excellent follow-up capability shown.

REFERENCE: *Magnetic Resonance Imaging in Medicine,* Volume I, 5/29/84, Bydder.

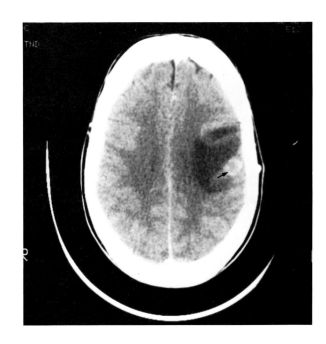

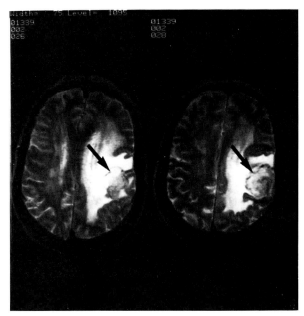

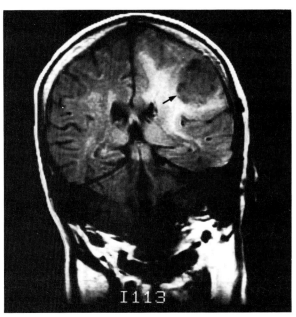

7: Craniopharyngioma (.6T)

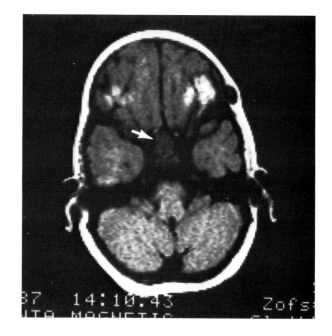

EXAM: MRI of the calvarium.

CLINICAL INFORMATION: Supersellar mass discovered incidentally at time of CT for head trauma.

TECHNIQUE: Axial, coronal, and sagittal views were obtained with both T1- and spin density weighting (500/34; 1000/34,70).

FINDINGS: Mass arising from the sella and extending in the supersellar cistern measures approximately 3 cm in vertical dimension, 2.5 cm in anterior posterior dimension, and 3 cm in maximum transverse dimension. This is extraaxial, and signal characteristics show hypointensity to CSF on the more T1- or spin-density-weighted images and a slight hyperintensity on the more spin-density- to T2-weighted image. The optic chiasm is markedly displaced upward, and the mass is lobulated and evaginates into the hypothalamic region with deformity of the third ventricle. There is nothing to suggest hydrocephalus at this time. Although no evidence of signal void to suggest calcification can be identified by this exam alone; the patient's age and location make the diagnosis of craniopharyngioma most likely.

IMPRESSION: Craniopharyngioma.

DISCUSSION: Fairly dramatic portrayal of this large supersellar mass which is self-evident. Craniopharyngiomas tend to have focal areas of calcification which are not well-demonstrated on this exam alone.

The central nervous system is the most common site of solid neoplasms in the pediatric patient. The increased sensitivity and better evaluation of total tumor volume should add to the management of pediatric tumors. The need for sedation is obvious, but also required, with CT and angiography for workup of tumors.

REFERENCE: Kucharczyk et al.: *Radiology* **155**:131, 1985.

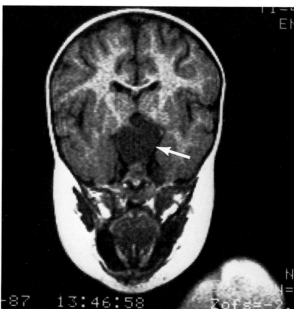

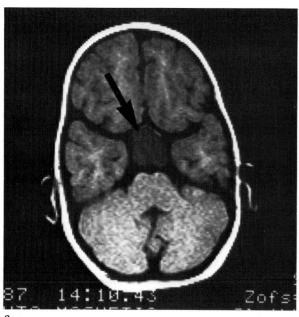

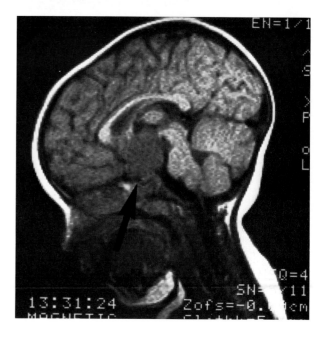

8: Brainstem Glioma (.6T)

EXAM: MRI of the head.

CLINICAL INFORMATION: 20-year-old with brainstem lesion identified on CT.

TECHNIQUE: Axial, coronal, and sagittal images were employed, using spin echo technique (2000/34,68; 1200/32).

FINDINGS: There is increased signal involving the middle cerebral peduncle and extending into the pons with marked mass effect and displacement and flattening of the fourth ventricle. This has the characteristics of an intraaxial lesion as compatible with a diffuse infiltrating mass, such as a brainstem glioma.

IMPRESSION: Brainstem glioma

DISCUSSION: Although the abnormality is identified with the associated mass effect on the contrast CT, the further extent of the lesion is better and more easily demonstrated on the MRI. This remains, in our opinion and in those of our reference-article authors, the modality of choice for evaluation of the brainstem. However, because of the lack of detection of small amounts of calcification, CT is considered a valuable adjunctive modality.

REFERENCE: Han et al.: *Radiology*, **150**:705, 1984.

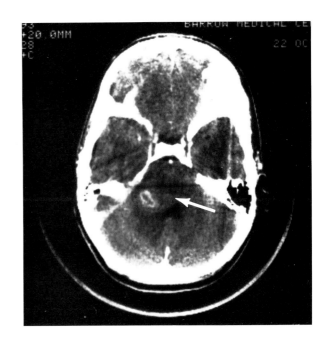

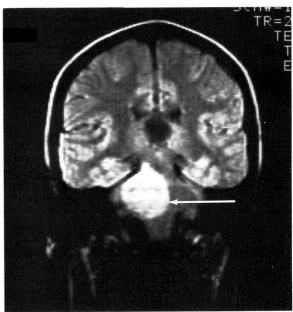

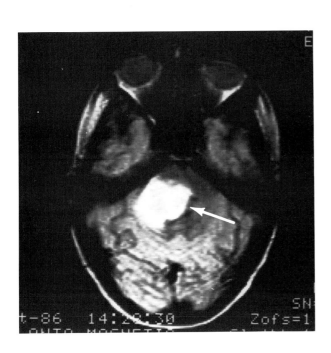

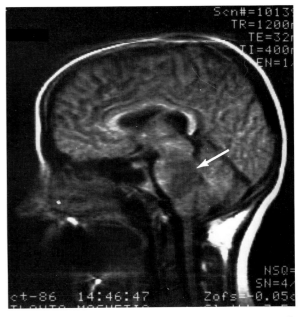

9: False Negative MR/CT Positive for Brainstem Glioma   (.6T)

EXAM: MRI of the head.

CLINICAL INFORMATION: 28-year-old female with a calcified pons glioma. MR requested for futher evaluation.

TECHNIQUE: Axial cuts with spin echo technique were employed (2000/40, 80).

FINDINGS: The study by MR criteria is normal. The calcifications that are well-demonstrated on the CT scans are not identified. Specifically no asymmetry of the pons, cerebellar peduncle, or medullary segment is identified. No hydrocephalus is seen.

IMPRESSION: Normal.

DISCUSSION: Calcification in small amounts without mass effect is repeatedly missed on MR examination. Larger focal pieces of calcification present as areas of absent signal. Despite missing small amounts of calcium it should be noted that MR is usually superior to CT scanning. The calcification, if associated with a mass, is well-detected. Though a case such as this confirms our belief that CT will remain a valuable tool in CNS investigations.

REFERENCE: Holland et al.: *Radiology* **157**:353, 1985.

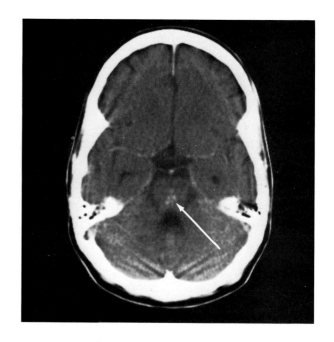

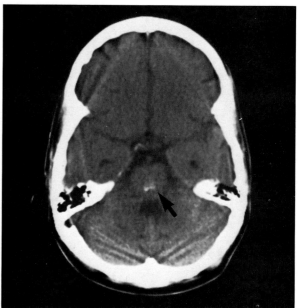

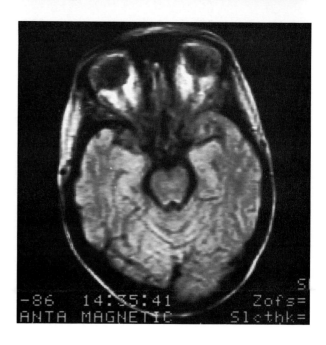

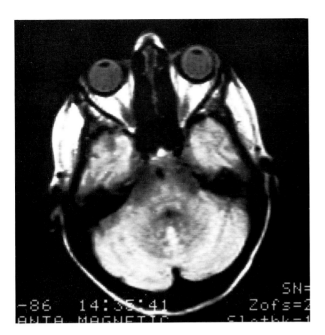

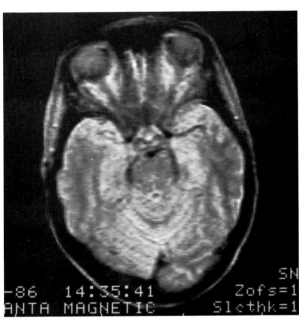

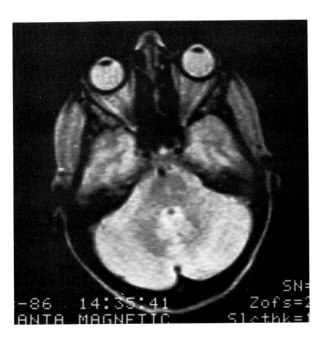

11

10: Glioblastoma Multiforme (.6T)

EXAM: MRI of the head.

CLINICAL INFORMATION: 69-year-old female with left hemispheric lesion.

TECHNIQUE: Axial double-echo and inversion recovery coronal images were obtained (2000/40,80; 1400/34/400).

FINDINGS: A large intraaxial mass is seen arising from the temporal lobe, with increased signal surrounding the mass and representing edema. Marked compression of the ventricular system on the left side with some mild left-to-right shift is identified. No evidence of active hydrocephalus is seen at this time. There are several low-signal-intensity rounded areas within the mass, probably representing cystic areas. Large size, marked edema, and suggestion of cysts raise the possibility of a very aggressive glioma, such as glioblastoma multiforme. Exclusion of a solitary large metastases is not possible.

IMPRESSION: Glioblastoma multiforme.

DISCUSSION: The aggressive nature, marked edema, and presence of cysts within this tumor suggest a more aggressive lesion. The presence of only one very large lesion is more in favor of a primary brain tumor, such as glioblastoma, rather than metastases. Note the cyst within the posterior portion of the tumor which correlates with the CT scan (arrow—image 2).

REFERENCE: Drayer et al.: Paper 96 presented at the meeting of the American Society of Neuroradiology, 1987.

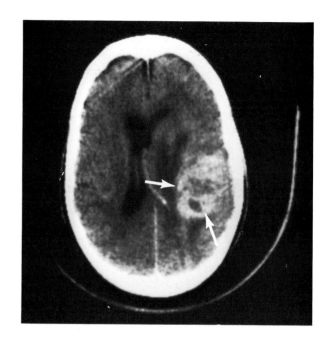

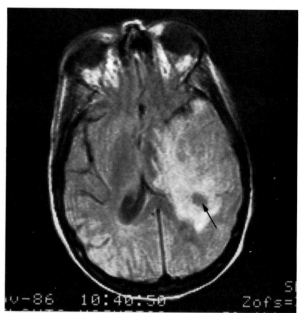

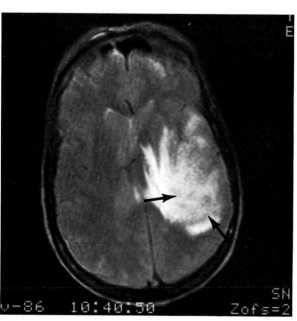

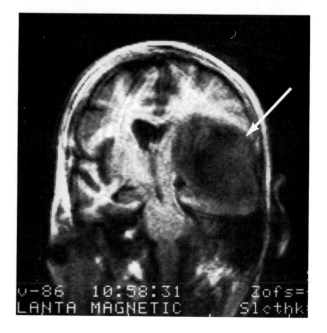

11: Planum Sphenoidal Meningioma (.6T)

EXAM: MRI of the Head.

CLINICAL INFORMATION: 54-year-old female with extremely poor vision in the left eye. CT scan shows a giant cribiform plate or planum sphenoidal meningioma.

TECHNIQUE: Axial and coronal scans were obtained using spin echo technique with a TE40/80 and TR2000 in the axial plane with a TE of 32 and TR of 500 in the coronal plane.

FINDINGS: There is large extradural mass arising to the immediate left of midline from the planum sphenoidal. There is considerable mass effect and a large amount of left frontal lobe edema. The mass has a well circumscribed edge. There are several areas centrally of decreased signal consistent with focal areas of calcification.

   The signal characteristic of the mass is certainly compatible with that of a meningioma. Given the appearance and location of the mass, this confirms a meningioma.

   There is edema involving the basal ganglia and temporal tip as well as the anterior portion of the parietal lobe on the left.

IMPRESSION: Large planum sphenoidal meningioma.

NOTE: The obvious easy visualization of a large mass in relationship to the important structures, such as the anterior cerebral artery and the bony floor of the anterior fossa, is useful for the neurosurgeon as preliminary investigation before resection. Early articles suggested the meningiomas would not lend themselves well to MR imaging. It is true that a very small meningioma with calcium content will appear isointense and sometimes, with even careful scrutiny, the meningioma is invisible with MR screening. It is probably also important to add that meningioma that are small and exert no mass effect are usually of no clinical significance. In contrast, large meningiomas such as this example demonstrate their presence by the related mass effect and surrounding edema.

FOLLOW UP: A meningioma was confirmed at surgery.

REFERENCE: Zimmerman et al.: *AJNR* **6**(2):149, 1985.

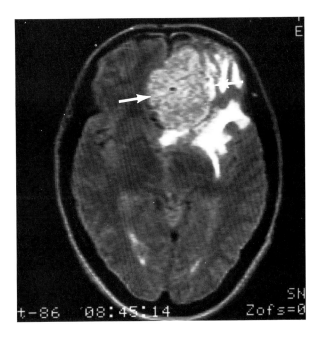

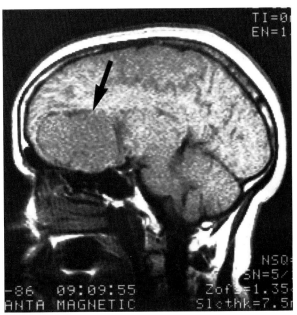

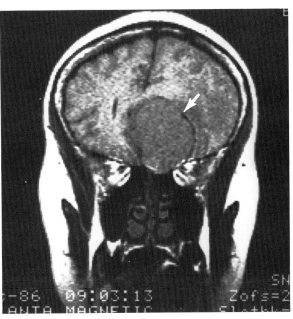

13

12: Thalamic Glioma (.6T)

EXAM: MRI of the head.

CLINICAL INFORMATION: Rule out mass in 69-year-old female with headaches for 3 years. Patient status postplacement of shunt for hydrocephalus.

TECHNIQUE: Axial and coronal T1- and T2-weighted images were acquired (2000/45,90; 1400/34/400).

FINDINGS: A mass is seen in the posterior midbrain on the right which extends into the quadrigeminal plate and superiorly into the thalamic pulvinar. This is slightly hyperintense on the more spin density images and hypointense on the T1-weighted images. There is marked increase in signal intensity with suggestion of small areas of low signal within the mass on the more T2-weighted image. A shunt is also identified and in satisfactory position.

IMPRESSION: Mass involving the right midbrain and thalamus is most consistent with glioma.

Shunt in place. Increased paraventricular signal probably represents altered water content of paraventricular white matter from active hydrocephalus that is now being treated.

DISCUSSION: The coronal view helps sort out the somewhat complicated axial images and demonstrates the entire cranial caudad extent of mass. Note also the ease with which the ventricular shunt device can be identified. Following active hydrocephalus, increased signal may persist in the paraventricular region for months to years. At this time, the size of the ventricles may be a more valuable indicator of the successful treatment of hydrocephalus. We also feel that the high-signal intensity becomes irregular and interrupted in places once the hydrocephalus has been treated, where as in active hydrocephalus, contiguous high-signal intensity surrounding the ventricles is seen.

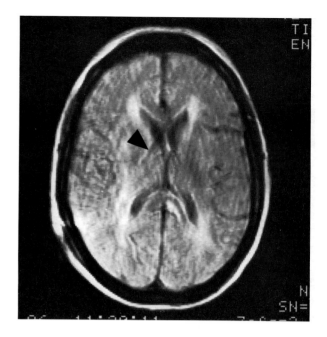

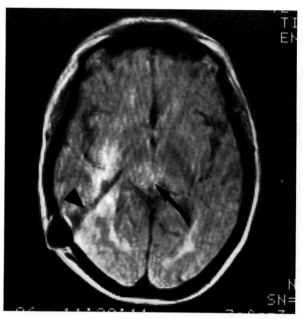

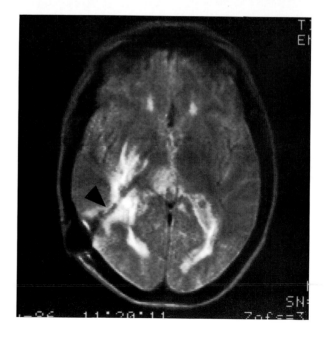

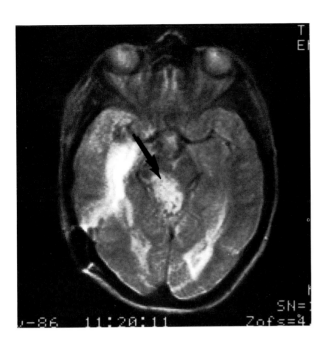

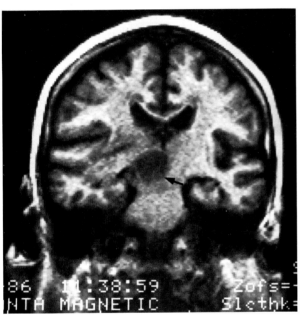

13: Petrous Apex Meningioma (.6T)

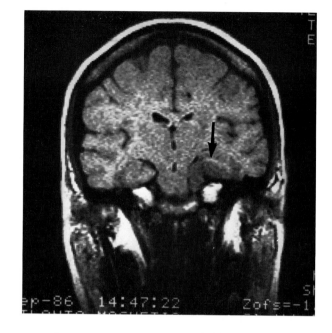

EXAM: MRI of the head.

CLINICAL INFORMATION: 46-year-old female with left-field peripheral vision decrease over past 6 weeks. Rule out brainstem tumor or compression of cranial nerves on the left.

TECHNIQUE: Axial and coronal T1- and T2-weighted images were acquired (500/34; 2000/45,90).

FINDINGS: There is a fairly large dural-based mass arising from the medial aspect of the left petrous bone. This invaginates up into the inferior aspect of the temporal lobe, slightly compressing the left-sided ventricular system. No shift is noted. The mass also produces some mass effect upon the middle cerebral peduncle and midbrain. There is a small rim of increased signal surrounding this mass, which appears to be extraaxial. This increased signal is felt to represent some edema. The mass remains fairly isointense with the gray matter on most of the sequences used.

IMPRESSION: Large meningioma arising from the petrous apex.

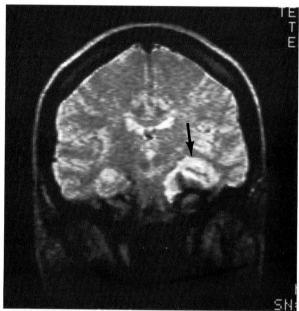

DISCUSSION: On first review, particularly of the axial images, the findings are somewhat difficult to localize. The sagittal and coronal views aid in easy localization of the tumor. The relatively low-signal intensity suggests, but is not diagnostic, of a more benign tumor, such as neurofibroma or meningioma.

The meningiomas account for approximately 15 percent of all intracranial neoplasms and are a common benign intracranial tumor. We feel that most meningiomas are easily detected with MR, despite early literature to the contrary. We agree with our reference article authors in that the tumors are typically iso- or hypointense and that separation of the tumor from the brain is easily made.

REFERENCE: Spagnoli: *Radiology* **161**:369, 1986.

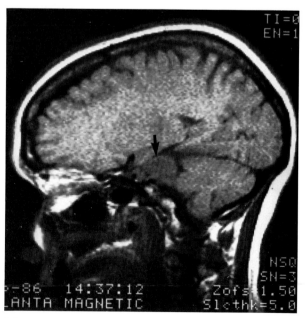

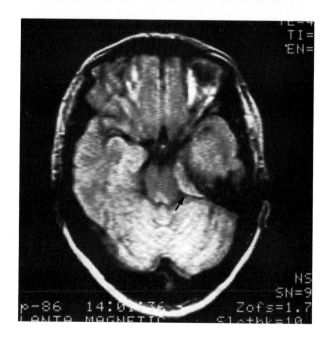

14: Subfrontal Meningioma (.6T)

EXAM: MRI of the head.

CLINICAL INFORMATION: 70-year-old male with dull headaches in the temporal regions and blackout spells.

TECHNIQUE: Axial and coronal T1- and T2-weighted images were acquired (2000/34,68).

FINDINGS: There is an extraaxial mass in the subfrontal region on the right. This is surrounded by high-signal intensity that represents surrounding edema. The mass is seen on coronal views to abut the dural surface of the floor of the anterior fossa.

IMPRESSION: Findings most consistent with a subfrontal meningioma.

DISCUSSION: Aside from a more accurate overall appreciation of the total tumor volume and its relationship to the hemispheres, there is significant information about the major arterial and venous structures and their relationship to the meningioma. Of particular use is the evaluation of the superior sagittal sinus and demonstration of its patency in convexity meningiomas. We feel that many of the points brought up by this reference article, which studies meningiomas only with the high-field-strength magnet, are borne out with our midfield experience.

REFERENCE: Spagnoli: *Radiology* **161**:369, 1986.

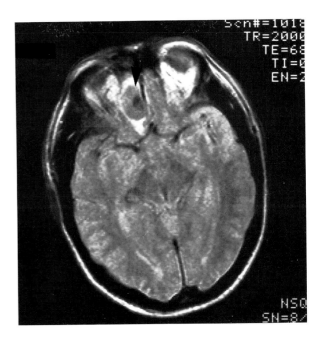

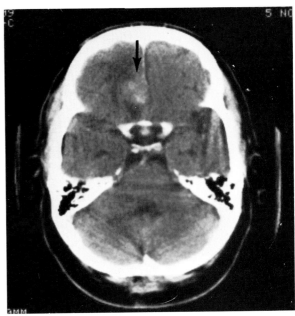

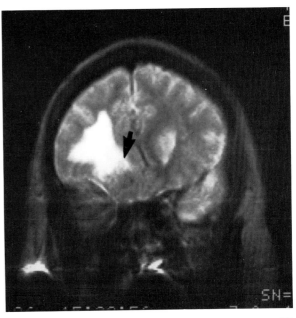

15: Cerebellar Pontine Angle Mass (.6T)

EXAM: MRI of the head.

CLINICAL INFORMATION: 37-year-old female with right sixth, seventh and eighth cranial nerve deficits.

TECHNIQUE: Axial and coronal spin density and T2-weighting were acquired (600/35; 1500/40,80).

FINDINGS: Large extraaxial mass is seen in the cerebral pontine angle on the right. This shows marked mass effect and displacement of the cerebellar peduncle and fourth ventricle from right to left. There is also a significant portion of the mass which invaginates into the anterior portion of the cerebellar hemispheres. Note is made, however, of relative sparing or nonenlargement of the acoustical canal. Also, no hydrocephalus is identified.

IMPRESSION: Large cerebellar pontine angle mass. Differential would include an acoustic neuroma or meningioma. Signal characteristics do not suggest an epidermoid or dermoid lesion. An exophytic glioma is possible, but felt to be unlikely. Important in the differential is a relative sparing of the acoustic canal, suggesting that this, in fact, is most likely a meningioma rather than an acoustic neuroma.

DISCUSSION: We feel, as do the authors of our reference article, that this should be the modality of choice as a primary imaging screen with patients of suspected cerebellar pontine angle tumors. Excellent delineation of the entire tumor size in relationship to the posterior fossa contents is well-displayed in this case. Our experience also parallels that of the reference article authors in that the size, shape, location, and morphologic features are of more help in the differential diagnosis than the various signal intensities on the different T1- and T2-weighted parameters.

REFERENCE: Gentry et al.: *Radiology* 162:513, 1987.

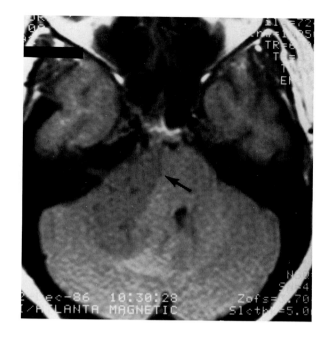

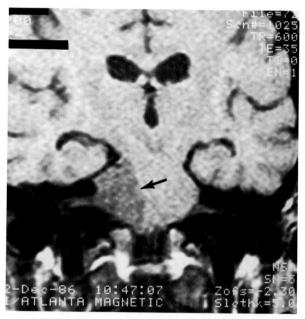

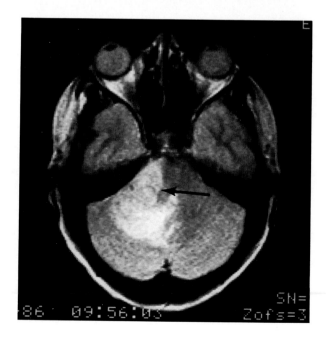

16: Sphenoid Wing Meningioma (.6T)

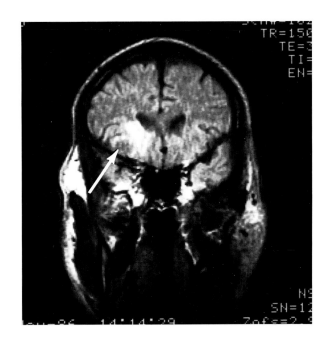

EXAM: MRI of the head.

CLINICAL INFORMATION: 49-year-old male with headaches for 3 weeks and throbbing in the right temporal region.

TECHNIQUE: Axial, coronal, and sagittal T1- and T2-weighted images were obtained (1500/40,80; 1400/34/400).

FINDINGS: An extraaxial lesion arising from the sphenoid bone is seen with associated surrounding high signal, representing edema. The mass is demonstrated on coronal and sagittal views to be extraaxial and invaginates into the overlying frontal lobe. There is some mild mass effect on the right lateral ventricle but no significant midline shift.

IMPRESSION: The findings are most consistent with a sphenoid wing meningioma and surrounding edema.

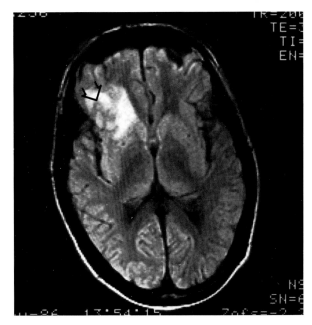

DISCUSSION: As per our reference article and our example, the inversion recovery sequence shows the meningioma as a hypointense mass, and there is good display of the meningioma in relation to the sphenoid wing or dural surface. Meningiomas represent a common, benign intracranial neoplasm. Early MR literature suggests that meningiomas avoid detection because of the amount of calcium causing them to remain isointense to the brain matter. We feel, as do the reference authors, that tumors of clinical significance are easily detected with MR because of the associated mass effect and edema. Small meningiomas creating no mass effect are usually incidental and of no clinical significance.

REFERENCE: Zimmerman et al.: *AJNR* **6**:149, March/April 1985.

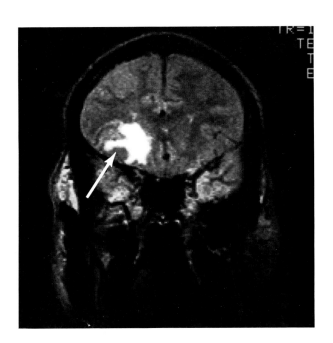

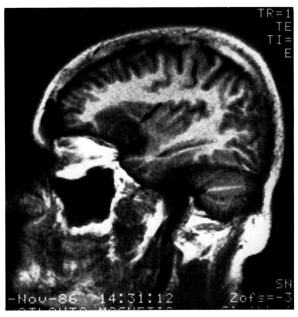

17: Calcification in Brainstem—Probable Glioma (.6T)

EXAM: MRI of the calvarium.

CLINICAL INFORMATION: 60-year-old with sudden inability to walk.

TECHNIQUE: Axial T1- and T2-weighted images were obtained (3000/32,64).

FINDINGS: Within the right brainstem, there is a lobulated area of low signal involving the pons and right middle cerebral peduncle. There is a small amount of enlargement of the brainstem. Differential between a heavily calcified brainstem glioma and a heavily calcified AVM.

IMPRESSION: Large calcification within the brainstem most likely representing a glioma versus a heavily calcified AVM.

REFERENCE: Bydder et al.: *JCAT* **9**:690, July/August, 1985.

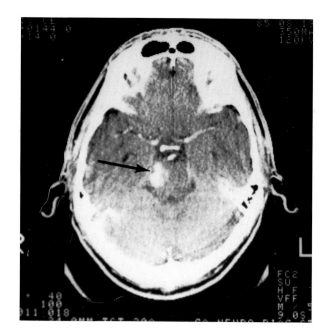

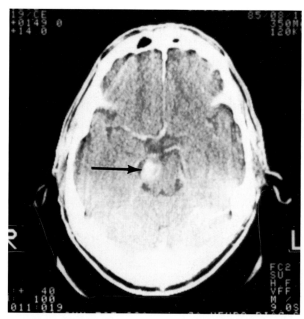

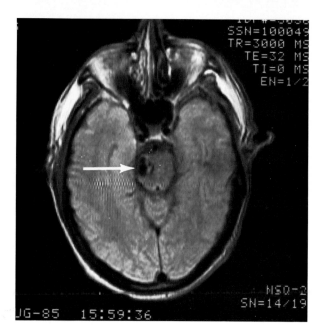

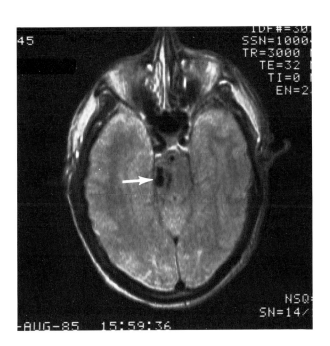

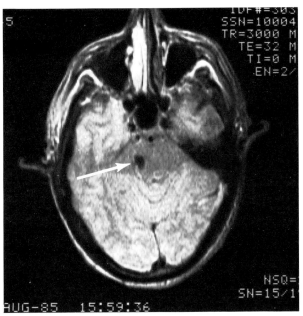

18: Angiosarcoma of the Frontal Lobe (.6T)

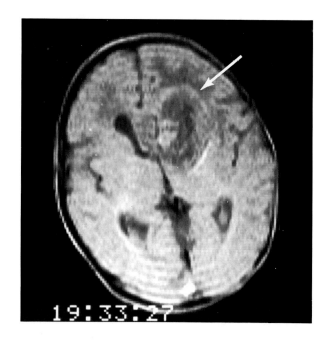

EXAM: MRI of the calvarium.

CLINICAL INFORMATION: 8-week-old male infant. Rule out intracranial mass.

TECHNIQUE: (2000/45,90; 1200/38/400; 600/32).

FINDINGS: A large left frontal mass with marked mass effect upon the ventricular system is identified. The large size of this mass raises the possibility of a neuroectodermal tumor or other primary glioma. Suspect very aggressive tumor histologically secondary to large size.

IMPRESSION: Large left frontal mass with peripheral areas of increased signal consistent with large primary tumor, probably with areas of hemorrhage. This shows marked mass effect. This correlates well with CT scan done 2 days earlier. Findings are of most concern for a very aggressive brain glioma or possibly a primitive neuroectodermal tumor. A gliosarcoma should also be included in the differential.

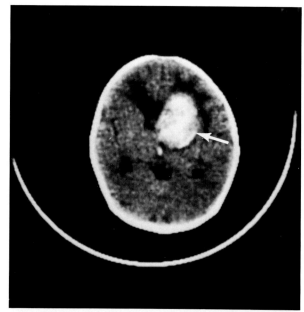

CONFIRMATION: Angiosarcoma was removed. The features of the postop intracranial study demonstrate a large CSF-filled space where the tumor was resected. On the coronal images, there was development of a subdural hematoma.

Surgical and autopsy specimen again confirm the diagnosis of an angiosarcoma.

REFERENCE: New et al.: *AJR* **147**:985, November 1986.

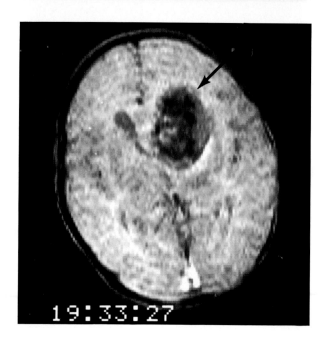

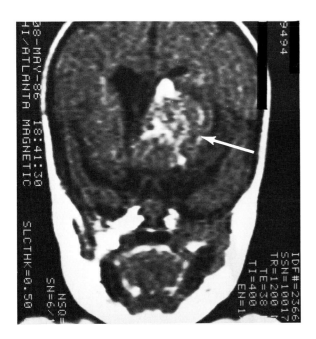

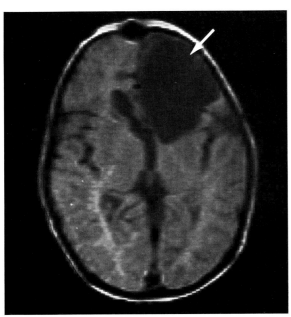

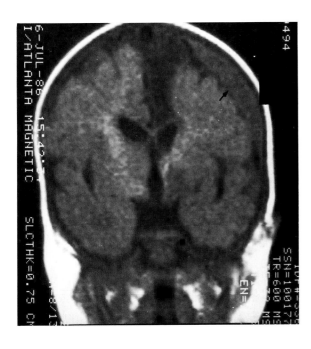

19: Temporoparietal Meningioma (1.5T)

EXAM: MRI of the calvarium.

CLINICAL INFORMATION: Evaluation of a right-sided mass in a 62-year-old female.

TECHNIQUE: Axial and coronal T1- and T2-weighted images were acquired (2000/20,70; 2100/30,100).

FINDINGS: A dural-based mass, very low signal similar to that of the cortical bone, is identified in the right temporoparietal region. There are some peripheral increased signals suggesting some surrounding edema. Finding is consistent with a meningioma.

IMPRESSION: Right temporoparietal meningioma.

DISCUSSION: Gadolinium-DTPA is a promising experimental contrast agent; however, the authors have compared sensitivities and emphasize the usefulness of an inversion recovery sequence with or without contrast to increase detection when a clinical diagnosis of meningioma is suspected. The authors also suggest that there are two groups of meningiomas: the "soft tumor" with a high level of contrast on T1- and T2-weighting and a "hard tumor" group showing the best contrast between tumor and brain on the inversion recovery sequences.

REFERENCE: Altman et al.: *AJNR* **6**:15, January/February, 1985.

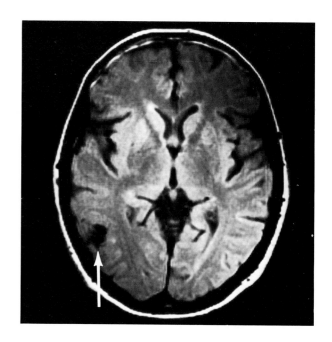

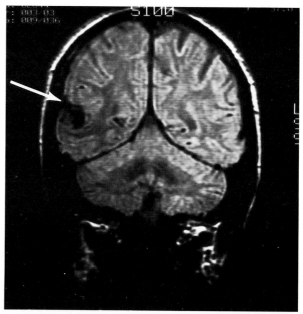

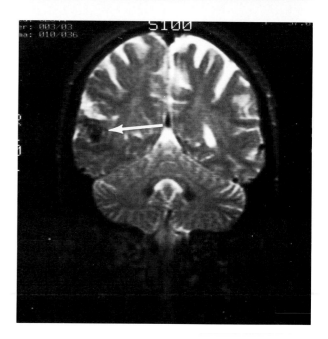

20: Anterior Falx Meningioma   (1.5T)

EXAM: MRI of the cranium.

CLINICAL INFORMATION: 39-year-old female evaluated for right hemifacial pain.

TECHNIQUE: Axial T1- and T2-weighted images were acquired (2000/20,40).

FINDINGS: A focal area of increased signal intensity is seen adjacent to the anterior medial falx on the right side. This is abnormal and correlates with an area of enhancement on CT.

IMPRESSION: Findings are consistent with an anterior falx meningioma.

DISCUSSION: This is a case in which the conspicuity of the lesion is greater on CT than MRI. The initial examination of the MRI failed to detect this lesion; however, with the CT scan and re-review, the lesion is apparent.

REFERENCE: Bydder et al.: *JCAT* **9**:690, July/August, 1985.

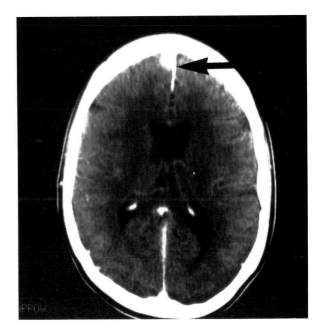

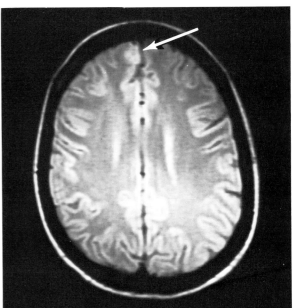

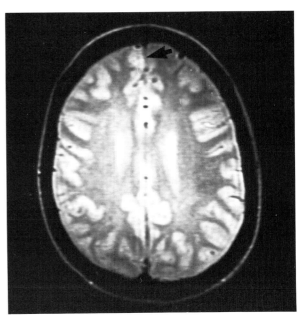

21: Cystic Glioma   (1.5T)

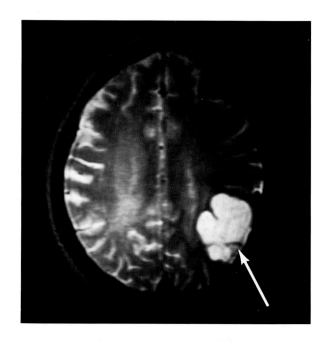

EXAM: MRI of the calvarium.

CLINICAL INFORMATION: This is a 60-year-old female with a predominantly cystic mass identified on CT.

TECHNIQUE: Coronal and axial T1- and T2-weighted images were acquired (2000/40,80).

FINDINGS: Predominantly cystic lesion with areas of lower intermediate signal radiating through and consistent with septations. In addition, there is a small area of solid structure in the posterior aspect of the cystic structure, suggesting a mural thrombus. Findings are most consistent with a cystic glioma. Hydatid disease was considered but excluded by history.

IMPRESSION: Cystic parietal mass with a small amount of soft tissue in the posterior area. Findings consistent with low-grade cystic glioma.

CONFIRMATION: A CT-guided biopsy yielded only CSF from the cystic component of the tumor.

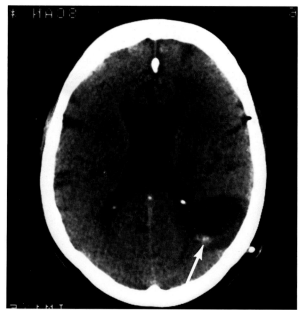

DISCUSSION: The T1- and T2-weighted images of cystic lesions in the cranium can be studied and used to increase specificity. Our reference article and example show that arachnoid and postoperative cysts remain isointense to that of the cerebral spinal fluid and that this cerebral spinal fluid within the ventricles and cisterns can be used as a ready reference. There is increased signal or prolongation of T2-weighting when there is increased protein within the cyst. These can represent inflammatory or tumoral change.

REFERENCE: Kjos et al.: *Radiology* **155**:363, 1985.

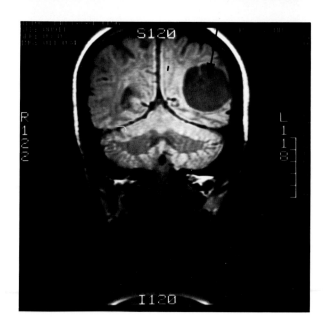

22: Intracranial Lymphoma (.6T)

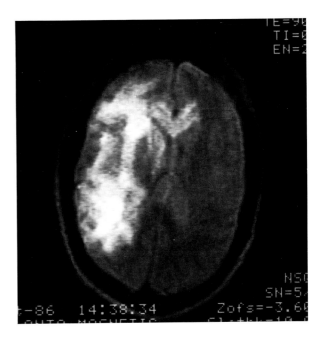

EXAM: MRI of the calvarium

CLINICAL INFORMATION: 39-year-old with 3-week history of dropping objects with left hand. Inability to lift left foot.

TECHNIQUE: Axial T1- and T2-weighted images were obtained (2000/40,90).

FINDINGS: Diffuse increased signal throughout the white matter with sparing of the peripheral cortical matter is identified in the frontal, parietal, and temporal regions on the right side. This is associated with mass effect and midline shift of the ventricular system. Finding is consistent with a diffuse infiltrating malignancy. No focal malignancy can be separated from the increased signal of edema.

IMPRESSION: Findings consistent with a diffuse infiltrating process, such as a glioma.

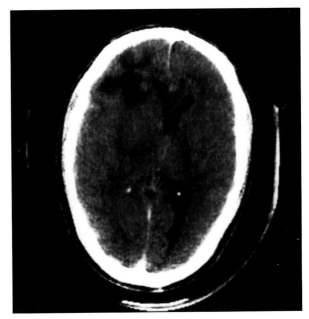

DISCUSSION: CT and MR are nonspecific; however, the relative sparing of the gray matter, better shown on MR, helps in confirming the suspicion of an infiltrative process. By history, patient had no findings to suggest inflammatory change, such as cerebritis, which would be hard to differentiate from the images submitted.

CONFIRMATION: Intracranial lymphoma was found following resection of the right frontal lobe.

REFERENCE: Lee et al.: *AJNR* 7:599, July/August, 1986.

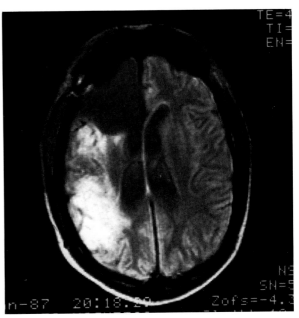

23: Left Temporal Glioma (.6T)

EXAM: MRI of the calvarium.

CLINICAL INFORMATION: Rule out intracranial mass in a male patient with left-sided weakness and abnormal CT.

TECHNIQUE: Coronal, axial, and sagittal T1- and T2-weighted images were acquired (2000/60; 700/32; 500/32).

FINDINGS: Intraaxial mass which sits within the right temporal region can be separated more easily on the spin density T1-weighted images. There is a marked amount of edema and mass effect with shift of the uncus toward the midline. Extensive amount of edema is seen extending through the white matter of the temporal, parietal, and occipital regions. The presence of an intraaxial mass, which is quite large with large amount of surrounding edema, is consistent with glioma. The size, degree of edematous change, and mass effect suggest a more malignant grade of glioma, such as a glioblastoma multiforme.

IMPRESSION: Left temporal glioma, probably glioblastoma multiforme.

DISCUSSION: Although the CT scan clearly defines abnormally swollen temporal and parietal lobes, the MR, particularly on coronal and sagittal Images, finds the intraaxial mass. The separation of the tumor mass and edema is more difficult on the T2-weighted images.

REFERENCE: Claussen et al.: *AJNR* **6**:669, September/October, 1985.

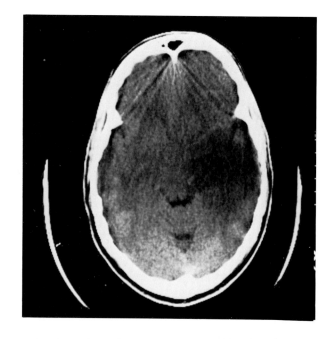

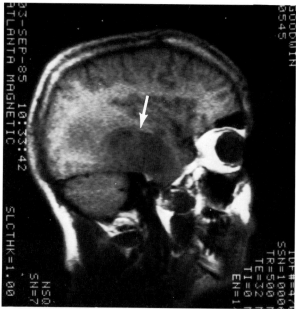

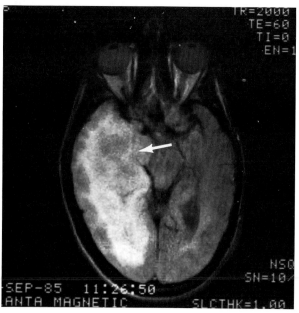

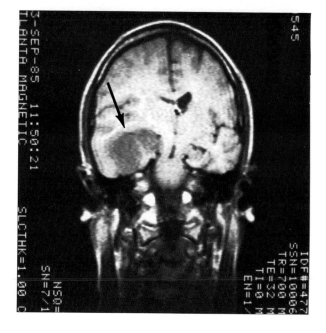

24: Medulloblastoma   (.6T)

EXAM: MRI of the calvarium.

CLINICAL INFORMATION: This is a 2-year-old with a posterior fossa mass.

TECHNIQUE: The images include a pre- and postoperative study, approximately 1 year apart. Axial and sagittal T1- and T2-weighted images were acquired (2000/45,90; 1500/38; 1200/32/400).

FINDINGS: A midline posterior fossa mass arising from the vermian region with marked compression of the fourth ventricle is identified. There is also a rounded mass in the suprasellar cistern. This is consistent with a medulloblastoma given the location and patient's age. A second suprasellar mass represents a CSF metastasis.

   The postop follow-up shows the more normal appearance of the posterior fossa with reexpansion of the fourth ventricle following resection. Note the placement of a shunt prior to surgery.

CONFIRMATION: Medulloblastoma removed at surgery.

REFERENCE: Kucharczyk et al.: *Radiology* **155**:131, 1985.

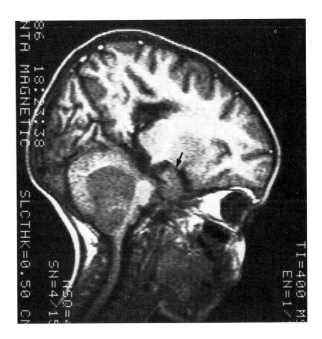

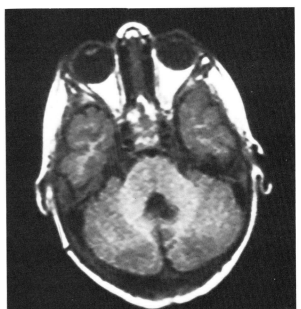

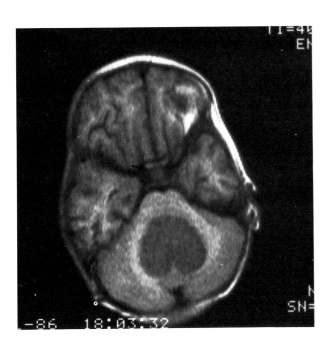

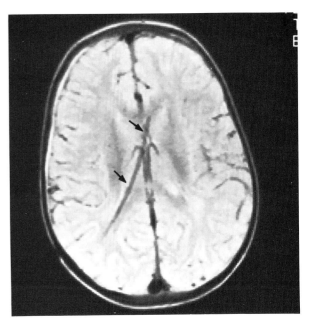

25: Facial Neuroma   (.6T)

EXAM: MRI of the head.

CLINICAL INFORMATION: 57-year-old male with right facial twitching for 3 years.

TECHNIQUE: Axial and coronal thin sections were obtained with spin density weighting (1500/30,60; 1000/35).

FINDINGS: The intracranial portion of the study was normal; however, in the petrous bone along the expected course of the descending facial nerve canal, there is definite asymmetric signal on the right side. There is a very high signal intensity identified. This is round and extends down into the stylohyoid foramina. The signal intensity follows along the expected descending canal of the facial nerve.

IMPRESSION: Right-sided abnormal signal consistent with small neuroma along the descending portion of the facial nerve. Maxillary sinusitis also noted.

DISCUSSION: The normal structures of the petrous bone show very little or no signal intensity, allowing abnormalities to stand out as in this case. Confirmatory high-resolution thin-section computer tomography for bone detail is felt to represent a prudent complementary study.

REFERENCE: Teresi et al.: *AJR* **148**:995, May, 1987.

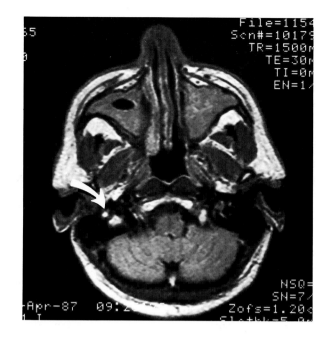

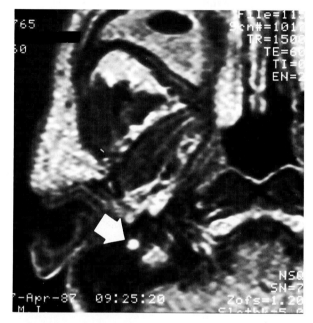

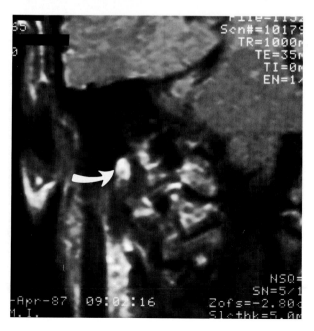

26: Glomus Jugulare Tumor (.6T)

EXAM: MRI of the head.

CLINICAL INFORMATION: 35-year-old female with signs and symptoms of posterior fossa mass.

TECHNIQUE: Axial and coronal imaging were acquired (2000/20,40; 2000/35,70).

FINDINGS: A large mass which has destroyed and invaded the medial petrous bone, and extended out into the cerebral pontine angle with marked evagination of the cerebellar peduncle and the anterior portion of the right cerebellar hemisphere, is identified. There is a separate focal rounded mass posterior to the larger extraaxial mass which shows high-signal intensity and a fluid level. No other lesions are seen and no evidence for hydrocephalus is identified.

Differential includes that of a very large acoustical neuroma or extensive meningioma with areas of bleeding and cyst formation. Also epidermoid or dermoid tumors could not be excluded. Because of the course, location, and extensive bony destruction, glomas jugulare tumor should also be considered.

DISCUSSION: The obvious ease of demonstrating a cerebral pontine angle tumor in relation to the bone is seen here.

The glomus jugulare tumor is a glomus tumor arising from the periganglianic cells or glomus body present along the jugular bulb which follows along the course of Jacobson's nerve. These patients usually complain of a pulsing tinnitus and hearing loss. These tumors tend to grow along the plane of least resistance, but can be associated with marked bony destruction.

The cystic formation posterior to the mass with the fluid level represents old hemorrhage. The dens are a black inferior portion representing the now separated heme with its iron molecule and the bright superior portion is the high-protein liquid portion of the clot.

REFERENCE: Daniels et al.: *AJNR* **6**:669, September/October, 1985.

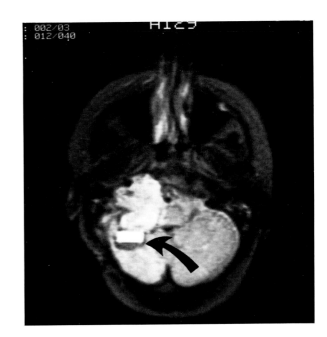

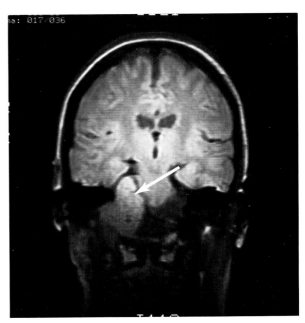

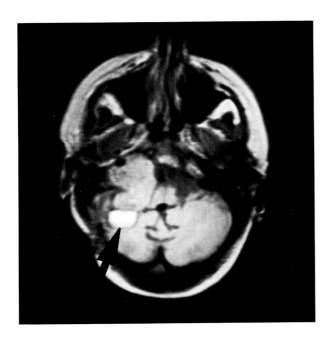

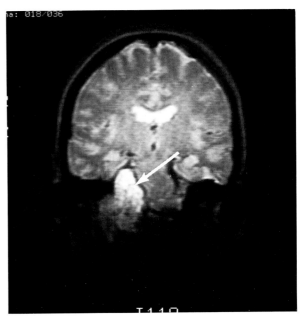

27: Petrous Apex Cholosteatoma (1.5T)

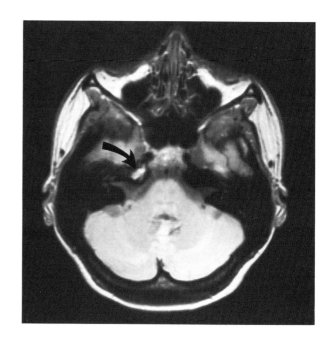

EXAM: MRI of the cranium.

CLINICAL INFORMATION: 47-year-old female with evaluation to rule out cause of headaches.

TECHNIQUE: Coronal and axial T1- and T2-weighted images were acquired (2000/20,40; 2000/40,80).

FINDINGS: Incidental note is made of a well-circumscribed area of increased signal in the right petrous bone tip. This is well-surrounded by low-signal intensity suggesting intact bone. Internal auditory canals are also well-displayed and appear intact and symmetric. The area of increased signal within the petrous apex is most consistent with a small cholesteatoma.

IMPRESSION: Right temporal bone petrous apex cholesteatoma.

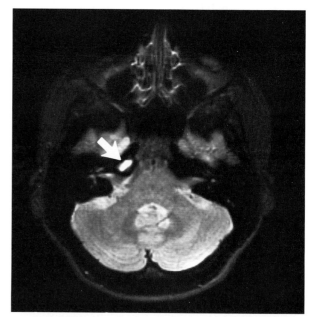

DISCUSSION: Small benign tumors typically found within the petrous apex include epidermoids, which are predominantly masses of epithelium. Dermoids, another common tumor in this region, include both the epithelium as well as hair follicles and other components of the skin. Both types of tumors exhibit increased signal intensity on both T1- and T2-weighting. This mass can be confirmed on the coronal views as well as on examining the T2-weighted images which depress the bone marrow signal within the clivus and condylar regions.

REFERENCE: Latack et al.: *Radiology* **157**:361, 1985.

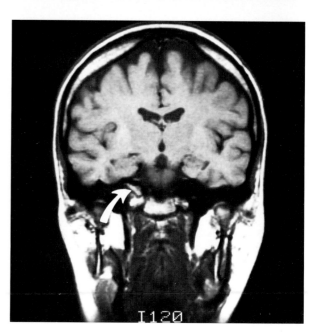

28: Small Acoustic Neuroma (.6T)

EXAM: MRI of the internal auditory canals.

CLINICAL INFORMATION: 41-year-old with left facial paralysis. Rule out left acoustic neuroma.

TECHNIQUE: Thin section and routine double-echo axial and coronal views were obtained through the calvarium and region of the internal auditory canals.

FINDINGS: There is a focal area of increased signal in the internal auditory canal on the left side. This is identified on both axial and coronal views. This region shows slight increase in signal intensity on the T2-weighted images.

IMPRESSION: Findings consistent with a small intercanalicular left acoustic neuroma.

DISCUSSION: The removal of the bone-averaging artifact and need for contrast injection either of air- or water-soluble contrast highlight the desirability of MR in this area of imaging. In addition, the inherent high-signal intensity of the tumor contrasts nicely to the low or absence of signal seen in the region of the petrous bones. The preferred technique by most investigators now is to accentuate the CSF-brain contrast and forgo the need for any T2-weighted images.

REFERENCE: New et al.: *AJNR* **6:**165, March/April, 1985.

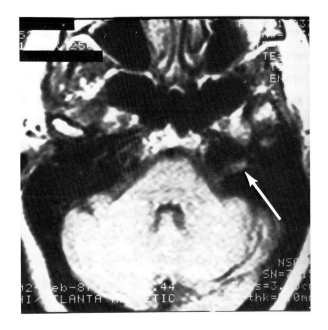

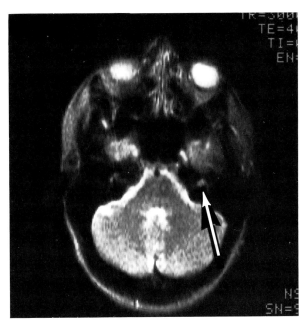

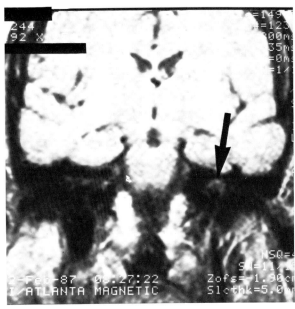

29: Gliosarcoma   (.6T)

EXAM: MRI of the calvarium

CLINICAL INFORMATION: 3-year-old with a partially resected gliosarcoma.

TECHNIQUE: Axial and sagittal views were obtained (2000/45,90; 525/34).

FINDINGS: A large parietal tumor ranging from 5 to 6 cm and extending into the left cerebral peduncle and midbrain is identified. Superior to the tumor is a 4-cm cyst like area. This represents the area of prior tumor resection. In addition, a subdural collection along the left parietal occipital region is noted.

IMPRESSION: Partially resected tumor by histologic specimen proven to be a gliosarcoma.

DISCUSSION: The cystic area can be separated from the residual tumor. The cystic region of resection stands out well, but the tumor is poorly seen on the sagittal T1-weighted images. Note made of the subdural collection in the region of prior surgery.

REFERENCE: Jack et al.: *AJNR* 8:117, January/February, 1987.

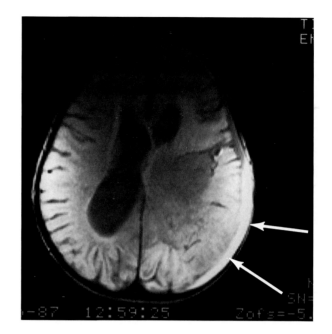

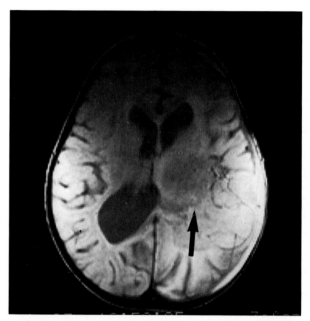

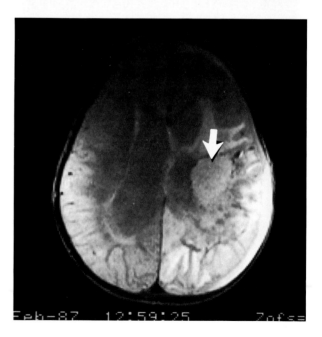

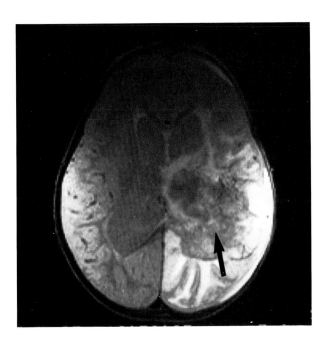

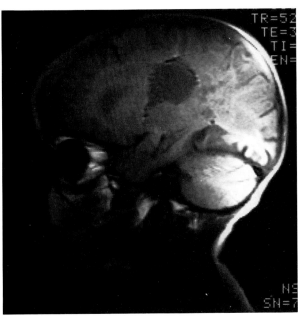

30: Carbon Monoxide Poisoning (.6T)

EXAM: MRI of the cranium.

CLINICAL INFORMATION: This is a 25-year-old male with schizophrenic behavior. Patient has had a history of carbon monoxide poisoning.

TECHNIQUE: Axial T1- and T2-weighted imaging was obtained (2000/20/90).

FINDINGS: Paired areas of increased signal in the globus pallidus are identified. The remainder of the exam is normal. The presence of paired increased signal in the basal ganglia is consistent with damage to it. The location and symmetry is consistent with an anoxic episode, such as seen in carbon monoxide poisoning.

IMPRESSION: Paired infarctions to the globus pallidus are consistent with an acute anoxic event, commonly seen in carbon monoxide poisoning.

DISCUSSION: Carbon monoxide toxicity can be seen as areas of necrosis—as in our case, in the globus pallidus. Additionally, lesions in the white matter or hippocampus can be identified. The symmetry of these lesions helps rule out differential consideration of other forms of inflammatory or demyelinating disease. Our case agrees with that of our reference article in that MR is very sensitive to the early changes from such anoxic events.

REFERENCE: Horowitz et al.: *Radiology* **162**:787, 1987.

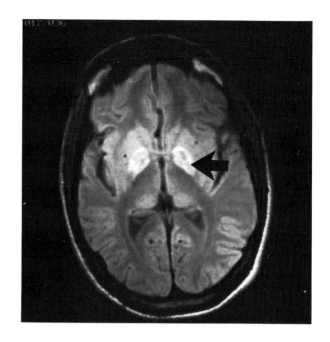

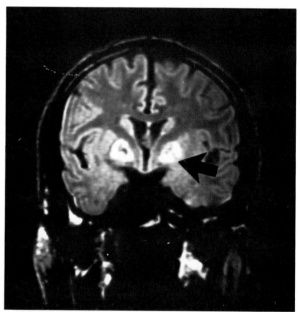

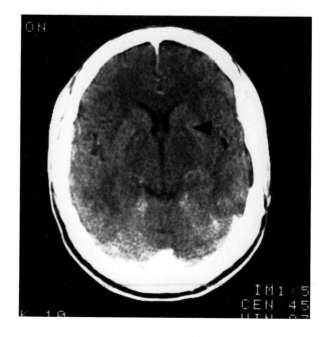

31: Chronic Left Frontal Hematoma (.6T)

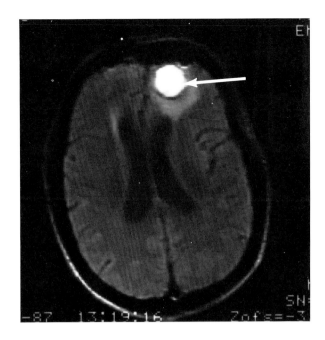

EXAM: MRI of the calvarium.

CLINICAL INFORMATION: 26-year-old with visual problems following severe head injury 2 months earlier.

TECHNIQUE: Coronal, sagittal, and axial T1- and T2-weighted images were obtained (2000/45,90; 550/34; 800/34).

FINDINGS: There is an area of high-signal intensity which is rounded and located within the medial anterior portion of the left frontal lobe. This is surrounded by a very low signal periphery and also by altered signal in the surrounding brain tissue, probably representing edema. This is seen to involve both frontal lobes to a degree.

IMPRESSION: Findings are consistent with chronic left frontal hematoma.

DISCUSSION: This reference offers a way to demonstrate intracranial hemorrhage in a midfield magnet by utilizing a partial saturation technique. The changes encountered in the acute, subacute, and chronic phases of hematoma have already been well-described in high-field articles.

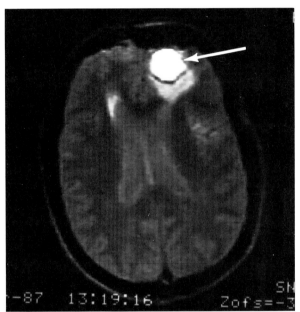

REFERENCE: Edelman et al.: *AJR* 7:751, September/October, 1986.

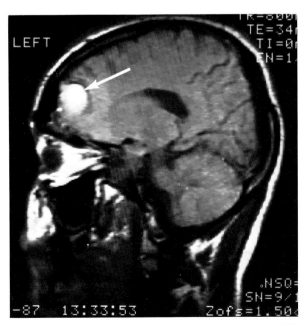

32: Subacute Hemorrhage (.6T)

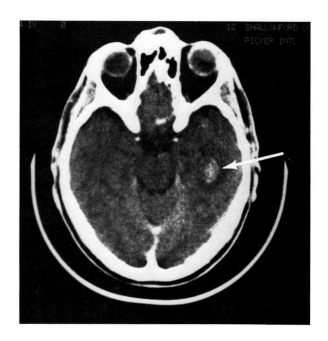

EXAM: MRI of the calvarium.

CLINICAL INFORMATION: CT demonstrates nonenhancing density in the left temporal region. Rule out tumor.

TECHNIQUE: Coronal and axial T1- and T2-weighted images were acquired in addition to sagittal inversion recovery (T1-weighted).

FINDINGS: In an area in the left temporal lobe, there is seen an increased signal intensity with a very low signal intensity center on the spin-density-weighted images. There is a suggestion of an even more peripheral low-signal rim on the more T2-weighted images. This area of abnormality is surrounded by an area of increased signal representing edema. The findings are most consistent with a subacute hemorrhage.

IMPRESSION: Subacute hemorrhage in the left temporal region.

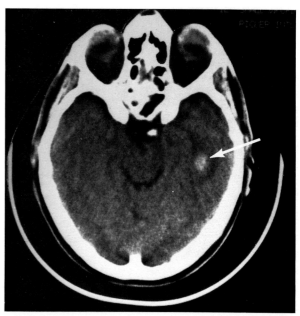

DISCUSSION: These images demonstrate the acute hematoma low signal surrounded by the changes of the high-intensity rim as the hematoma ages into the subacute stage. Images 3 and 4 show the increased signal intensity periphery. The eventual evolution to a low-signal rim is suggested on Image 5.

REFERENCE: Grossman, Robert: *MR Clinical Symposium* Vol. II, #5, 1986.

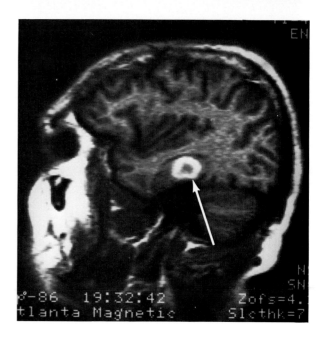

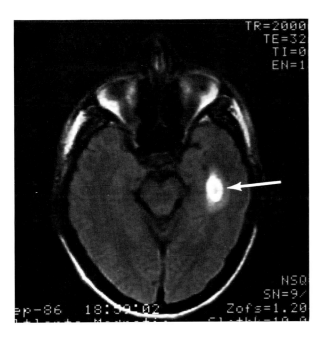

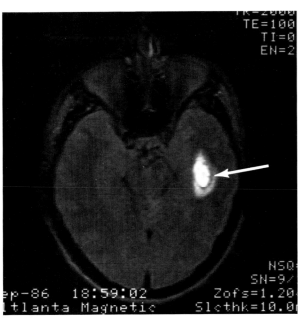

33: Frontal Parietal Contusion (.6T)

EXAM: Magnetic resonance imaging of the calvarium.

CLINICAL INFORMATION: 43-year-old male in a motor vehicle accident. Doing well on discharge. Now with profound alteration sensorium. Exclude late developing subdural hematoma.

TECHNIQUE: Axial, coronal, and sagittal spin density and T1-weighted images were acquired (1400/40; 850/34; 575/34).

FINDINGS: There are bilateral parietal areas of increased signal extending from the cortical surface deep into the white matter tracks. These correlate with areas of contusion demonstrated on CT; however, the extent of the contusion is much larger than that shown on CT scan.

IMPRESSION: Left frontal parietal contusion with small subdural and right parietal contusion.

DISCUSSION: MR can be a useful adjunct to the evaluation of severe head-trauma patients. Our experience has rendered several impressive cases of much more extensive damage than were initially expected following CT scanning.

   Note also the ease with which small subdural collections can be identified.

REFERENCE: Zimmerman et al.: *AJR* **147**:1215, December, 1986.

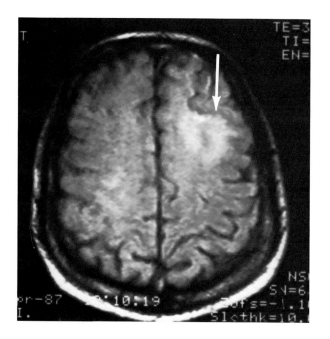

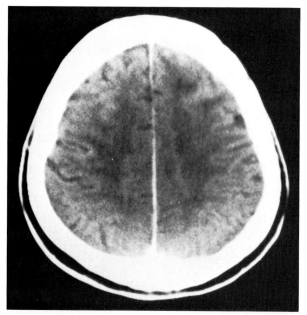

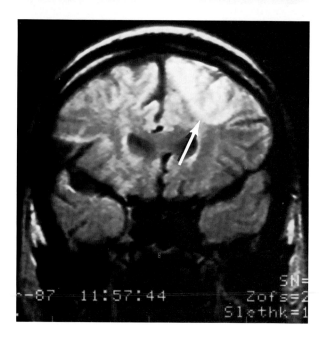

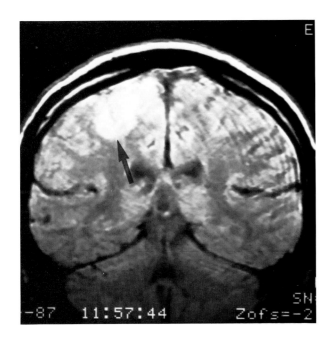

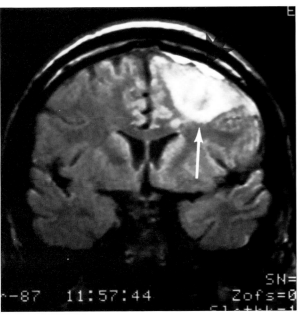

34: Chronic Right Cerebellar Hematoma (.6T)

EXAM: MRI of the calvarium.

CLINICAL INFORMATION: Rule out infarction in 75-year-old male. CT scans demonstrate a low density in the right cerebellar hemisphere.

TECHNIQUE: Coronal T1- and T2-weighted images were acquired (2000/45,90).

FINDINGS: There is marked increase in signal seen in a large mass in the right cerebellar hemisphere with mass effect upon the fourth ventricle. Findings are most consistent with a large chronic hemorrhage in the right cerebellar hemisphere.

DISCUSSION: Hemorrhaged blood within the parenchyma goes through three stages which are appreciated by MR imaging. The behavior of the blood or the signal given relates to the amount of deoxygenation and the freeing of the heme from the red blood cell membranes. The acute stage of clot within the first 10 to 14 days shows a decrease in the central signal of the clot on the MR scan image. The subacute, or second to fourth, week shows a high-signal center by a low-intensity ring. The transition between acute and subacute is the conversion of the ring to a dark or very low signal following a very high signal intensity stage. In all cases, the hematoma may be surrounded by increased signal, representing edema within the surrounding brain.

The final, or chronic, stage, greater than 3 to 4 weeks, shows the hematoma to have increased signal on both T1- and T2-weighted images, as in our case.

REFERENCE: Mori: *Radiology* **157**:87, 1985.

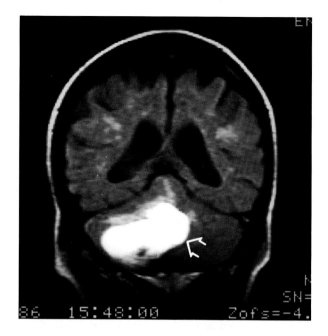

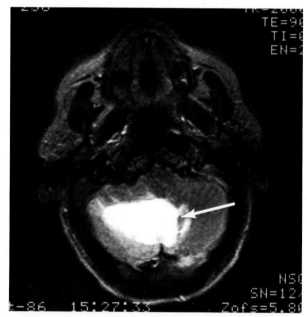

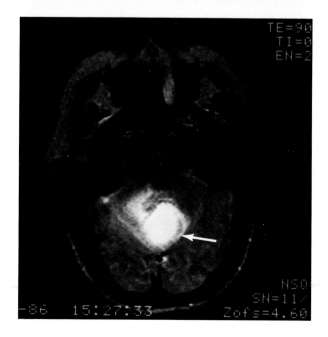

35: Small Parietal AVM   (1.5T)

EXAM: MRI of the calvarium.

CLINICAL INFORMATION: 7-year-old male. Question of an AVM in the right parietal-occipital region.

TECHNIQUE: Spin echo axial T1- and T2-weighted and coronal T1-weighted images were acquired (2000/25,80; 400/25).

FINDINGS: A tangle of vessels with flow-void phenomenon is seen in the posterior parietal-occipital lobe. There is slight increased signal surrounding this area, reflecting a small amount of edema. Centrally, a focus of high-signal intensity is identified within the tangle. This may represent some small amount of hemorrhage.

IMPRESSION: Small parietal-occipital AVM.

DISCUSSION: MRI shows increased sensitivity to the so-called cryptic AVM. In addition, good vascular anatomy can be demonstrated on MR while this is sometimes just suggested or poorly illustrated on CT. In the latter, the visible AVM may show up as a diffuse, nonspecific area of enhancement. In our case, the feeding and draining vessels are well-identified, and their relationship within the cortex is easily identified. In addition, a small amount of edema and hemorrhage associated with AVMs can be demonstrated. We have also had several cases of nonspecific so-called spontaneous hemorrhage in which visualization of small arterial vascular structures within the hemorrhage explains its presence.

REFERENCE: Lemme-Plaghos et al.: *AJR* **146**:1223, June, 1986.

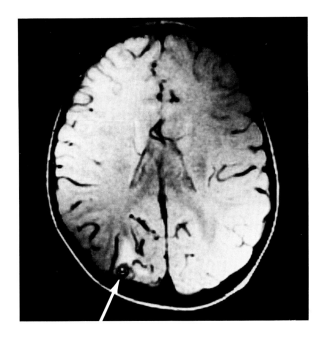

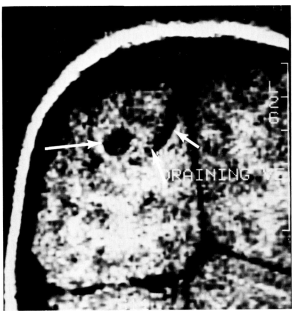

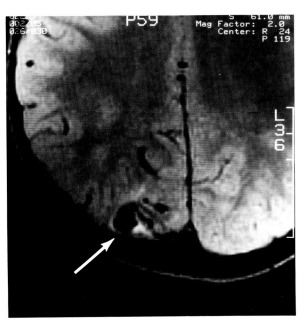

36: Thrombosis of the Superior Sagittal Sinus (.6T)

EXAM: MRI of the calvarium.

CLINICAL INFORMATION: 20-year-old with meningitis complaining of pressure-type headaches with loss of speech and numbness in the right arm and leg.

TECHNIQUE: Coronal and axial T1- and T2-weighted images were acquired.

FINDINGS: There is a persistent increased signal in the region of the transverse sigmoid and superior sagittal sinus on both T1- and T2-weighted images. The persistence of increased signal intensity in a vascular compartment is consistent with thrombosis.

IMPRESSION: Thrombosis of the superior sagittal, transverse, and sigmoidal sinuses.

DISCUSSION: MR can demonstrate the presence of clot within vascular structures, making the need for intraarterial angiography unnecessary when superior sagittal sinus thrombosis is a clinically raised question. Thrombosis contrasts to the normal signal void of flowing blood. There is some paradoxical enhancement and this necessitates the inspection of both the T1- and T2-weighted images; confirmation in two planes is helpful to exclude the presence of a flow phenomenon, paradoxically enhancing blood, versus a true, clot. If there has been paradoxic enhancement of the flowing blood rather than a true clot, the T1-weighted or spin-density-weighted images will show absence of signal. In our case, increased signal was seen on both T1 and T2 axial and coronal views, substantiating a suspicion of thrombosis.

REFERENCE: *JCAT* **10**:10–15, January/February, Virapongse et al.: *Radiology* **162**:779, 1987.

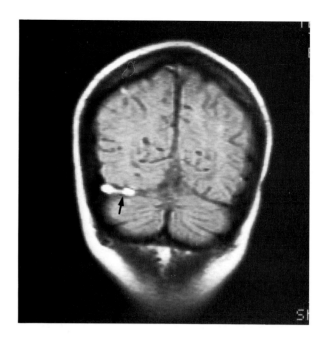
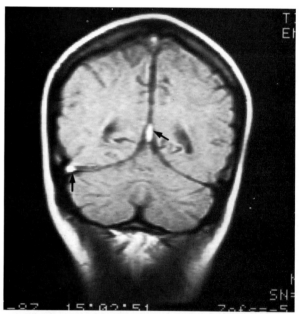
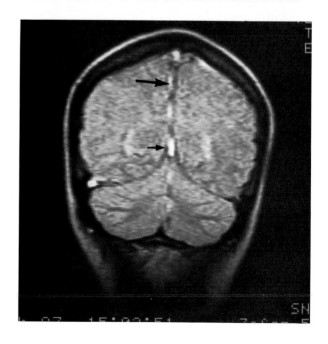

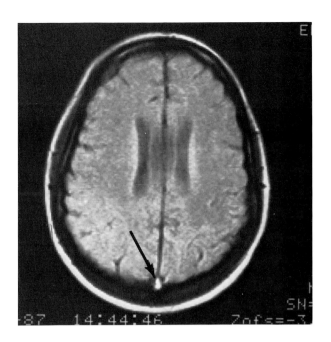

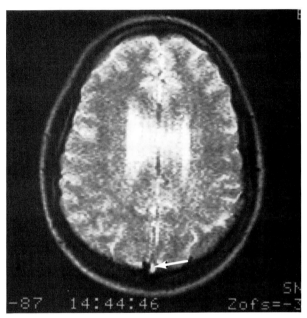

37: Venous Angioma (.6T)

EXAM: MRI of the head.

CLINICAL INFORMATION: A venous angioma demonstrated on prior arteriography. Rule out associated hydrocephalus in a 3-year-old male.

TECHNIQUE: Coronal and axial T1- and T2-weighted images were acquired (2000/32,64; 1000/60).

FINDINGS: Small tubular structure exhibiting absence of signal, or signal void, is seen extending from the deep frontal region superiorly and posteriorly to the midline superior sagittal sinus. This exhibits the findings typical of venous angioma. There is no associated mass effect or hemorrhage.

IMPRESSION: Venous angioma.

DISCUSSION: Venous angiomas are somewhat characteristic on MRI exam and help in differential between the simple congenital anomalous drainage and the more worrisome AVMs.

REFERENCE: Scott et al.: *AJNR* **6**:284, March/April, 1985.

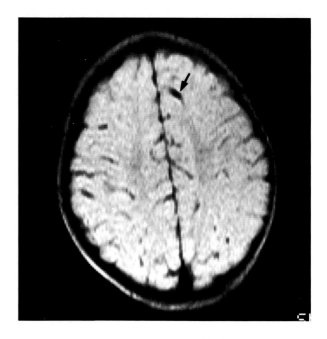

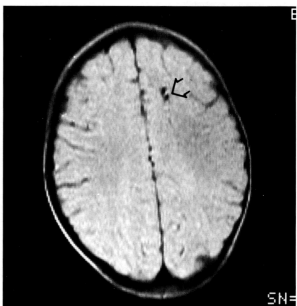

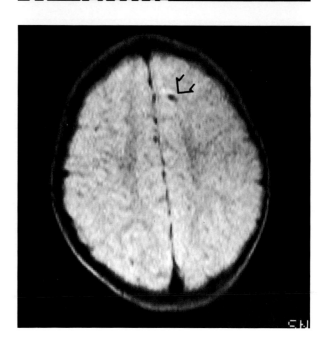

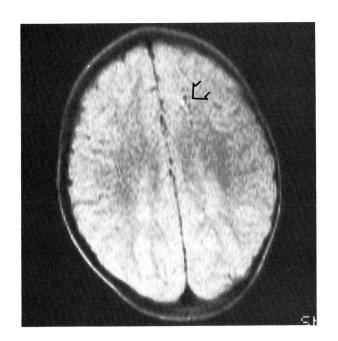

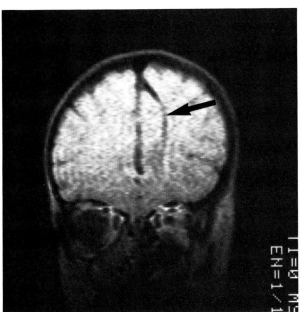

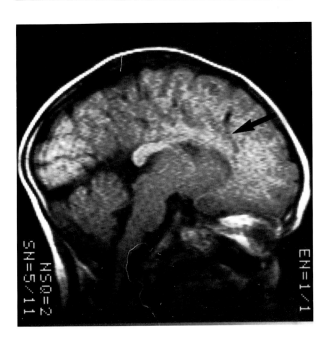

47

38: Subdurals   (.6T)

EXAM: MRI of the head.

CLINICAL INFORMATION: Confirmed subdural suspected on a scan done earlier and degraded by motion.

TECHNIQUE: Axial and coronal T1- and T2-weighted images were acquired (1500/30,60; 1200/30,60).

FINDINGS: Again, increased areas of signal are seen in subdural collections which bilaterally cover the temporal and parietal regions. The ventricular system is normal to small for patient's age.

IMPRESSION: Subdural collections bilaterally over the temporal, parietal, and occipital regions.

DISCUSSION: Despite motion on the first series (Image 1), a definitely increased signal is seen within the subdural region bilaterally. MR was successful in imaging the subdurals again on a repeat study several days later. These were of value since, in this particular patient, numerous CT scans, with and without contrast, had failed to delineate these collections.

REFERENCE: Zimmerman et al.: *AJNR* 7:757, September/October, 1986.

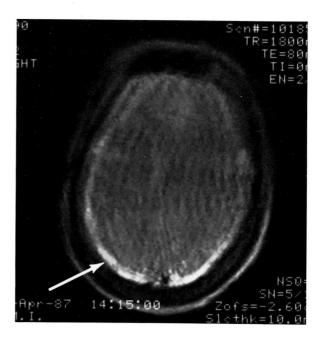

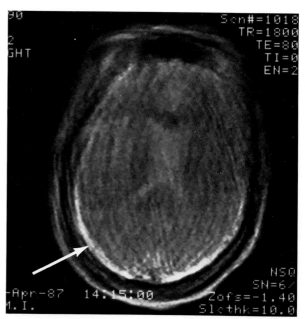

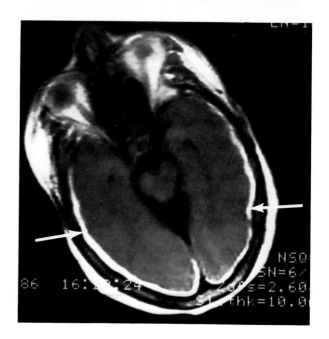

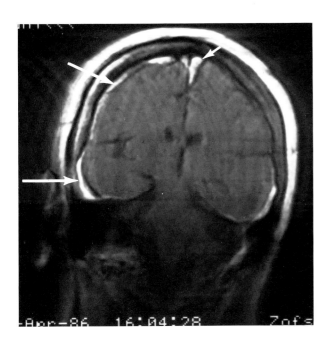

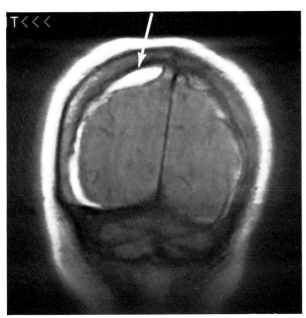

39: Acute Hemorrhage   (.6T)

EXAM: MRI of the head.

CLINICAL INFORMATION: 78-year-old with headaches. Evaluated for mass in the frontal region.

TECHNIQUE: Axial and coronal T1- and T2-weighted images were obtained (2000/40,80).

FINDINGS: There is an area of very low signal, similar to that of the cortical bone, seen in the right parietal lobe. This is small and produces no significant mass effect. Characteristics are consistent with an acute intracerebral hemorrhage. This correlates with an area of increased density on a noncontrast CT scan done at the same time.

IMPRESSION: Acute intracerebral hemorrhage.

REFERENCE: Nose et al.: *JCAT* **11**:184, January/February, 1987.

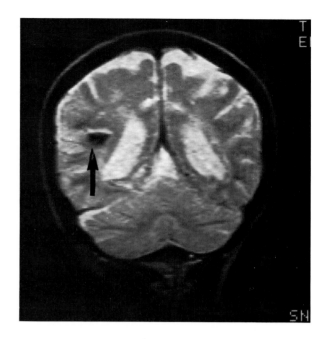

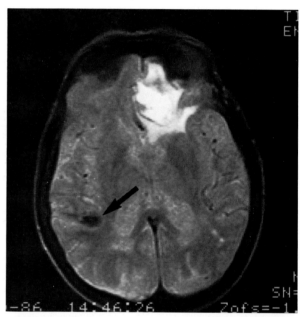

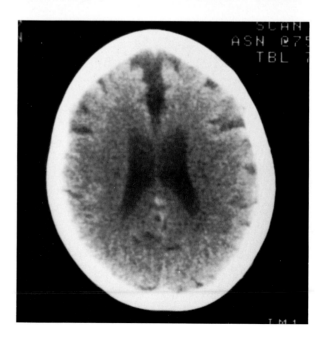

40: Chronic Subdural (1.5T)

EXAM: MRI of the calvarium.

CLINICAL INFORMATION: 67-year-old male with a history of depression.

TECHNIQUE: Coronal and axial T1- and T2-weighted images were acquired (200/20,80).

FINDINGS: A parietal convexity subdural is identified. There is a signal void between the subdural collection and cortices. This suggests calcification within a chronic subdural hematoma. These findings are right-sided. A smaller, but definite, collection is also noted in the left parietal region. These are associated with flattening of the sulci.

DISCUSSION: There is a marked increase in sensitivity to small chronic subdural collections which is shown above. The small arrows delineate the collections and are also adjacent to the low-signal area felt to represent the calcification which is a common finding in more chronic subdurals. On the axial studies, at first glance, the CSF enhancement, particularly with the T2-weighted images, may cause the subdural to be less apparent. The subdural on the axials has a sheetlike appearance, and there is distortion of the normal sulci architecture.

REFERENCE: Han et al.: *Radiology* **150:**71, 1984.

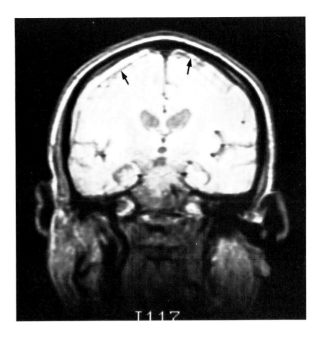

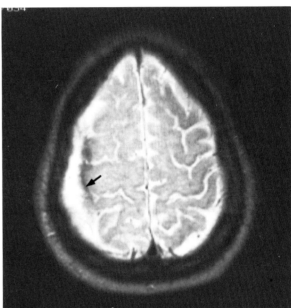

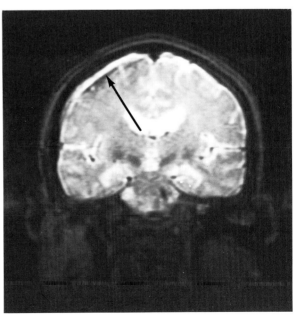

41: Middle Cerebral Artery Aneurysm (.6T)

EXAM: MRI of the calvarium.

CLINICAL INFORMATION: 67-year-old male. Rule out right middle cerebral aneurysm.

TECHNIQUE: T1 and T2 axial images were obtained (2200/45,90).

FINDINGS: An area of definite aneurysmal expansion is seen in the region of the middle cerebral trifurcation (Image 1—arrow). This correlates with an area of calcification and contrast enhancement on the contrast CT done 1 month earlier.

IMPRESSION: Findings most consistent with a middle cerebral artery aneurysm in the trifurcation.

DISCUSSION: Although MR, like CT, may miss a small aneurysm, the diagnosis of aneurysm in this case is quite specific. The use of low signal within the flowing blood and calcification and its intimate relationship to the normal arterial anatomy exclude diagnosis of a heavily calcified glioma.

REFERENCE: Olsen et al.: *Radiology* **163**:431, 1987.

This case is courtesy of Al Alexander Lancaster Magnetic Imaging.

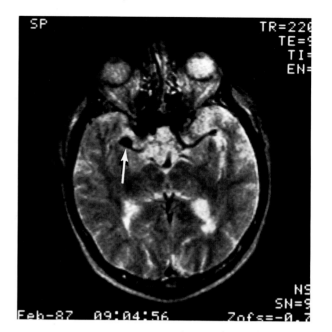

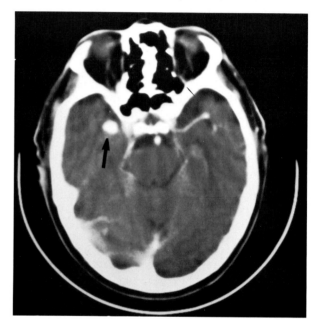

42: Toxo-Plasmosis   (1.5T)

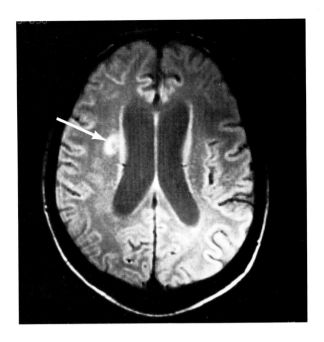

EXAM: MRI of the head.

CLINICAL INFORMATION: This is a 46-year-old male with AIDS. Change in mental status prompted this investigation to rule out space-occupying mass.

TECHNIQUE: Axial scans were obtained with spin echo technique (2000/40,80).

FINDINGS: These are compared to CT scan done 3 days earlier. There is a single right paraventricular area of increased signal with central decreased signal consistent with a target lesion. No other focal signal abnormality detected. The remainder of changes show widening of the ventricular system and sulci consistent with a moderate generalized atrophic change.

IMPRESSION: Solitary mass lesion in right paraventricular region of most concern for toxoplasmosis. Intracranial infections cannot be totally excluded.

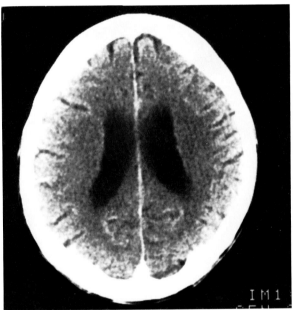

DISCUSSION: The alarming spread of AIDS necessitates our familiarity with various parasitic infestations. The number of agents proven with AIDS has increased. Statistically, however, toxo-plasmosis remains the most usually encountered. Infections with intracranial lymphoma being the most usual neoplastic agent, investigators Hesselink et al. presented a paper at the ASMR and proposed four different patterns of abnormality seen with various infestations. These range from atrophic changes to numerous areas of increased signal. The investigators have preliminary statistics concerning the likelihood of various organisms being categorized in each of the classifications. At this time, the results report that 70 percent of the San Francisco gay population has converted or been exposed to the AIDS virus.

REFERENCE: Hesslink et al.: **8**: *MRI pattern of brain involvement with pathologic correlation.* Paper presented at the meeting of the ASMR, 1987.

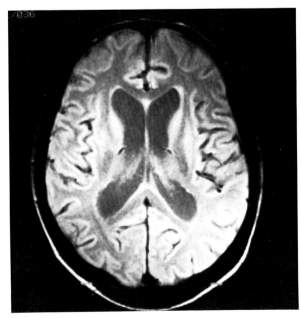

43: Cryptococcal Meningitis (1.5T)

EXAM: MRI of the calvarium.

CLINICAL INFORMATION: This is a 28-year-old male with proven cryptococcal meningitis.

TECHNIQUE: Axial scans were obtained (2000/40,80). These were compared to CT scans obtained 2 days earlier with contrast.

FINDINGS: Numerous areas of increased signal are identified in the basil ganglia, middle cerebral peduncle. These all show increased signal and rounded well-marginated borders with some apparent focal mass effect. When compared with CT, more numerous lesions can easily be appreciated. Retrospectively, the right middle cerebral peduncle may be somewhat enlarged and abnormal (arrow).

Numerous masslike areas of abnormality in the brainstem and middle cerebral peduncle correlate with a proven meningitis. This may represent vasculitis and infarction; however, intercranial infestation from cryptococcal meningitis or other possible agents, such as tuberculosis, toxoplasmosis, or lymphoma, cannot be excluded.

DISCUSSION: Although the CT is positive and the differential between infection and vasculitis with infarction is not resolved, the MRI demonstrates more numerous lesions than those appreciated with CT as well as a larger extent of involvement than that appreciated with CT.

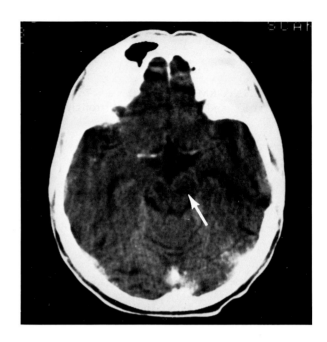

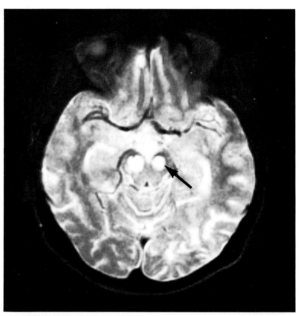

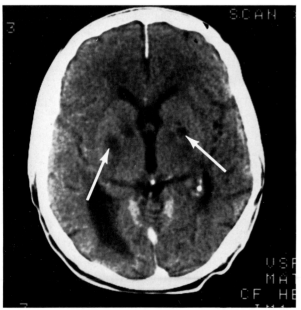

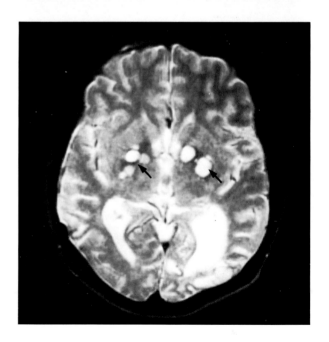

44: Sarcoidosis   (.6T)

EXAM: MRI of the calvarium.

CLINICAL INFORMATION: This is a 51-year-old male with fever, increased cells, and protein. Findings strongly supportive of a diagnosis of neurosarcoidosis.

TECHNIQUE: Axial and coronal T1- and T2-weighted images were obtained (200/40,80; 2000/60,120).

FINDINGS: A single focus of increased signal is identified involving and mildly expanding the left middle cerebral peduncle. Small area of increased signal is seen in the left centrum semiovale on the coronal view. Small areas of increased signal are quite nonspecific; however, with a history of neurosarcoidosis, this is certainly consistent with the diagnosis.

IMPRESSION: Abnormal area of increased signal of the left centrum semiovale and larger area involving the left middle cerebral peduncle.

DISCUSSION: Sarcoidosis can involve the central nervous system in 3 to 5 percent of cases. It usually involves the pituitary gland, hypothalamus, and suprasellar cistern. These can present as focal intraparenchymal or meningeal masses. The nonspecific major of these areas of increased signal is seen with the comparative cut from a different patient with clinically presumed MS (Image 3).

REFERENCE: Reed et al.: *AJR* **146**:819, April, 1986.

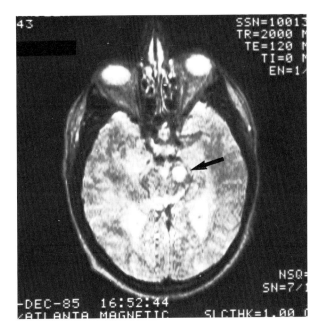

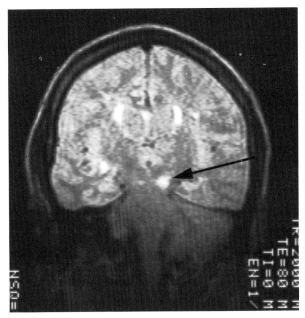

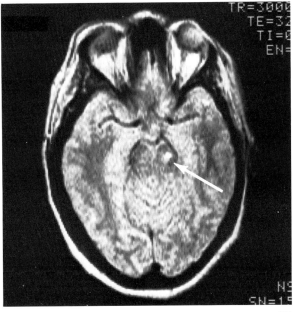

45: Subcortical Arterial Sclerotic Encephalopathy (.6T)

EXAM: MRI of the calvarium.

CLINICAL INFORMATION: 75-year-old male with right cerebellar hemisphere infarct finding.

TECHNIQUE: Axial T1- and T2-weighted images were acquired (2000/45,90).

FINDINGS: Diffuse increased signal in patchy confluent lesions are identified in the white matter of both hemispheres. There are also numerous small separate areas of increased signal throughout the white matter in both hemispheres. The right cerebellar hemisphere reveals a lesion (not shown) consistent with chronic clot.

IMPRESSION: Diffuse increase in the periventricular white matter consistent with numerous areas of demyelination presumably, by history, secondary to old infarction.

DISCUSSION: The presence in older age groups of periventricular areas of increased signal is a nonspecific, but frequent, finding encountered with MRI. The increased signal may be secondary to MS; however, subcortical arteriosclerotic encephalopathy, infarction, hydrocephalus, and chemotherapeutic and radiation changes may mimic the appearance of severe MS. Much depends on the clinical history, findings, and age of the patient when diagnosing this somewhat nonspecific finding. As our reference article points out, some degree of increased signal with aging is normal.

REFERENCE: Zimmerman et al.: *AJNR* **7**:13, January/February, 1986.

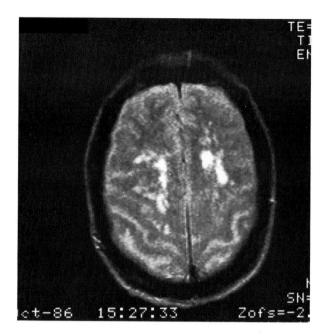

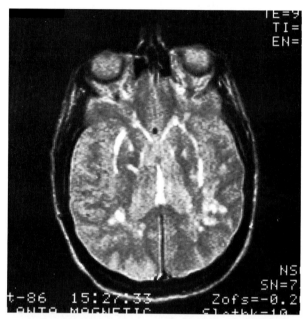

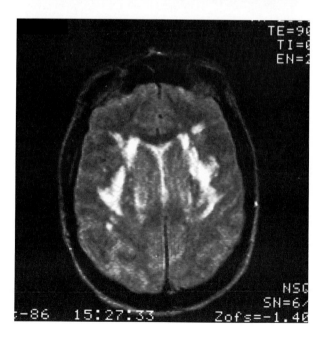

46: Infarction Secondary to Vasculitis (1.5T)

EXAM: MRI of the calvarium.

CLINICAL INFORMATION: This is a 66-year-old female with proven temporal arteritis. Rule out intercranial pathology.

TECHNIQUE: T1- and T2-weighted axial images were obtained through the calvarium (2000/20,80).

FINDINGS: Small areas of increased signal are seen involving the right basal ganglia and right centrum semiovale. These are nonspecific but, with history supplied, are certainly compatible with small areas of gliosis from vascular infarction.

IMPRESSION: Small areas of increased signal secondary to vascular infarct, presumably related to vasculitis.

DISCUSSION: Small areas of increased signal such as this depend heavily on any additional history of physical findings supplied by the clinicians. Without the history of temporal arteritis proven by biopsy, the differential would be more broad-based, including arteriosclerotic vascular disease, inflammation, or gliosis secondary to old trauma.

REFERENCE: Zimmerman et al.: *AJR* 7:13, January/February, 1986.

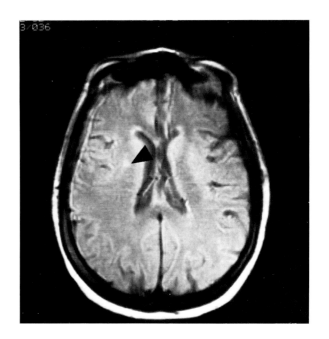

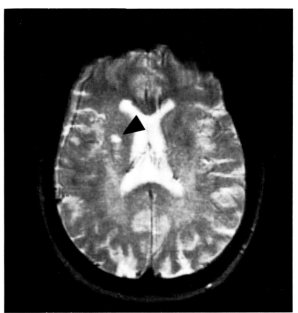

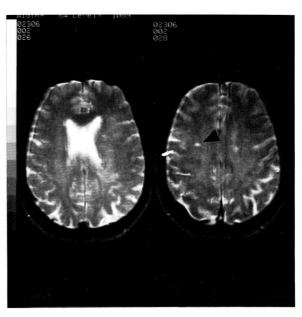

47: Posterior Cerebral Artery Infarction (.6T)

EXAM: MRI of the head.

CLINICAL INFORMATION: Rule out a brain tumor in 58-year-old female with inability to read and numbness involving the right foot and fingers.

TECHNIQUE: Coronal T1- and T2-weighted images were acquired (2000/40,80; 1500/34,68).

FINDINGS: In both views, there is increased signal intensity involving the vascular distribution supplied by the left posterior cerebral artery. There is no suggestion of a mass within this area of increased signal, and there is only limited mass effect upon the adjacent ventricular system. In addition, numerous areas of increased signal are seen on other cuts (not shown). This correlates well with the CT scan and is also consistent with an infarction.

IMPRESSION: Left posterior cerebral artery infarction.

REFERENCE: Savoiardo et al.: *AJNR* **8**:199, March/April, 1987.

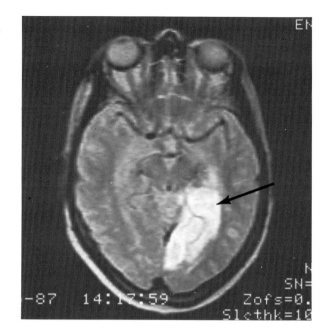

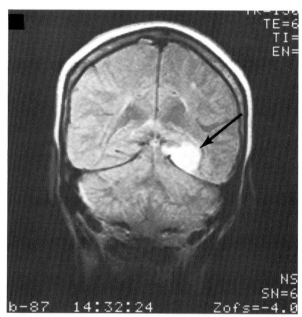

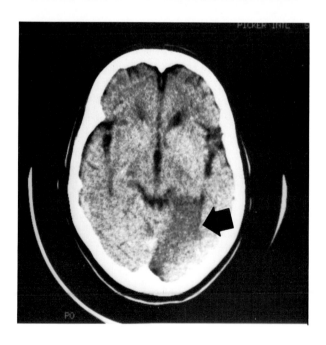

48: Superior Cerebellar Artery Infarction (.6T)

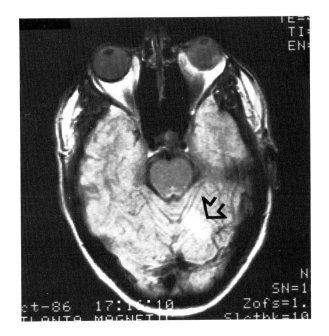

EXAM: MRI of the calvarium.

CLINICAL INFORMATION: 40-year-old who awoke with dizziness and numbness in the left arm and leg, persisting for 1 week. Angiography showed abnormality in the superior vermian artery. CT scan consistent with an enhancing infarction.

TECHNIQUE: Axial and coronal T1- and T2-weighted images were acquired (2000/40,80).

FINDINGS: An area of increased signal is seen in the region of the cerebellar hemisphere on the left side. This involves the gray matter up to the tentorium but shows no evidence of a mass effect. Findings, because of distribution and lack of mass effect, are most consistent with that of an infarction.

IMPRESSION: Superior cerebellar artery infarct involving the left hemisphere.

DISCUSSION: This is the most consistent vascular territory seen in the posterior fossa. It involves the superior aspect of the hemisphere, the superior vermis, and a large part of the deep white matter tract.

REFERENCE: Savoiardo et al.: *AJNR* 8:199, March/April, 1987.

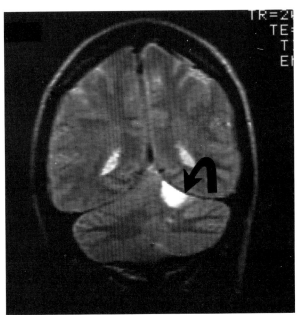

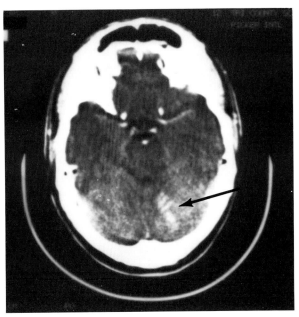

49: Nonspecific Leukoencephalopathy (.6T)

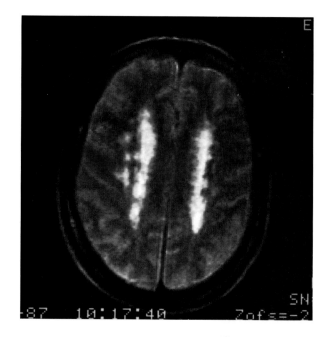

EXAM: MRI of the calvarium.

CLINICAL INFORMATION: 69-year-old female with weakness and ataxia.

TECHNIQUE: Axial T1- and T2-weighted images were acquired (2000/40,80).

FINDINGS: Pattern of paraventricular T2-signal prolongation is noted with a lumpy, bumpy pattern of increased signal, particularly along the paraventricular roof of the lateral ventricles. There is, in addition, matching areas of increased signal in the more posterior aspect of the pons. Differential here between severe MS or vascular disease and some superimposed changes of aging is difficult.

IMPRESSION: Suspect changes are secondary to ischemia and leukoencephalopathy of aging. MS cannot be totally excluded, but is not suggested on the basis of patient's age or history.

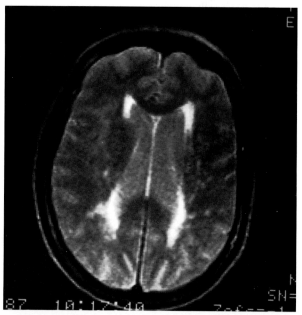

DISCUSSION: Twenty to thirty percent of patients over the age of 65 demonstrate patchy areas of white-matter increased signal. The differential between aging changes versus infarction or even demyelination is difficult. The increase of these lesions correlate with a higher degree of dementia, but this is also seen in normal patients of advanced age. In addition, when the areas of signal are confluent and homogeneous, the exclusion of hydrocephalus cannot be made. In our reference case, disturbing matched lesions in the pons provide further difficulty in making an ultimate diagnosis.

REFERENCE: Brant-Zawadzki et al.: *AJNR* **6**:675, September/October, 1985.

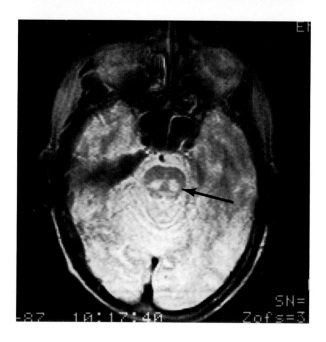

50: Multiple Sclerosis (Grade III)   (.6T)

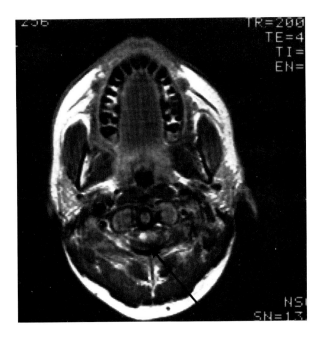

EXAM: MRI of the calvarium.

CLINICAL INFORMATION: 25-year-old with dizziness and nausea. Rule out foramen magnum lesion, neuroma, or MS.

TECHNIQUE: T1- and T2-weighted coronal, sagittal, and axial images were acquired (2000/40,80).

FINDINGS: Numerous areas of increased signal intensity in the paraventricular region, particularly in the occipital horns and roof of the lateral ventricles, are identified. In addition, in the right superior cervical cord at the level of the dens, there is a persistent area of focal increased signal involving the right hemicord. This is seen on both the T1- or spin density and T2-weighted axial images.

IMPRESSION: Findings consistent with multiple sclerosis, Grade III classification. Right cervical cord lesion consistent with a focus of demyelination.

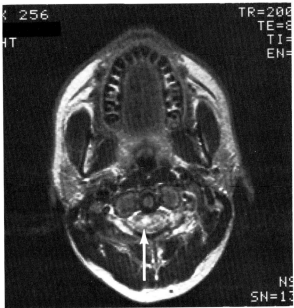

DISCUSSION: The spinal cord can show involvement in approximately 5 to 10 percent of patients being screened for MS. This high cervical cord lesion was included incidentally on the routine cranial study. Sagittal and coronal views were obtained (not shown) to exclude any extraaxial explanation for patient's deficits. Caution must be used when examining the most inferior cord of a sequence secondary to flow phenomenon at that level. If there is a question, we typically rescan with the area of abnormality centered in the reacquisition. In this particular case, there were several slices below this area of abnormal signal. This is also confirmed as being present on both sequences of the double-echo series.

REFERENCE: Maravilla et al.: *AJR* **144**:381, 1985.

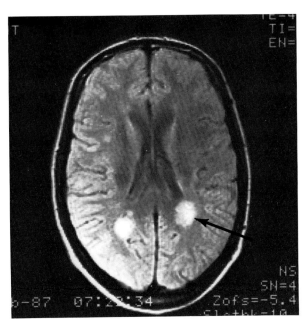

51: Multiple Sclerosis
(Grade IV)   (.6T)

EXAM: MRI of the calvarium.

CLINICAL INFORMATION: Rule out demyelinating disease in 48-year-old male.

TECHNIQUE: Coronal and axial T1- and T2-weighted images were acquired (2000/45,90; 2000/32, 64).

FINDINGS: Twelve areas of white matter and paraventricular-based increased signal intensity are seen. These are not associated with mass effect. The ventricular system and remainder of study are normal.

IMPRESSION: Findings are most consistent with multiple sclerosis.

DISCUSSION: Number of lesions seen places this within a Grade IV classification on the Edwards, Farlow, and Stephens scale. MS is a diagnosis previously based most heavily on clinical criteria. MR offers an excellent paraclinical modality which, at this time, replaces the need in large part for CT, CSF studies, and urinary dynamics. In our reference article, the authors reviewed over 100 patients. Those with MS showed the following distribution: 84 percent in supratentorial white matter, 8 percent in cortical gray matter, 5 percent in brainstem, and 2 percent in cerebellum. This is a fairly useful breakdown of the locations of the lesions and helps in a greater appreciation of the various appearances of MS.

REFERENCE: Stewart et al.: *Mayo Clin Proc* **62**:174, 1987.

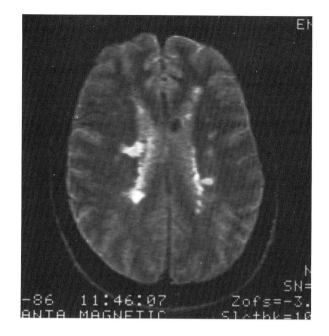

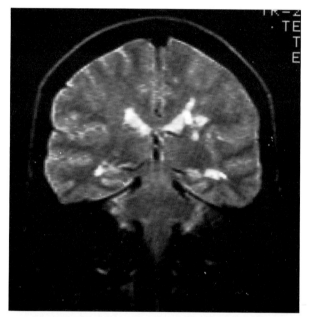

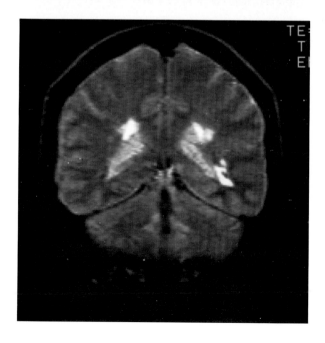

52: Multiple Sclerosis (Grade III) (.6T)

EXAM: MRI of the head.

CLINICAL INFORMATION: Rule out demyelinating disease in 36-year-old female.

TECHNIQUE: Axial and coronal T1- and T2-weighting were acquired (2000/45,90; 1400/35/400).

FINDINGS: There are numerous areas of increased signal intensity involving the white matter of both hemispheres. The largest of these is in the midright centrum semiovale, and, on the T1-weighted images, this shows marked hypointensity compared to the white-matter tracks. Findings are consistent with a demyelinating process such as multiple sclerosis.

IMPRESSION: Multiple sclerosis.

DISCUSSION: Characteristic appearance of areas of increased signal intensity involving predominantly the white matter (most typically the centrum semiovale, paraventricular regions) has proven to be one of the earliest and strongest utilities of the MR imager. The diagnostic sensitivity to demyelinating areas with MR far exceeds that of CT scanning. There is some difficulty or overlap between MS and infarction. However, in the correct clinical situation, with the characteristic distribution of lesions the differential can be reliably sorted out. We consider the early sixties to be a good cutoff point for decreased likelihood of the areas of increased signal to represent MS when there is a new onset of symptoms. In addition the predominantly white-matter-based lesions particularly if they populate the roof of the lateral ventricles or occipital region also favor diagnosis of MS over infarction. Although the gray-white and gray matter can be involved in MS in approximately 10 percent of cases, the localization of most lesions in the gray-white region or the gray cortex, or the demonstration of a definite vascular area of involvement, heavily favors the diagnosis of infarction over MS.

REFERENCE: Runge et al.: *Radiographics* **6**(2): March, 1986.

This case is a Grade III, and the total number of lesions was between four and eight. This is based on a grading scale offered by Edwards, Farlow and Stephens in *AJR* **147**:571, September, 1986.

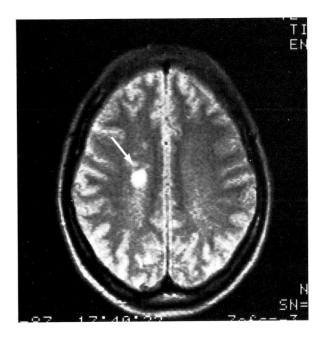

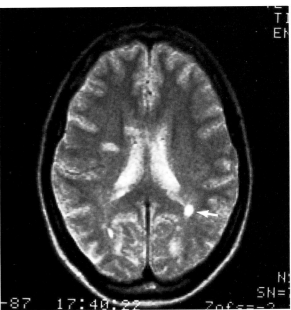

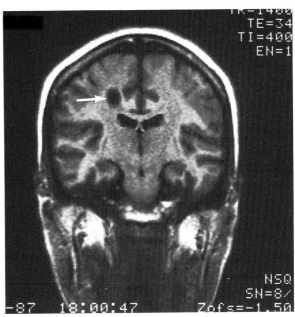

53: Multiple Sclerosis
(Grade V) (1.5T)

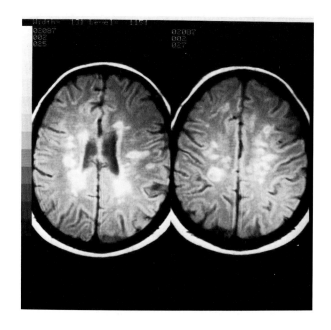

EXAM: MRI of the calvarium.

CLINICAL INFORMATION: This includes three females from ages 30 to 38 presenting with symptomatology consistent with multiple sclerosis.

TECHNIQUE: Axial T1- and T2-weighted images were acquired (2000/20,90).

FINDINGS: Numerous confluent patches in the periventricular region are noted in both hemispheres. No evidence of mass effect is seen. The remainder of the study is normal.

IMPRESSION: Findings consistent with multiple sclerosis. The numerous confluent patches place this in a Grade V category. Severe MS in three separate patients.

DISCUSSION: This case is submitted for comparative purposes to the Point 6 cases included, demonstrating that the lesions of MS are well-identified and evaluated on both mid- and high-field strengths.

REFERENCE: Sheldon et al.: *AJNR* **6**:683, September/October, 1985.

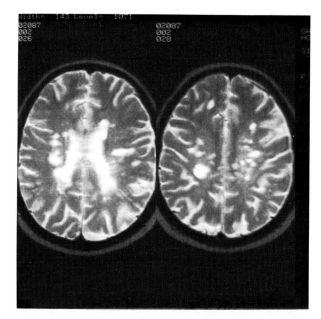

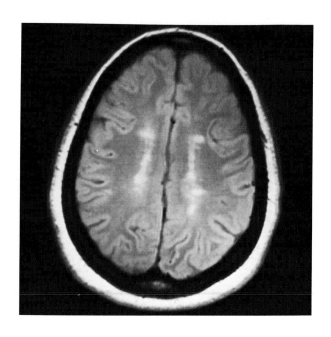

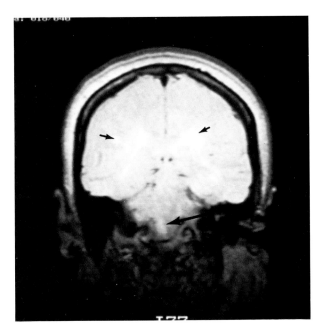

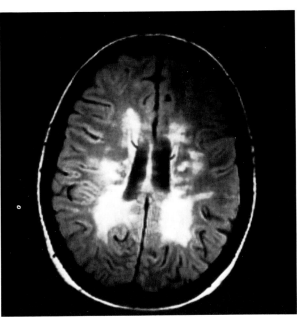

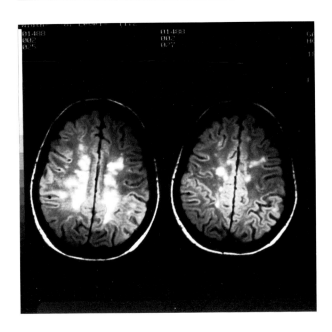

65

54: Multiple Sclerosis Versus Infarction (1.5T)

EXAM: MRI of the calvarium.

CLINICAL INFORMATION: 50-year-old female. Rule out multiple sclerosis.

TECHNIQUE: Spin echo (2000/20,80).

FINDINGS: Axial scans demonstrate numerous areas of white matter and periventricular signal. Some of the lesions involve the cortices (not shown). The differential between MS and multiple areas of infarction must be made clinically.

IMPRESSION: Numerous areas of increased signal, certainly consistent with a demyelinating process; however, a vascular etiology cannot be excluded.

DISCUSSION: Old MS plaques may be apparent on the CT scans. Contrast may enhance or show the presence of plaque as well. However, the sensitivity of CT has been, at best, up to 50 percent, whereas MRI is clearly more sensitive. There is some overlap in specificity as it relates to the possibility of MS versus vascular infarction. In a case such as this, the exclusion of vascular lesions, without the clinical findings, would be difficult.

REFERENCE: Sheldon et al.: *AJNR* **6:**683, September/October, 1985.

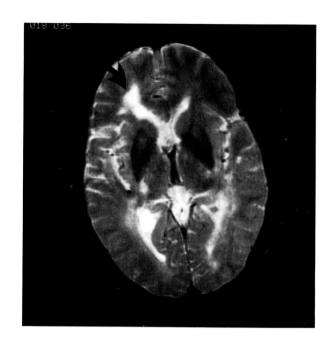

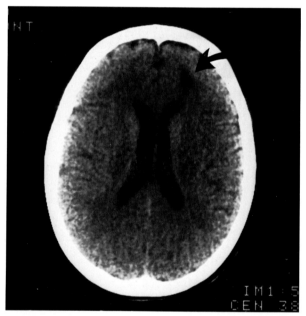

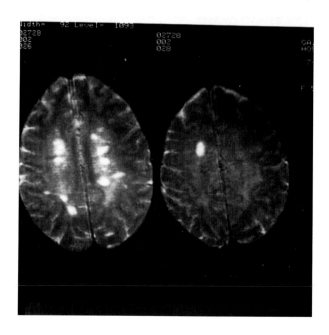

55: Hamartoma (.6T)

EXAM: MRI of the head.

CLINICAL INFORMATION: Fourteen-year-old male mildly retarded with seizure disorder. Rule out neoplasm.

TECHNIQUE: Spin echo technique was employed (2000/32,64).

FINDINGS: There is an extracerebral cystic collection posterior to the occipital horn. There is, however, dysmorphic enlargement of both ventricles and a large irregular mass showing isointense signal characteristics to that of the normal surrounding brain located in the right frontal region. There is no recognizable normal caudate or basal ganglia on the right side. There is deviation of the ventricular system from right to left. There is no surrounding edema.

IMPRESSION: Numerous congenital malformations are detected; however, a large conglomerate mass in the right frontal region with similar signal characteristics to that of more normal-appearing left-hemisphere white and gray matter suggests that this represents a large hematomous mass, rather than glioma.

DISCUSSION: Numerous cerebral abnormalities in the pediatric population are well-identified with MR. Lack of any radiation is certainly one of the more favorable features of MR. In younger children, safe sedation can be obtained using oral chlorahydrate (50 mg/kg).

REFERENCE: Han et al.: *JCAT* **9**:103, January/February, 1985.

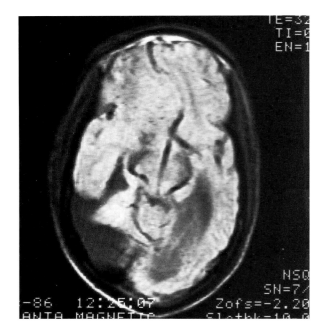

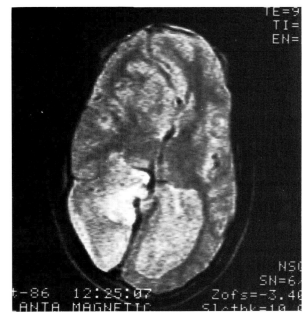

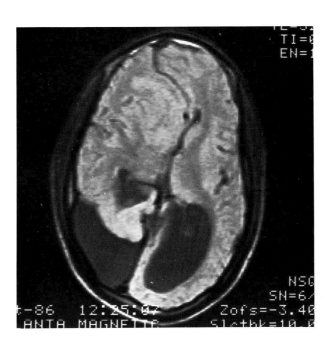

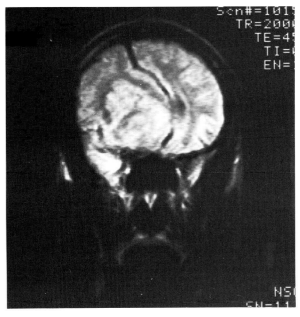

56: Hydrocephalus　(.6T)

EXAM: MRI of the head.

CLINICAL INFORMATION: 56-year-old with lapses in memory involved in trauma.

TECHNIQUE: Axial and coronal T1- and T2-weighting and sagittal T1-weighting were acquired. (2000/30,60; 500/25).

FINDINGS: There is mass dilatation of the lateral ventricles and third ventricular cavity. There is also pronounced signal void in the aqueduct. The fourth ventricle is slightly enlarged but within top normal limits for size. There is evidence for signal void in both the aqueduct and in the base of the fourth ventricle (arrow). The presence of the signal characteristics in the aqueduct and base of the fourth ventricle suggests that the level of the obstruction may be over the convexities and the region of the arachnoid villi.

Note is also made of a homogeneous thin area of increased signal surrounding the ventricle.

IMPRESSION: Marked hydrocephalus, level of obstruction probably in the region of the convexity.

DISCUSSION: The morphologic enlargement of the ventricles can be easily demonstrated on MR. Sagittal view offers a good assessment of the aqueduct. The characteristics of demonstrating flow signal in areas of CSF turbulence allow for good assessment in areas of potential obstruction and exclusion or demonstration of level of obstruction. Our case demonstrates fairly significant flow at the aqueduct and the base of the fourth ventricle. Signal void can be seen with CSF pulsation or flow. The combination of such signals seen both in the aqueduct and in the base of the fourth ventricle suggests that the obstruction is beyond the ventricular system itself.

In addition, at this time increased signal surrounding the ventricles is felt to represent good corroborative evidence that the hydrocephalus is still active. Note should be made, however, that the increased signal may persist in these regions following treatment because of the gliosis resulting from the previous abnormal migration of CSF through the neural tissue.

REFERENCE: Bradley et al.: *Radiology* **159:**611, 1986.

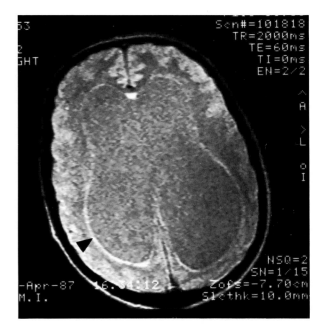

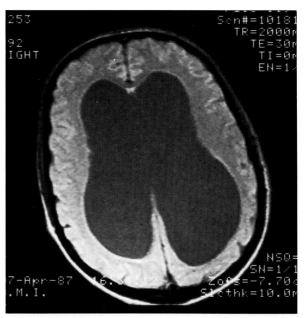

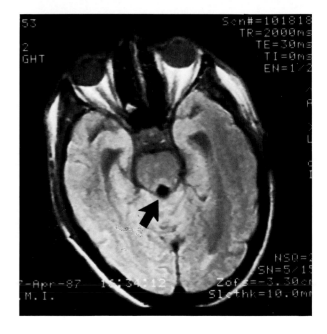

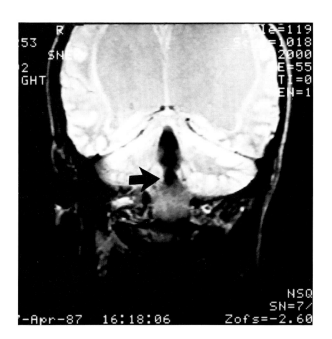

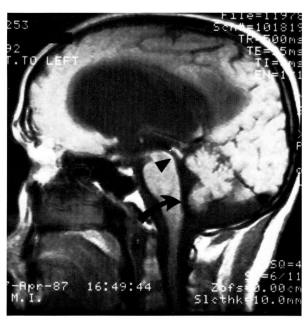

57: Shunted Hydrocephalus (.6T)

EXAM: MRI of the head.

CLINICAL INFORMATION: 73-year-old female previously shunted, Paraplegia and pain in legs. Previous bladder cancer.

TECHNIQUE: Axial and coronal images were obtained through the calvarium (2000/40,80; 2125/30,60).

FINDINGS: Midline dilated ventricular system noted with identification of a ventricular decompression device entering from the right parietal region. The shunt tubing apparently crosses the midline with the tip of the shunt catheter in the region of the left frontal horn (see small arrow). There is increased paraventricular signal, particularly in the frontal and occipital regions of the ventricles. Numerous other areas of other nonmass-producing increased signal are identified in the white matter of both hemispheres. The lack of any significant focal mass effect suggests that these areas of altered signal are most likely the residual gliosis from marked hydrocephalus. The irregular nonhomogeneous signal suggests that the hydrocephalus has been treated. This is also confirmed by identification of ventricular shunt.

IMPRESSION: Shunted hydrocephalus with residual numerous areas of increased signal in paraventricular region, probably representing postshunted gliosis.

DISCUSSION: The ability to do both axial and coronal images leads to more accurate identification of the location of shunt devices. There is some difficulty in separating out the effect of water change in the white matter from active hydrocephalus versus infarction or metastatic disease. The numerous areas of abnormality lacking any mass effect are the best indicators that this represents gliosis from prior hydrocephalus rather than metastatic disease. Some superimposed vascular insult cannot be excluded.

REFERENCE: Bisese et al.: MRI in the evaluation of shunt devices. Exhibit presented at the ASNR meeting, 1986.

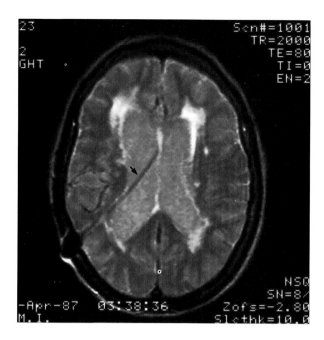

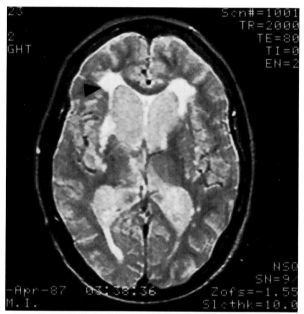

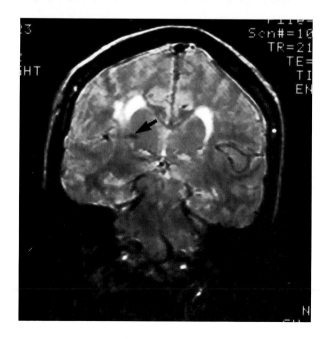

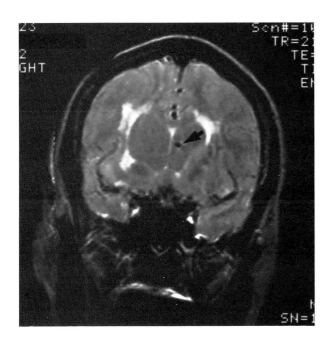

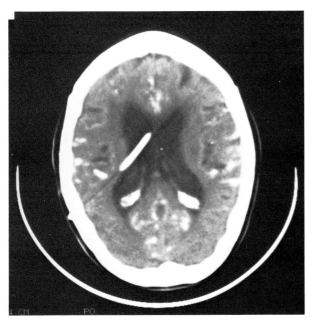

58: Dandy Walker Cyst   (.35T)

EXAM: MRI of the head.

CLINICAL INFORMATION: This is a young female for evaluation of brain dysmorphia.

TECHNIQUE: T1-weighted axial and sagittal images were acquired through the calvarium (500/30).

FINDINGS: Characteristic posterior fossa midline cleft from failure of vermis to develop is identified with a large posterior cystic mass. Note the excellent demonstration on the sagittal view (Image 3) of the enlarged posterior cystic mass as it protrudes superiorly through the tentorial hiatus.

IMPRESSION: Findings consistent with dandy walker cyst.

DISCUSSION: Pediatric brain dysmorphia is easily evaluated with MR. The ability to image in several planes, particularly sagittal, allows for a good evaluation of the supratentorial structures, such as the corpus callosum, in the same sitting. The ventricular size is also easily evaluated during this imaging session.

REFERENCE: Han et al.: *JCAT* **9**:103, 1985. Hirsch: *Radiology* **155**:550, 1985.

Courtesy of William Bednartz, Williamsport Magnetic Imaging

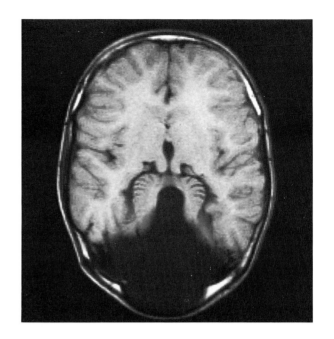

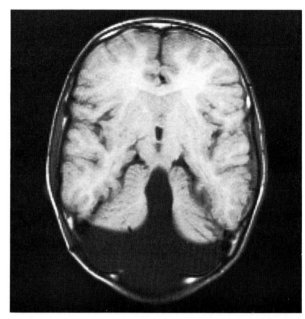

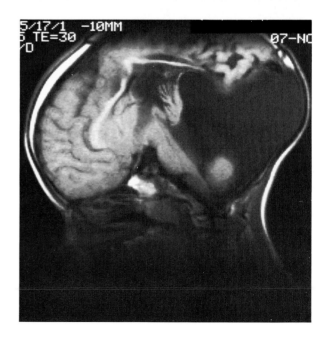

59: Subarachnoid Temporal Cyst (.6T)

EXAM: MRI of the calvarium.

CLINICAL INFORMATION: 54-year-old male with unsteady gait.

TECHNIQUE: Axial, coronal, and sagittal T1- and T2-weighted images were acquired (2200/45,90; 600/32).

FINDINGS: Intracranial study was considered normal. Note is made of a cyst within the pineal gland.

DISCUSSION: The pineal gland arises from a diverticulation and proliferation of cells within the roof of the third ventricle, early in fetal development. The closing of the distal aspect of the diverticulum is cut off, allowing small cavities to arise within the pineal gland. The lining of these cavities consist of ependymal or neuroglilial cells. Larger cysts within the pineal gland are referred to as *hydrops*. The cysts were easily overlooked with CT because of the content being isodense with that of CSF in the peripineal subarachnoid space. The cysts are more easily appreciated on the sagittal and coronal views.

REFERENCE: *AJNR* 7:1081, November/December, 1986.

Special thanks to Al Alexander Lancaster Magnetic Imaging

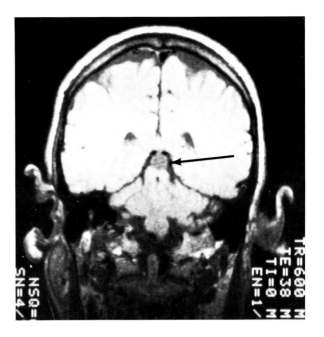

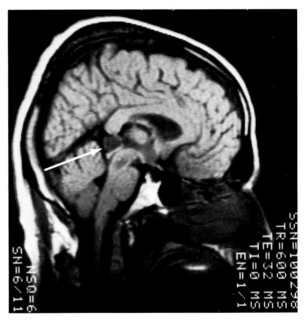

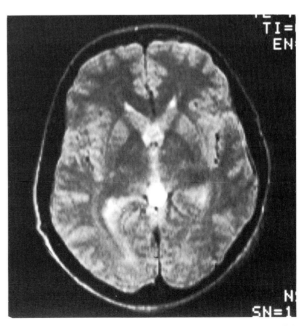

60: Aqueduct Stenosis with Hydrocephalus   (.6T)

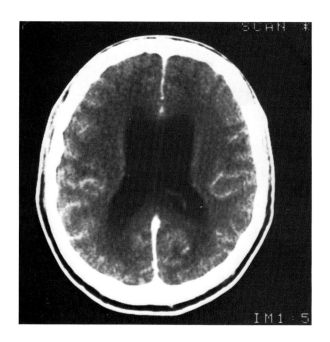

EXAM: MRI of the calvarium.

CLINICAL INFORMATION: 27-year-old male with mental confusion and headache.

FINDINGS: Marked enlargement of the ventricular system is identified with increase in the periventricular signal. The aqueduct is poorly visualized and shows an increased signal intensity; no definite lumen was identified. The fourth ventricular system is small and midline.

IMPRESSION: Aqueductal stenosis with active hydrocephalus.

DISCUSSION: In addition to the findings of increased signal intensity around the ventricles, recent literature suggests that hydrocephalus reduces the thickness of the corpus callosum. The normal thickness has been stated in our reference article as 6 mm. A measurement below this, taken at the level of the foramen of Monro, is consistent with the diagnosis of hydrocephalus, although some overlap with atrophic patients does occur.

REFERENCE: El Gammal et al.: *AJNR* **8**:591, July/August, 1987.

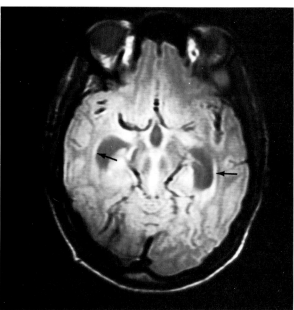

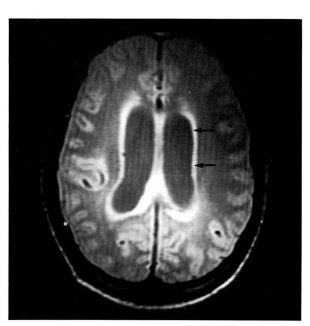

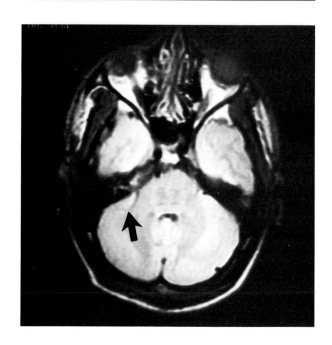

61: Subarachnoid Cyst in the Ambient Cistern (.6T)

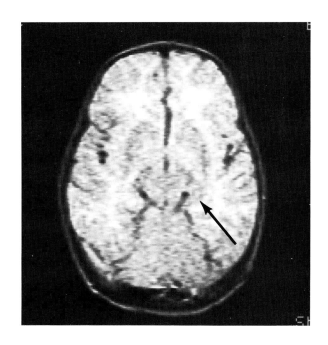

EXAM: MRI of the calvarium.

CLINICAL INFORMATION: 7½-month-old with cyst on CT. MRI to confirm.

TECHNIQUE: Axial and coronal T1- and T2-weighted images were acquired (2000/45,90; 2000/34,68).

FINDINGS: In correlation with the CT scan done at the same time, there is focal enlargement of the lateral recess of the ambient cistern. This area shows homogeneous signal which remains isointense with the CSF on both spin density and T2-weighted images. No suggestion of any solid content is seen, and no associated mass effect is identified. The finding is most consistent with a small subarachnoid cyst.

IMPRESSION: Subarachnoid cyst in the ambient cistern.

DISCUSSION: Arachnoid cysts, usually supratentorial, are thought to arise secondary to trauma or inflammation of the meninges. The more rare infratentorial cysts have been described as arising in the retrocerebellar or cerebellar pontine angle. Our reference article reports two large quadrigeminal subarachnoid cysts which would occur in a more midline location than does our ambient cistern cyst. The ability to compare the behavior of this area to the surrounding CSF helps confirm the impression that this should represent an incidental cyst.

REFERENCE: Choi et al.: *AJNR* 7:725, July/August, 1986.

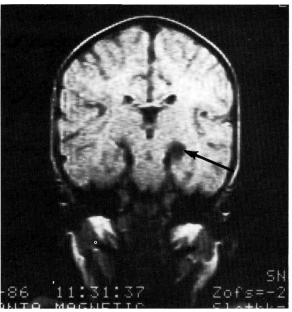

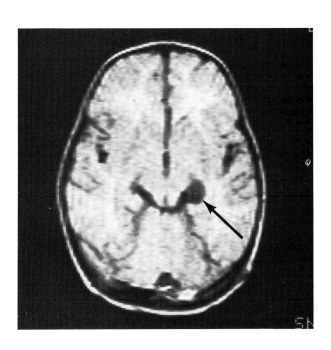

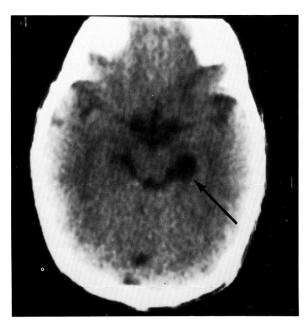

62: Subarachnoid Cyst Adjacent to the Pineal Gland (.6T)

EXAM: MRI of the head.

CLINICAL INFORMATION: 49-year-old female evaluated for headaches. CT scan demonstrated a right parapineal abnormality. Rule out tumor.

TECHNIQUE: Axial and coronal scans were obtained through the calvarium (2000/31,62).

FINDINGS: There is a CSF-containing region which is asymmetric on the right side. This shows apparent displacement of the thalamic pulvinar and hibenular commissure. There is no evidence of any internal alteration of signal intensity or heterogeneity to suggest any solid component. The area of abnormal enlargement on the right behaves in isointense fashion to that of the interventricular CSF.

IMPRESSION: Asymmetric enlargement of the subarachnoid cyst adjacent to the pineal gland with mild mass effect suggests the presence of a small subarachnoid cyst. There is no evidence of a tumor. Pineal gland and associated structures are normal.

DISCUSSION: Small subarachnoid cysts can be easily identified, and suggestion on CT of a possible low-density tumor can be reevaluated with MR. This behavior, similar to that of other areas of CSF on the scan, offers an excellent internal comparison to exclude possible tumor. Also note the ease with which the adjacent structures in the region of the pineal gland can be evaluated.

REFERENCE: Kjos et al.: *Radiology* 155:363, 1985.

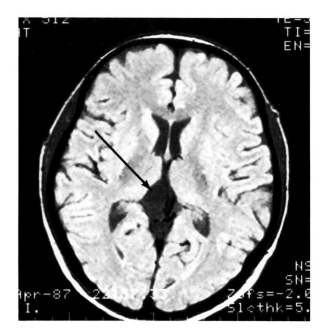

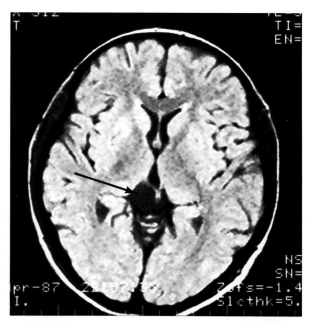

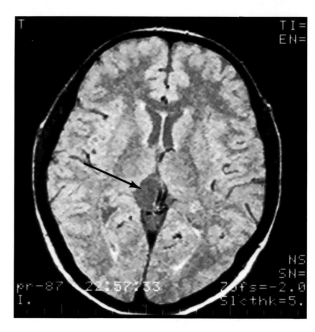

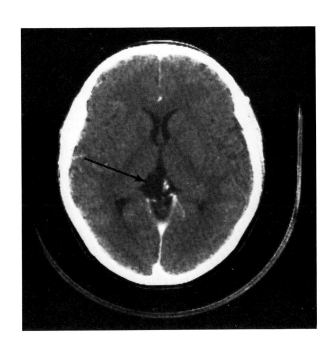

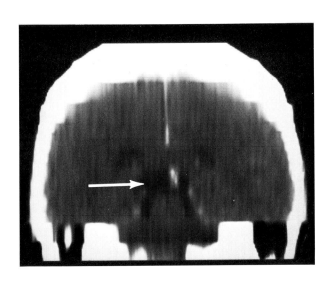

63: Active Hydrocephalus with Metastatic Disease of the Pineal Region   (.6T)

EXAM: MRI of the calvarium.

CLINICAL INFORMATION: 69-year-old with dementia and blurred vision. Known carcinoma of the lung. Question of hydrocephalus.

TECHNIQUE: Axial and coronal T1- and T2-weighted images were obtained (2000/40,80; 2000/31,62).

FINDINGS: Ventricular system is midline, but dilated, and surrounded with a homogeneous, increased signal intensity suggesting active hydrocephalus. In addition, the pineal gland shows as isointense to brain parenchyma on the more spin density or T1-weighted images with significant increase in signal intensity on the T2-weighted images. The gland also appears enlarged.

IMPRESSION: Active hydrocephalus. The enlarged pineal gland with increased signal intensity is abnormal and most likely represents a metastatic deposit to the pineal gland from a patient with known lung CA.

IMPRESSION: Pineal enlargement, probably secondary to metastases from known lung CA with active hydrocephalus.

DISCUSSION: This is an excellent example of the homogeneous increase in signal seen with active hydrocephalus. Metastatic disease to the pineal has been less published, and the normal pineal tumors seen in the pediatric and young-adult populations, such as the pineocytomas, pineoblastomas, and terratomas, are usually reported.

Also note the homogeneous increase in signal surrounding the ventricles on both echo sets. This is a particularly useful sign for active hydrocephalus.

REFERENCE: Naidich et al.: *AJR* **146**:1246, June, 1986.

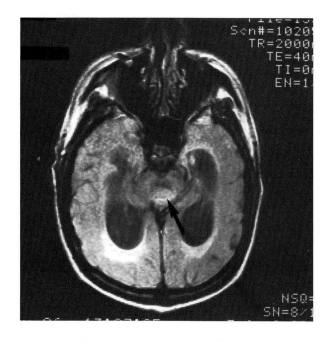

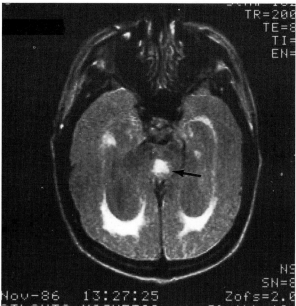

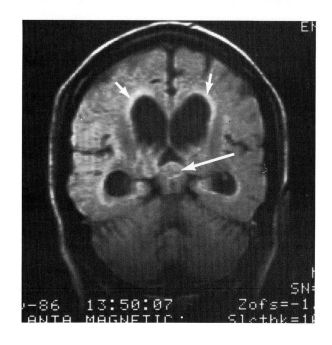

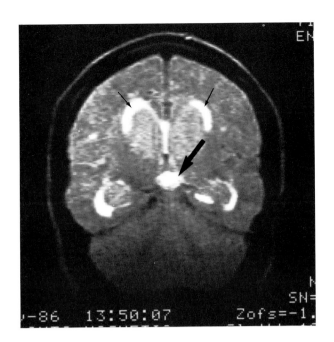

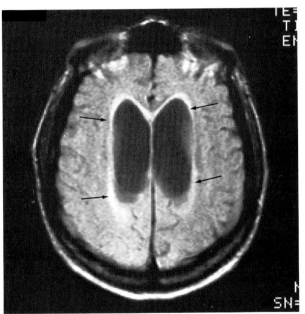

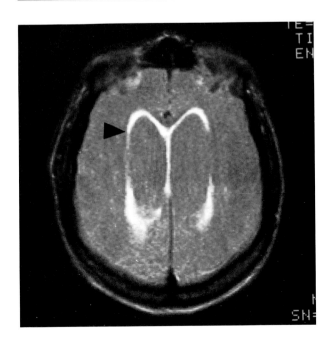

64: Cerebellar Pontine Angle Meningioma (1.5T)

EXAM: MRI of the calvarium.

CLINICAL INFORMATION: This is a 39-year-old male with right cranial nerve pathology, involving multiple cranial nerves.

TECHNIQUE: Axial and coronal T1- and T2-weighted images were acquired (200/20,40; 500/25).

FINDINGS: A large extraaxial mass in the right cerebral pontine angle is identified. This extends from the superior aspect of the clivus to the lower pons. There is marked invagination and distortion of the brainstem. The internal auditory canal is not widened and shows slightly different signal characteristics, suggesting that it has been spared. There are tubular areas of signal void surrounding the outer margins of this mass consistent with draping veins. Differential includes meningioma versus an acoustic neuroma. The sparing of the internal auditory canal suggests that this mass is a meningioma.

IMPRESSION: Right cerebral pontine angle meningioma.

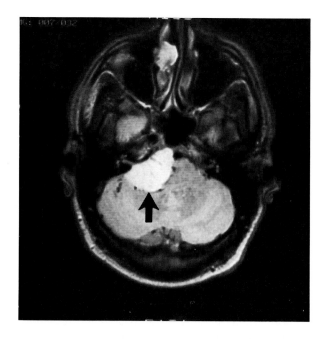

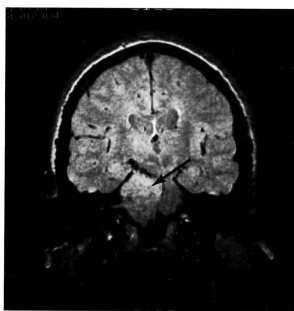

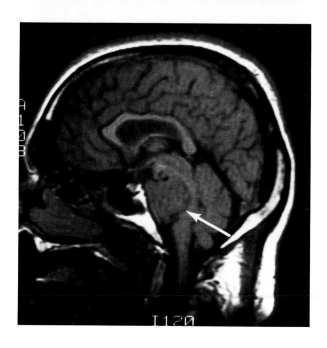

65: Cystic Encephalomalacia   (.6T)

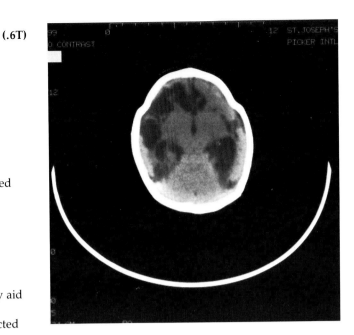

EXAM: MRI of the head.

CLINICAL INFORMATION: This is a 2-year-old with severe-damage anoxic insult from birth. This twin suffered a severe intrauterine transfusion insult.

TECHNIQUE: Coronal and axial T1-weighted images were acquired (900/34).

FINDINGS: Extensive cysts throughout both markedly atrophied hemispheres are identified. These represent a severe cystic encephalomalacia. However, certain structures, such as the posterior fossa, brainstem, and the midbrain, remain well-preserved as well as some of the inferior and lateral temporal cortices. Comparison to a CT scan done approximately 2 years earlier shows no progression of the atrophic changes.

DISCUSSION: The ability to do coronal and sagittal views may aid in the more accurate evaluation of residual cortex in severely damaged children. Small amounts of hemorrhage may be detected by the more sensitive MRI modality.

REFERENCE: McArdle et al.: *Radiology* **163**:395, 1987.

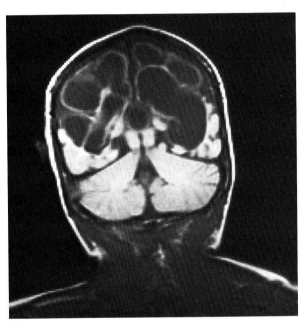

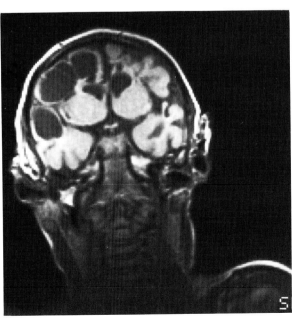

66: Subdural Hygromata (.6T)

EXAM: MRI of the head.

CLINICAL INFORMATION: 3-year-old with elevated intracranial pressure and abnormal CT.

TECHNIQUE: Spin echo sequences in the axial and coronal planes were obtained (2000/35,70; 1660/34,68).

FINDINGS: Bilateral subdural extracerebral collections are noted. These are slightly larger on the left and surround the temporal lobe as well as cover the frontal and parietal regions. There is some suggestion of mild mass effect upon the left temporal lobe, as well as the ventricular system, with very minimal left-to-right shift. There is, however, right-sided extracerebral collection which probably accounts for partial correction of the mass effect.

IMPRESSION: Bilateral extracerebral collections consistent with hygromata.

DISCUSSION: Although the CT and actual MRIs are equivalent, the additional coronal orientation increases the overall approximation of the collection size when compared with the axial images of either the MR or CT alone.

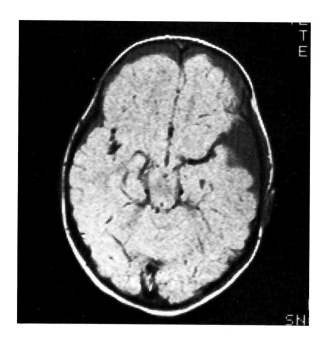

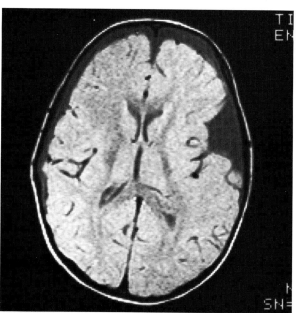

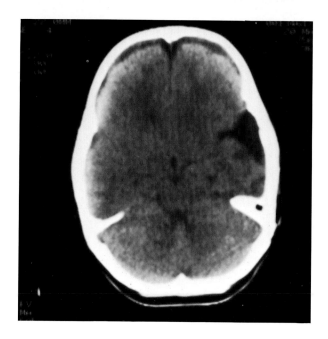

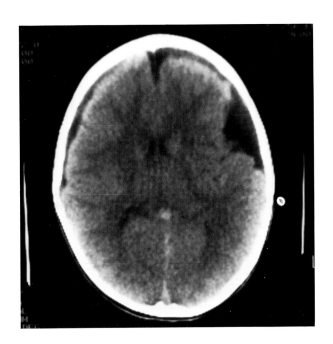

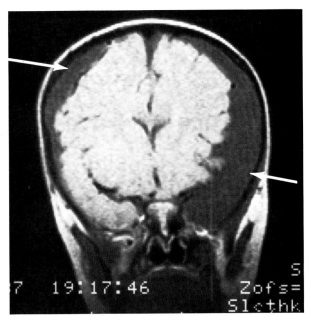

67: Megalocephaly   (.6T)

EXAM: MRI of the cranium.

CLINICAL INFORMATION: 2½-year-old male doing well clinically, but with increase in head size.

TECHNIQUE: Axial spin density images were obtained (700/32).

FINDINGS: The hemispheres are symmetric and normal. The ventricular system is normal and symmetric. The overall head size is increased for patient's age and disproportionate to body size. This finding is, however, made clinically with circumferential measurement of the cranial vault. No evidence of a mass or hydrocephalus is identified.

IMPRESSION: Megalocephaly.

DISCUSSION: Megalocephaly is a poorly understood term. The diagnosis, excluding active hydrocephalus, should differentiate between a primary megencephaly and a megencephaly of arrested hydrocephalus or a deposition disease.

REFERENCE: Lee et al.: *AJNR* **7**:605, July/August, 1986.

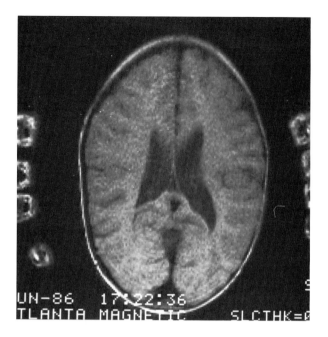
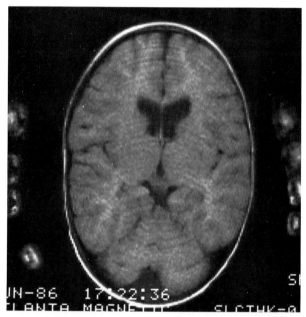
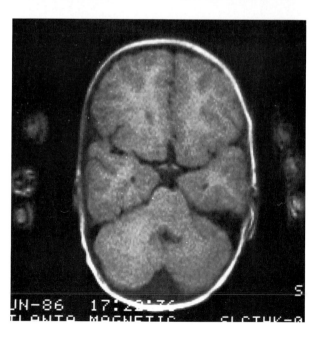

68: Frontal Parietal Arachnoid Cyst (.6T)

EXAM: MRI of the head.

CLINICAL INFORMATION: 64-year-old presenting with nondilating right pupil.

TECHNIQUE: Axial and coronal double-echo sequences were obtained (2000/32,64).

FINDINGS: Intracranial study is normal with the exception of a well-circumscribed cyst along the right frontal parietal convexity which behaves, in its signal intensity, similar to that of the surrounding CSF and the sulci and ventricular system. There is a slight scalloping of the internal table overlying this region. Findings are most consistent with a benign subarachnoid cyst. This does not appear to exhibit significant mass effect, and the ventricular system remains normal.

IMPRESSION: Frontal parietal subarachnoid cyst. An exophytic cystic glioma could not be totally excluded, but lack of any edema or mass effect is evidence against this diagnostic possibility.

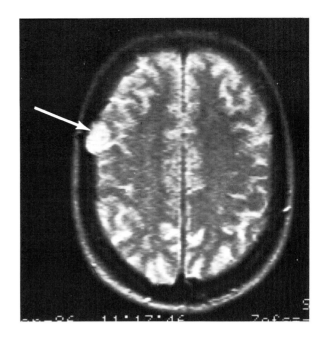

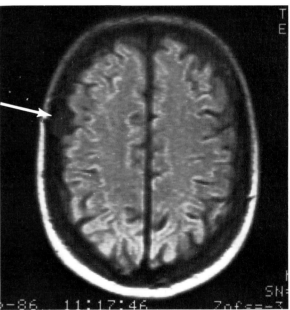

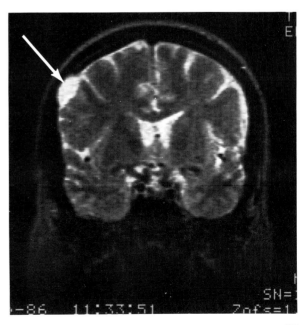

69: Adenocarcinoma of the Lacrimal Gland (.6T)

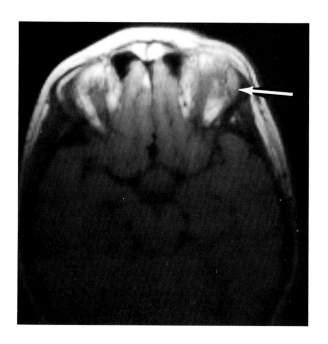

EXAM: MRI of the orbits.

CLINICAL INFORMATION: Female patient with a left swollen eyelid.

TECHNIQUE: T1-weighted images were acquired (1800/60; 600/38). These were oriented in the axial and coronal directions.

FINDINGS: Enlargement of the left lacrimal gland is associated with a small, but definite, amount of destructive change in the bony orbital roof. Findings of concern for a neoplastic involvement of the lacrimal gland.

IMPRESSION: Lacrimal gland enlargement with associated bony change, highly suspect for neoplastic change within the lacrimal gland. Consider adenocarcinoma of the lacrimal gland.

DISCUSSION: Excellent visualization of the lacrimal gland which is well-contrasted in its relation to the other orbital contents because of the intra- and extraconal fat available. In addition, the numerous planes allow for examination of any subtle bone change.

CONFIRMATION: Adenocarcinoma of the lacrimal gland was removed at surgery.

REFERENCE: Hyman et al.: *Applied Radiology* November/December, 1985.

Courtesy of Dr. Al Alexander/Paul Collura, Lancaster Magnetic Imaging

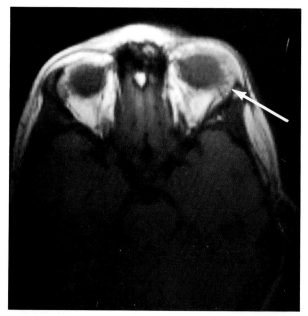

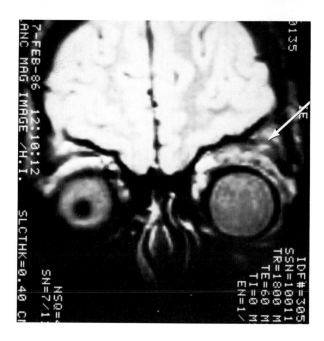

70: Graves' Disease   (.6T)

EXAM: MRI of the orbits.

CLINICAL INFORMATION: 43-year-old female with hyperthyroidism. Treated with Iodine 131. Now hypothyroid. Developing vertigo and dizziness. Rule out intracranial mass.

TECHNIQUE: Routine axial T1- and T2-weighted images were acquired (not shown); in addition, coronal spin density or T1-weighted images were obtained (650/38).

FINDINGS: Diffuse enlargement of the lateral, superior, medial, and inferior rectus muscles is identified. This diffuse muscle enlargement is consistent with Graves' Disease.

IMPRESSION: Diffuse enlargement of the rectus muscles consistent with patient's known Graves' Disease.

DISCUSSION: Our reference article demonstrates the use of various signal intensities with the combination of morphologic or CT-like features to increase the specificity of diagnosis of orbital pathology. As concerns our case, the most important differential made when encountering enlargement of the rectus muscles is the exclusion of a possible malignancy, such as a lymphoma. Graves' disease demonstrates a characteristically low signal on both T1- and T2-weighted imaging. Lymphoma demonstrates a characteristic increase in signal on the T2-weighted images.

REFERENCE: Sullivan et al.: *RadioGraphics* **7**: January, 1987.

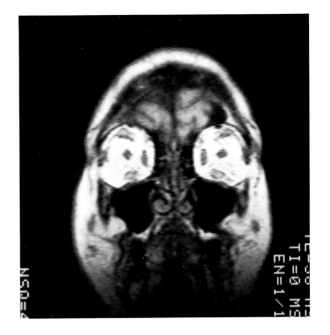

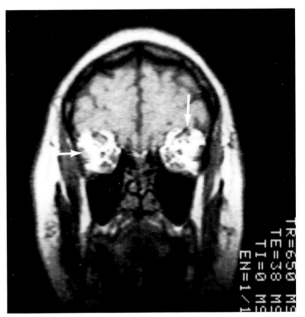

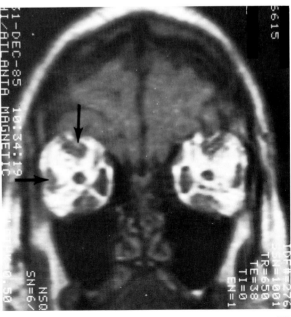

71: Multicentric Lymphangioma   (1.5T)

EXAM: MRI of the orbits.

CLINICAL INFORMATION: Patient is a 26-year-old female with obvious facial lymphangioma. Rule out intraorbital extension.

TECHNIQUE: Coronal and axial T1- and T2-weighted images were acquired (1500/20,60; 400/25).

FINDINGS: A medial supraconal, well-circumscribed mass with increased signal intensity on the T2-weighted images is identified. This has heterogeneous structure and appears to be somewhat cystic. This does not extend into the intraconal compartment of the orbit.

IMPRESSION: Lymphangioma.

DISCUSSION: This is a multicentric lymphangioma. There may be a small thread of attachment between the facial and infratemporal extension of the lymphangioma and the orbital mass, but these could not be demonstrated during our imaging session.

REFERENCE: Saint-Louis et al.: Paper presented at the meeting of ASNR, May, 1987.

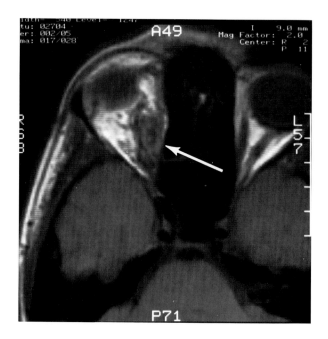

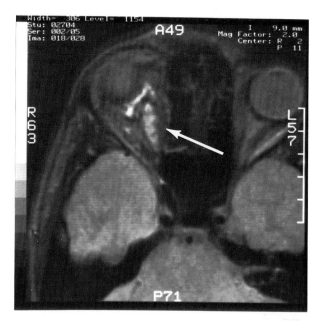

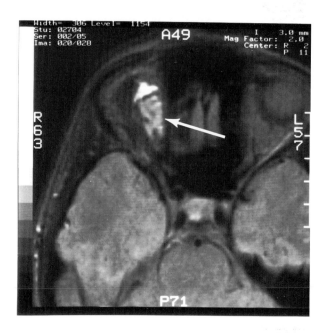

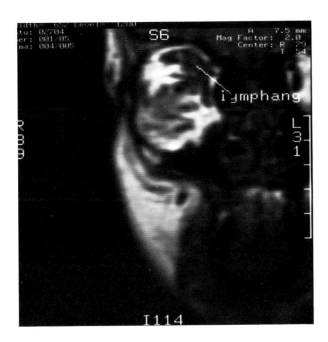

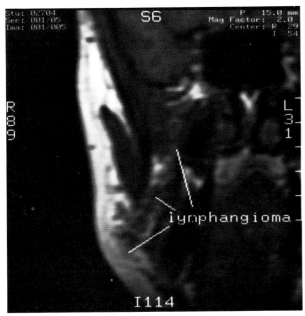

72: Pituitary Adenoma   (1.5T)

EXAM: MRI of the pituitary.

CLINICAL INFORMATION: 21-year-old female. Rule out pituitary tumor.

TECHNIQUE: Coronal, axial, and sagittal T1- and T2-weighted images were acquired (1500/25,70; 400/25; 2000/40,80).

FINDINGS: There is an 11-mm enlargement of the pituitary gland. This shows a diffuse isointense on the more T1 and T2 spin-density-weighted images and a definite increased signal on the T2-weighted images. This is a higher signal intensity than that of the CSF spaces, excluding an empty sella.

IMPRESSION: The findings are consistent with an adenoma of the pituitary.

DISCUSSION: The conventional CT coronal orientation is easily applied to the MR investigation of the pituitary. The relation to the optic chiasm is well-delineated. The sagittal orientation adds an additional understanding to the infundibular recess of the third ventricle and relation of the optic chiasm to the pituitary gland as well.

CONFIRMATION: Surgical removal of a pituitary adenoma was obtained approximately 1 week following this imaging session.

REFERENCE: *Radiology* **161**:761, 1986.

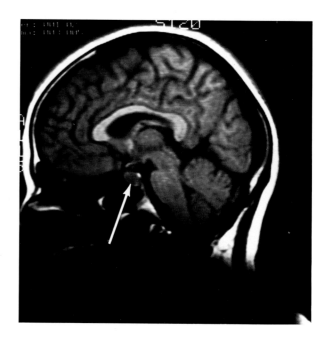

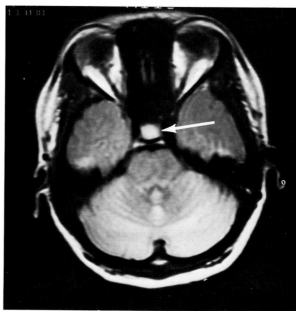

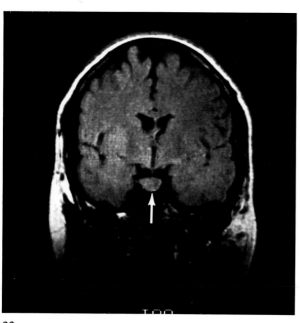

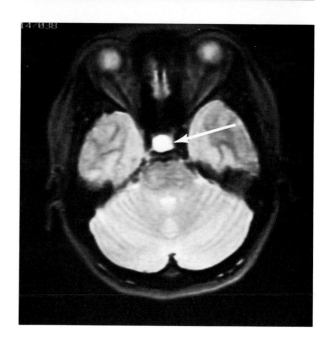

73: Empty Sella (1.5T)

EXAM: MRI of the pituitary gland.

CLINICAL INFORMATION: Multiple sclerosis.

TECHNIQUE: Axial and sagittal T1- and T2-weighted images were obtained (2000/40,80; 400/25).

FINDINGS: One small area of increased signal is identified in the left cerebellar hemisphere. Supratentorial images (not shown) were consistent with multiple sclerosis.

This study is included to show the cavernous expansion of the sella turcica with a flattened, smallish pituitary along the dependent portion of the sella turcica. The empty sella is presumed to be secondary to a defect in the diaphragm sellae, which allows the CSF to pulsate into the sella, causing expansion in a chronic fashion. The diagnosis of "empty" sella suggests absence of pituitary tissue. However, we suspect that the pituitary is merely compressed or atrophied because of the chronic CSF pulsation against it. The infundibulum commonly can be followed to the floor of the sella on CT axial cuts, as is also demonstrated. In addition, the axial image shows excellent extension of the infundibular recess of the third ventricle. This is identified as a small area of CSF density located centrally through the infundibulum.

IMPRESSION: Empty sella.

DISCUSSION: The diaphragm sellae is a dural membrane along the upper margin of the pituitary fossa. A defect or failure to fully form can allow CSF pulsation to be transmitted into the sella turcica. This chronic pulsation may cause the sella to enlarge as if containing a tumor. The enlarged sella with compressed, or possibly atrophied, pituitary gland has an empty appearance.

REFERENCE: Daniels et al.: *AJNR* 7:765, September/October, 1986.

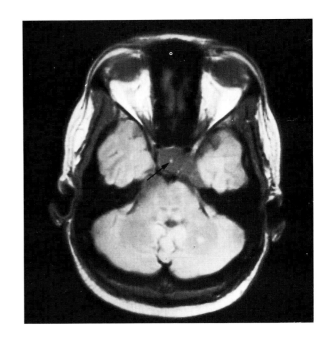

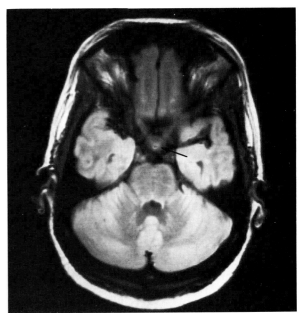

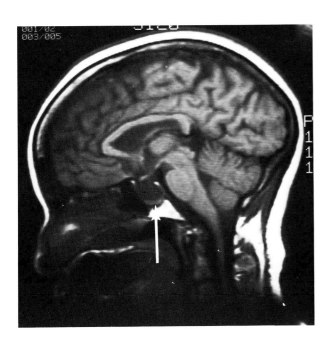

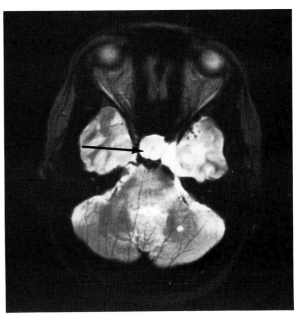

74: Macroadenoma (1.5T)

EXAM: MRI of the pituitary.

CLINICAL INFORMATION: Rule out a suprasellar mass in a 48-year-old male with optic difficulty.

TECHNIQUE: Coronal T1- and T2-weighted images were acquired (1200/25,60).

FINDINGS: There is a large sella tumor which extends and invades into the right cavernous sinus. Superior, lateral, and anterior to it are several large, rounded cystic cavities. The largest of these, to the left of midline and superior, extends into the suprasellar region and flattens the floor of the third ventricle. The increased signal intensity on both T1- and T2-weighted images suggests that these cysts contain products of chronic hemorrhage.

IMPRESSION: Large pituitary adenoma with large associated cyst, probably representing focal hemorrhages within the tumor.

DISCUSSION: The MRI offers an excellent demonstration of a tumor extension into the cavernous sinus. On contrast high-resolution CT, the cavernous sinus and the enhancing tumor overlap, and separation of these is not possible.

In addition, MR is unusually sensitive to the detection of hemorrhage and cysts within a tumor, as demonstrated here (curved arrow). Note the apparent small area of hemorrhage identified on the more T2-weighted images, which is virtually invisible on the first echo set (see small arrows—Image 2).

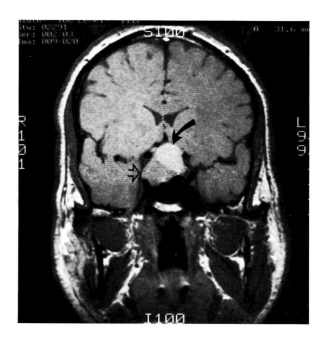

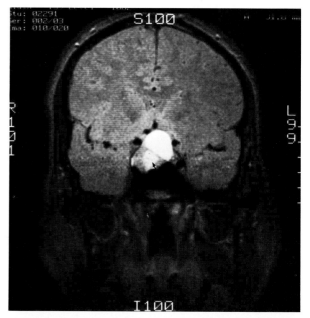

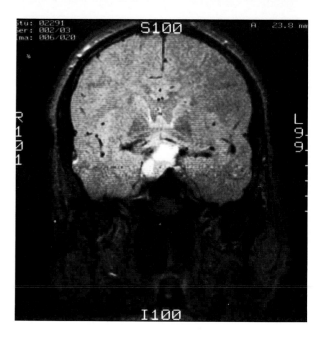

75: Macroadenoma   (.6T)

EXAM: MRI of the pituitary.

CLINICAL INFORMATION: 44-year-old male with possible pituitary tumor suggested on CT scan.

TECHNIQUE: Sagittal and coronal T1- and T2-weighted images were obtained (1700/38,64; 500/38).

FINDINGS: Macroadenomatous enlargement of the pituitary gland is identified. There is a near isointense signal from the tumor compared to brain tissue on the T1- and T2-weighted images. No extension in the sphenoid sinus is seen. The superior portion of the gland protrudes into the suprasellar cistern.

IMPRESSION: Macroadenoma.

DISCUSSION: Sagittal view offers unusual facial contour which suggests with the coarsened facial features, the presence of acromegaly. This was present clinically. The ability to scan the tumor in two dimensions should lead to a more accurate volumetric assessment of a tumor. This should be of particular usefulness to the endocronologist in evaluating the response of tumors to the chemotherapeutic regime.

REFERENCE: *ADNR* 7:209, March/April, 1986.

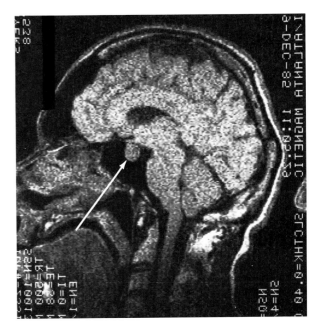

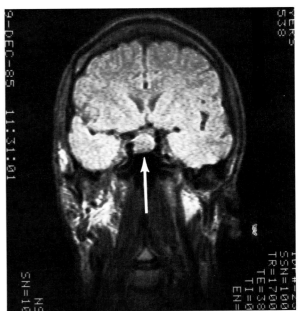

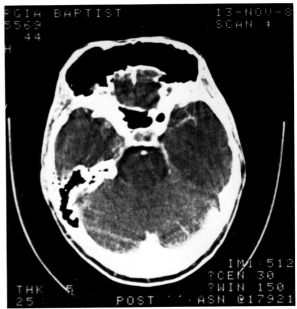

76: Macroadenoma Pre- and Postchemotherapy (1.5T)

EXAM: MRI of the pituitary gland.

CLINICAL INFORMATION: This is a 42-year-old male with findings consistent with a pituitary tumor.

TECHNIQUE: The images shown are on the initial study and on the two-month postchemotherapeutic checkup. These include T1- and T2-weighted images in the coronal and sagittal planes (2000/40,80; 400/25; 600/25).

FINDINGS: A mass measuring 2 to 3 cm in dimension extends from the sella with displacement of the optic chiasm. This is a midline mass with slight increase in signal intensity compared to brain on T1-weighted and definite increase on T2-weighted images. This apparently spares the cavernous sinuses with marked extension into the suprasellar cistern.

Follow-up study 2 months later shows marked loss of tumor volume with a slightly distorted third ventricle, but little evidence of tumor.

IMPRESSION: Large pituitary adenoma with marked response to two-month follow-up to a chemotherapeutic regime.

DISCUSSION: In our reference article, MR and CT were compared and MRI was proven superior in the evaluation of macroadenomas with regard to infundibular abnormality, cavernous sinus invasion, and optic chiasm compression. MR may underevaluate the bony erosion seen, but we contend this is a secondary finding and that MR is exquisitely sensitive to any extension of tumor into the sphenoid sinus.

In regard to the microadenomas, MR may miss a small adenoma which does not enlarge the pituitary gland, but recent advances in thin section capacity capabilities suggest that this limitation of MR, when compared to CT, will shortly be reversed.

REFERENCE: Davis et al.: *AJNR* 8:107, January/February, 1987.

Pre-Treatment

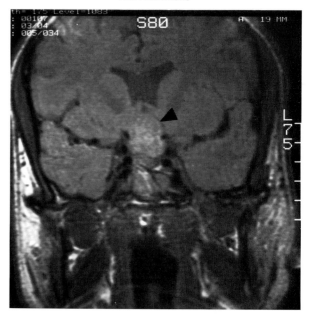

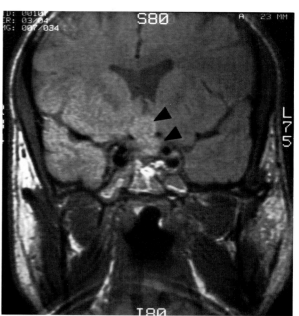

Pre-Treatment

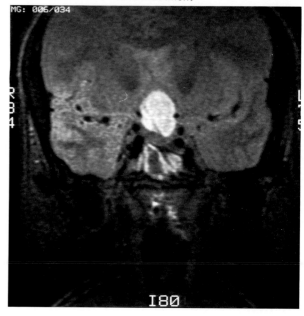

Post-Treatment

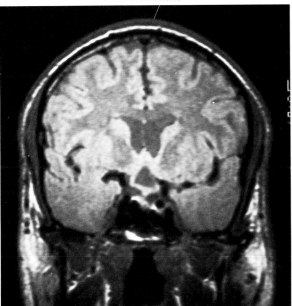

Pre-Treatment

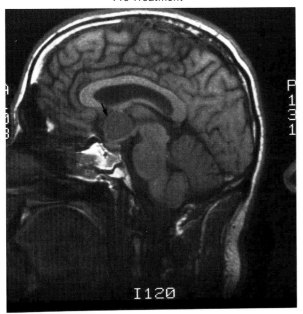

Post-Treatment

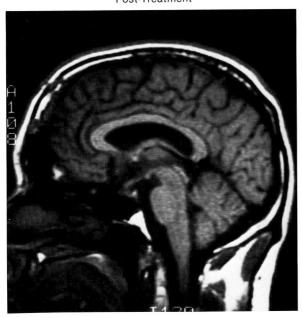

77: Adenoma with Hemorrhage (.6T)

EXAM: MRI of the pituitary.

CLINICAL INFORMATION: 21-year-old with known tumor of the pituitary gland discovered at 15 years of age. On medication. Doing well for 2 to 3 years. Two months ago, recurrent headaches with reappearance of symptoms, including lactation and blurred vision.

TECHNIQUE: Coronal and sagittal T1- and T2-weighted images were obtained (2000/35,80; 600/34).

FINDINGS: The enlarged gland, identified on the coronal images to the left and within the inferior portion of the gland, is a high-signal focus consistent with hemorrhage. The high signal suggests that this is probably a chronic hemorrhage.

IMPRESSION: Pituitary adenoma with chronic hemorrhage.

REFERENCE: Daniels et al.: *AJNR* **6**:187, March/April, 1985.

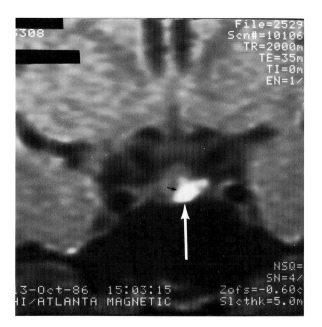

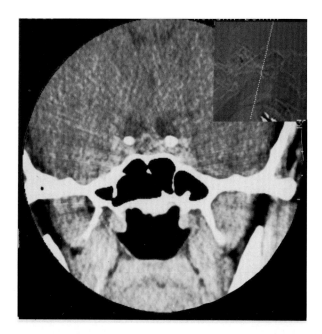

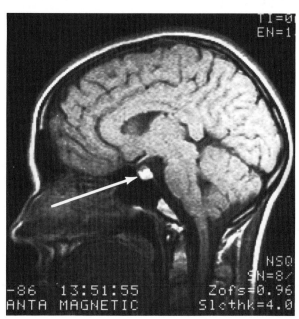

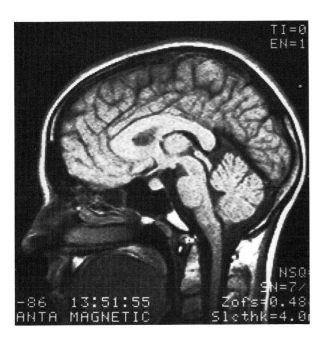

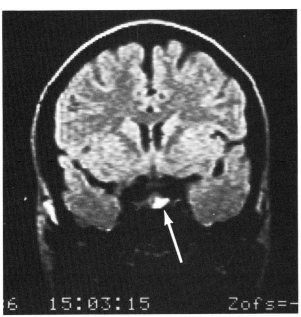

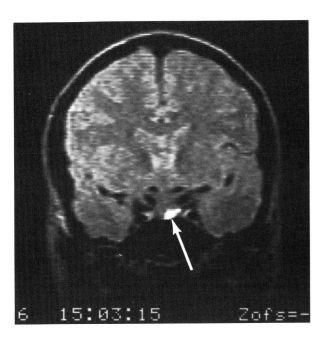

97

78: Lymphoma of the Parotid Gland with Extension into the Gasserian Ganglion   (1.5T)

EXAM: MRI of the calvarium.

CLINICAL INFORMATION: The patient is a 39-year-old female with diffuse severe right facial pain.

TECHNIQUE: Axial (2000/20,80; 800/20).

FINDINGS: There is marked asymmetric enlargement of the gasserian ganglion as well as the maxillary segment of the fifth cranial nerve. This is followed down into an abnormal-appearing parotid gland with irregular stellate margins. The findings are consistent with a diffuse neoplastic involvement. Question of a parotid gland tumor originating and growing in a retrograde fashion through the cranial fifth nerve versus a lymphoma.

IMPRESSION: Lymphoma in parotid gland with extention into gasserian ganglion.

CONFIRMATION: Surgical Rx of lymphoma.

DISCUSSION: Contrast resolution of the parotid gland is quite good and felt to be superior to that of CT. This allows for evaluation of parotid neoplasms in the parapharyngeal spaces. The sagittal and coronal views are particularly helpful in following the extent of the parotid tumors, as seen in this case. Note the incidental microadenoma in the left sella turcica (small arrow).

REFERENCE: Mandelblatt et al.: *Radiology* **163**:411, 1987.

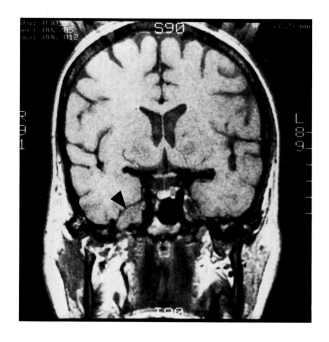

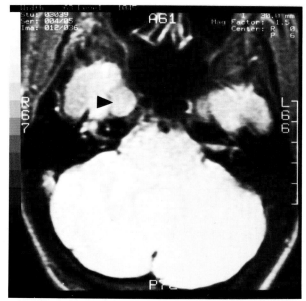

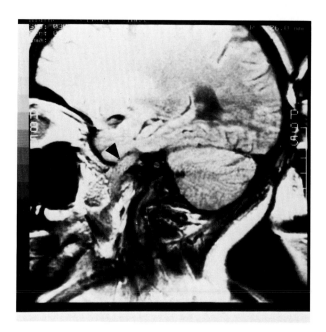

79: Nasopharyngealcarcinoma (1.5T)

EXAM: MRI of the head.

CLINICAL INFORMATION: Patient with known nasopharyngeal-carcinoma sent for evaluation.

TECHNIQUE: Sagittal T1-weighted images were acquired (500/25).

FINDINGS: There is diffuse expansion of the clivus with soft tissue extension filling the sphenoid sinus and extending out into the nasopharyngeal region and along the anterior or prevertebral soft tissue to the level of the body of C2 vertebra. The soft tissues extend anteriorly into about the midportion of the nasal passages. There is marked bony destruction and bulging of the clivus posteriorly without good evidence for direct extension into the prepontine cistern.

IMPRESSION: Findings consistent with a large nasopharyngeal-carcinoma as described.

CONFIRMATION: Epidermoid carcinoma has been biopsied.

DISCUSSION: Note the impressive amount of information demonstrated in the sagittal view. This is an excellent view for follow-up of this tumor in its post radiation course.

REFERENCE: Glazer et al.: *Radiology* **160**:343, 1986.

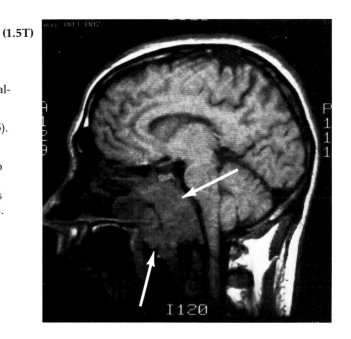

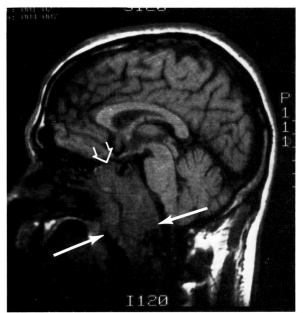

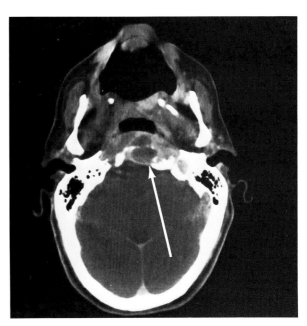

80: Cordoma of the Clivus   (.6T)

EXAM: MRI of the calvarium.

CLINICAL INFORMATION: This is a check on size of shunt in a 25-year-old female with proven cordoma.

TECHNIQUE: Axial and sagittal T1- and T2-weighted images were acquired (500/32; 3000/32,64).

FINDINGS: Large destructive mass is identified arising from the inferior portion of the clivus, extending to its interior portion, and anteriorly and superiorly through the C1 arch. A large soft tissue mass arising from the clivus markedly indents the medullary belly, and this places the brainstem and posterior fossa contents posteriorly.

IMPRESSION: Findings consistent with a large cordoma. Note made of the absence of the bony posterior elements of C1-2 and C2-3 from prior decompressive surgery.

DISCUSSION: The cordoma is a soft tumor thought to arise from notochord remnant cells. These are seen predominantly in the clival and cervical regions. The remainder are seen mostly in the sacral region. Cordomas have, however, been reported throughout the vertebral column.

REFERENCES: Amendola et al.: *Radiology* **158**:839, 1986. Han et al.: *Radiology* **150**:705, 1984.

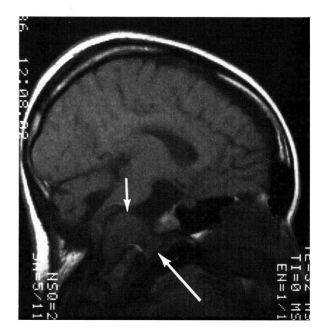

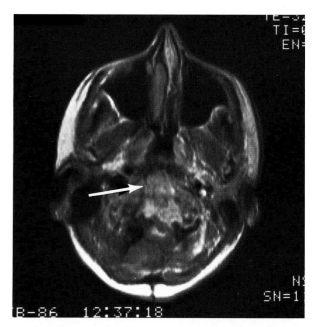

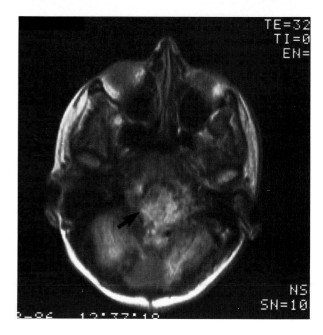

81: Thyroglossal Duct Cyst   (.6T)

EXAM: MRI of the neck.

CLINICAL INFORMATION: Evaluate a large anterior neck mass.

TECHNIQUE: Sagittal and coronal T1- and T2-weighted images were acquired (2200/30,90; 540/34; 450/34).

FINDINGS: A smooth marginated anterior neck mass in the infrahyoid region just anterior to the thyroid cartilage is identified. This measures approximately 3.8 × 3.9 cm. The tail-like posterior area projects from the mass and superiorly toward the base of the tongue. There is an increased homogeneous signal on the more T2-weighted images, suggesting that this is a cystic or fluid-containing mass. Location in the midline and the presence of what appears to be a well-marginated fluid-filled mass suggest that this is most consistent with a thyroglossal duct cyst.

IMPRESSION: Thyroglossal duct cyst.

REFERENCE: Dietrich et al.: *Radiology* **159**:769, 1986.

Courtesy Al Alexander of Lancaster Magnetic Imaging

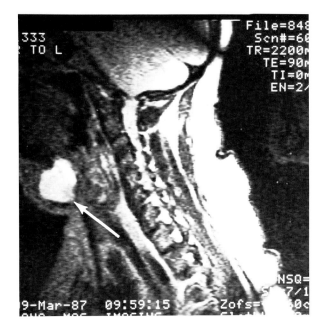

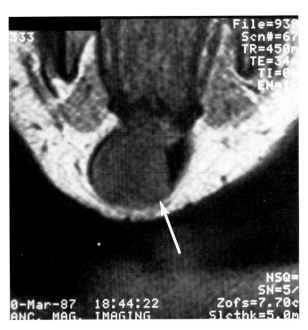

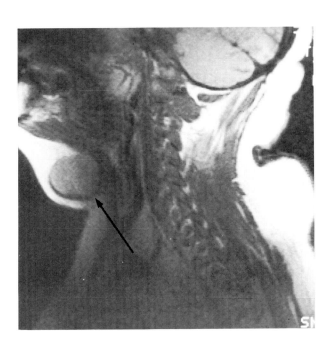

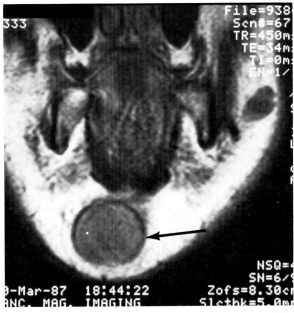

82: Rhabdomyosarcoma (.6T)

EXAM: MRI of the neck.

CLINICAL INFORMATION: 8-year-old female, status post chemotherapy, for rhabdomyosarcoma in the infratemporal fossa.

TECHNIQUE: T1- and T2-weighted images were obtained (2000/32,64; 2700/60,120).

FINDINGS: An area of abnormal intermediate signal intensity on the more T1 or spin density images seen is in the left side, replacing the normal pterygoid plate anatomy as well as extending through the pterygoid muscle. There is also a fluid filling the left maxillary sinus. This shows increased signal on the T2-weighted images. This is consistent with a soft tissue tumor arising from the muscle, such as a rhabdomyosarcoma.

IMPRESSION: Rhabdomyosarcoma.

DISCUSSION: This accounts for 4 to 8 percent of all malignancies in patients under the age of 15 years. Rhabdomyosarcomas are the most common soft tissue sarcomas of childhood.

REFERENCE: Latack et al.: *AJNR* **8**:353, March/April, 1987.

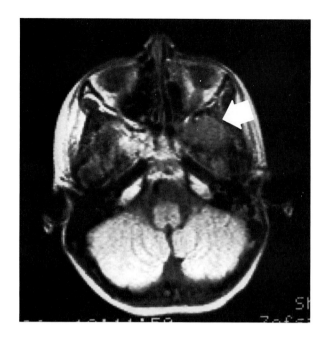

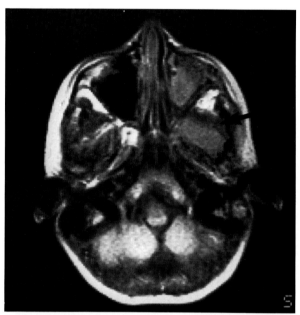

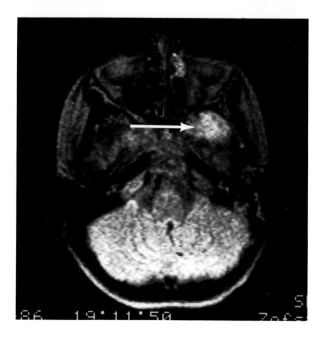

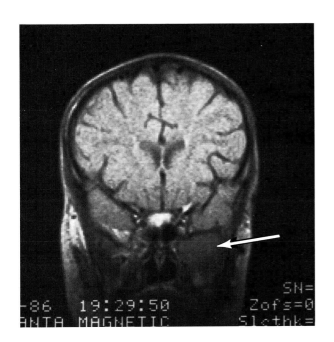

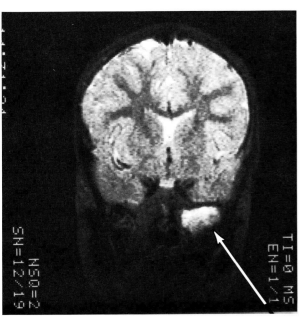

83: Scalp Lipoma   (.6T)

EXAM: MRI of the head.

CLINICAL INFORMATION: Evaluation of a 67-year-old female for amnesiac episodes. Rule out mass.

TECHNIQUE: Sagittal, axial, and coronal images were obtained (2000/40,80; 525/34).

FINDINGS: The images included show a small focal area of lipomatous material with increased or prolonged T1 signal which remains isointense with that of the other scalp fat. The focal collection of fat is considered to represent a small scalp lipoma. The remainder of the study is incidental.

DISCUSSION: Incidental scalp lipomas and sebaceous cysts are noted at times on evaluation. The signal void seen within the bone excludes any malignant characteristics of the incidental masses.

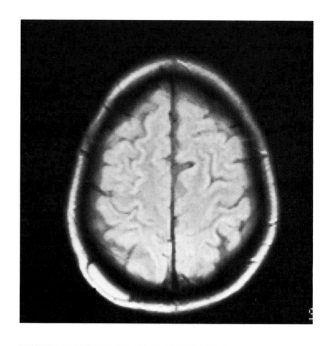

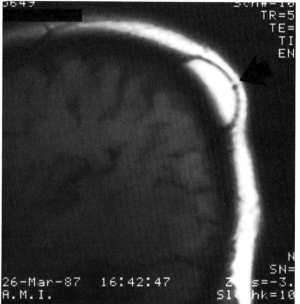

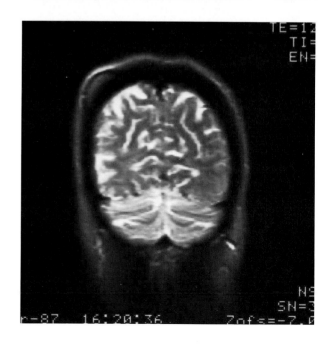

84: Cervical Neurofibroma (1.5T)

CLINICAL INFORMATION: The patient is a 39-year-old male with right upper-extremity symptomatology.

TECHNIQUE: Surface coil sagittal and axial T1- and T2-weighted images were obtained (1500/25,90; 1000/25).

FINDINGS: The dumbbell-shaped tumor was seen on the right side, extending through the C3-4 right neural foraminal canal. This deviates the cord from right to left, and there is associated bony widening of the canal. The location and tendency to grow through the neural foraminal canal in dumbbell-shaped fashion with associated chronic bone change suggests that this is a chronic benign lesion. This is a typical location and behavior for a neurofibroma.

IMPRESSION: Cervical neurofibroma.

REFERENCE: Hyman: *AJNR* **6**:229, March/April, 1985.

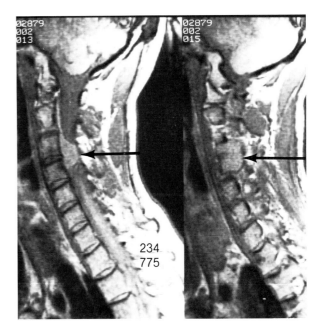

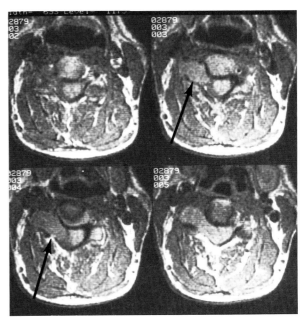

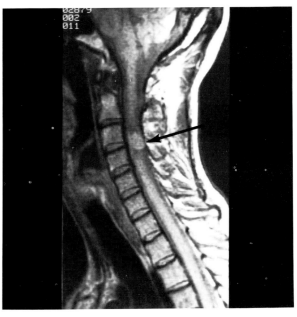

85: Metastatic Involvement in the Cervical Region (.6T)

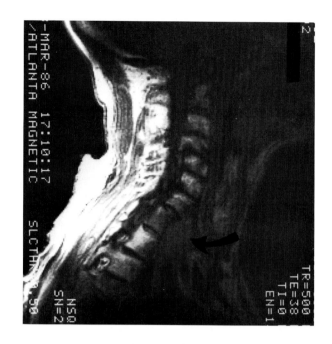

EXAM: MRI of the cervical spine.

CLINICAL INFORMATION: 76-year-old with a right apical pleural-based tumor and neck pain. Rule out metastatic disease.

TECHNIQUE: Surface coil T1-weighted sagittal images were obtained through the cervical spine (500/38).

FINDINGS: C7, T1, T2, and the posterior aspect of C6 all show decreased signal intensity within the vertebral bodies. These are quite characteristic of metastatic disease within the vertebral bodies. There is some retrolisthesis of several of the vertebral bodies, but no evidence of an epidural metastatic spread.

IMPRESSION: Diffuse metastatic involvement in the cervical and upper thoracic region.

DISCUSSION: The ability to demonstrate metastatic disease is shown well. In addition, peripheral to the central canal, metastatic involvement of the nerves as they exit the foramina can be identified (Image 2—small arrows). The tumor extends through the pleural mediastinal space, as well as lateral to the bony vertebral column, and probably catches the cervical and thoracic roots as they join the brachial plexus.

REFERENCE: Armington et al.: *AJNR* 8:361, March/April, 1987.

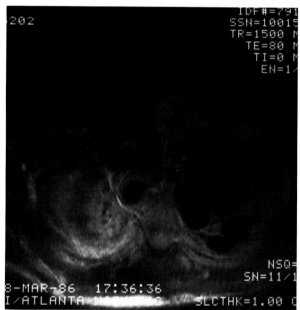

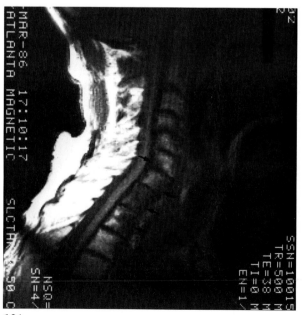

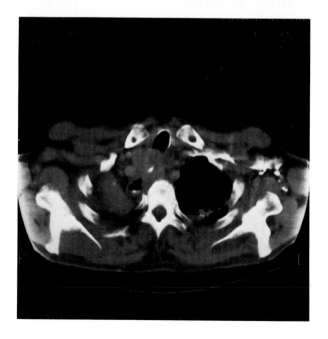

86: Old Traumatic Deformity to the Dens (.6T)

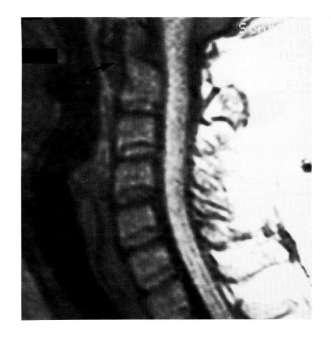

EXAM: MRI of the cervical spine.

CLINICAL INFORMATION: Rule out disc disease in a 38-year-old involved in a motor vehicle accident 6 years ago. Now, neck and right arm pain.

TECHNIQUE: T1- and T2-weighting were acquired in the sagittal orientation (1800/34,68).

FINDINGS: The dens has an unusual alignment and appears somewhat anterior to the normal position with respect to the body of C2. There is no evidence of any soft-tissue swelling, and the alignment and other findings in the cervical spine are normal.

IMPRESSION: Unusual configuration of the dens. Question an old fracture through the dens.

DISCUSSION: Note the unusual outline of the dens in the C2 body (tomography-midline tomogram submitted for comparison). Early articles suggested that bone detail was quite poor; however, the overall morphology as well as the medullary content, is excellently detailed on MRI, as evidenced by our case.

REFERENCES: Sze et al.: *Radiology* **161**:391, 1986. Lee et al.: *AJNR* **6**:209, March/April, 1985.

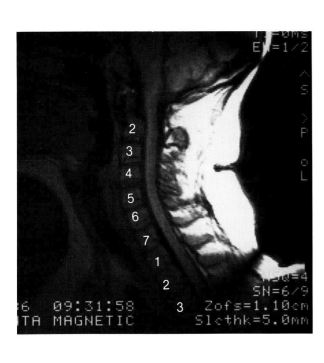

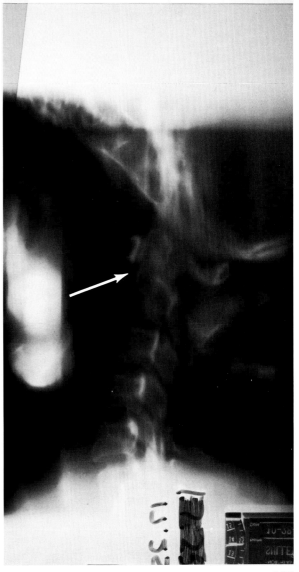

87: Cord Tumor   (.6T)

EXAM: MRI of the cervical spine.

CLINICAL INFORMATION: 53-year-old female with previous radiation for lymphoma and history of breast CA. Now clinically presents with Brown-Séquard's syndrome.

TECHNIQUE: Surface coil and axial T1- and T2-weighted images were acquired (500/38; 3000/38,76).

FINDINGS: There is diffuse enlargement of the cord from the C2 to C6 levels. Diffuse symmetric enlargement is consistent with a diffuse process, possibly inflammatory, but more suspect because of homogeneous signal on both sagittal and axial views for a neoplastic growth such as an ependymoma. There is a slight increase in signal intensity on the more T2-weighted images (Image 3).

IMPRESSION: Diffuse cord swelling, may be secondary to inflammation or radiation change; however, we suspect cord tumor such as ependymoma.

REFERENCE: Masaryk et al.: *JCAT* **10**:184, March/April, 1986.

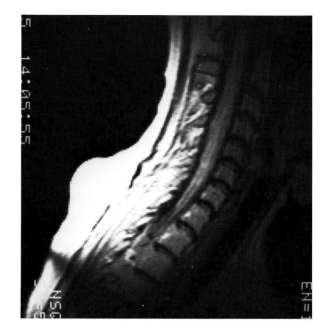

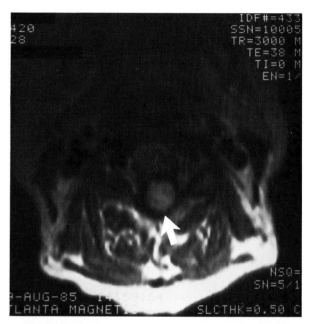

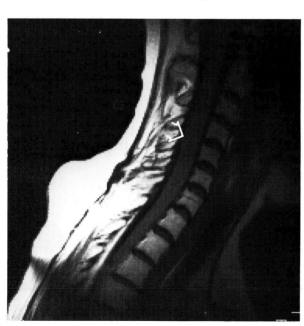

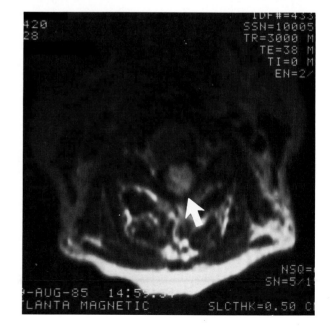

88: C4-5 Fusion (Normal Post Surgical Appearance) (.6T)

EXAM: MRI of the cervical spine.

CLINICAL INFORMATION: 43-year-old female involved in a motor vehicle accident, complaining of tingling and numbness in the right arm. Prior surgical fusion.

TECHNIQUE: Sagittal and axial T1- and T2-weighted images were acquired (1400/40; 1000/60).

FINDINGS: C4-5 postoperative fusion identified. No evidence of recurrent disc herniation identified.

IMPRESSION: Normal postoperative appearance of the C4-5 fusion.

DISCUSSION: Note the loss of the normal endplate anatomy and disc signal. The low signal located centrally in the site of surgery may be surrounded by high-signal-intensity foci. This is, in part, secondary to a metal artifact. Presumably the graft or small flecks of metal from the operating surgeon's instrument cause enough paramagnetic material to cause this defect. This should not be confused with the presence of infectious material, hematoma, or another abnormality.

REFERENCE: Heindel et al.: *JCAT* **10**:596, July/August, 1986.

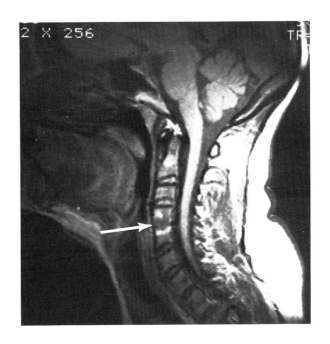

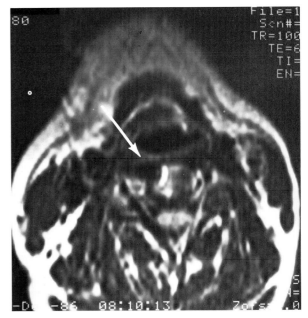

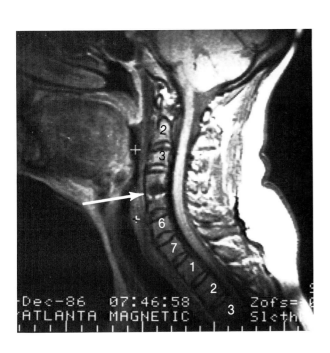

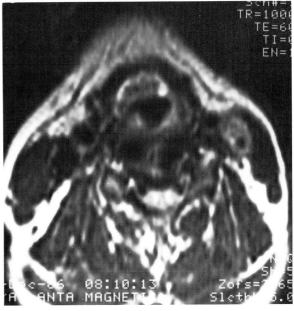

89: C5-6 Disc Herniation (.6T)

EXAM: MRI of the cervical spine.

CLINICAL INFORMATION: Rule out a C5-6 disc herniation, in a 46-year-old female involved in a motor vehicle accident previous. Now complains of neck, right arm, and finger pain with numbness. No left-sided symptoms.

TECHNIQUE: Sagittal T1- and T2-weighted images were acquired (1200/45,90).

FINDINGS: There is a large C5-6 disc herniation with mild to moderate degenerative change of the disc material. The herniation deviates the cord and slightly effaces it at this level. This is central and right-sided in location.

IMPRESSION: C5-6 disc herniation.

REFERENCES: Heindel et al.: *JCAT* **10**:596, July/August, 1987. Modic et al.: *Radiology* **161**:753, 1986.

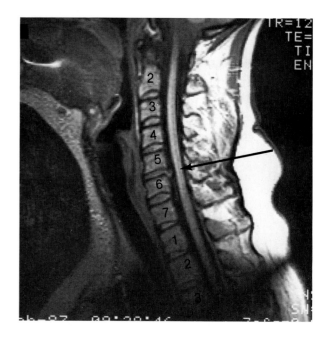

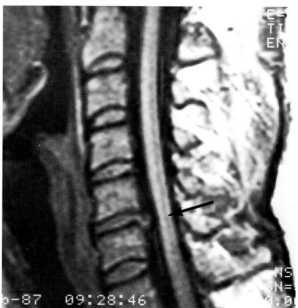

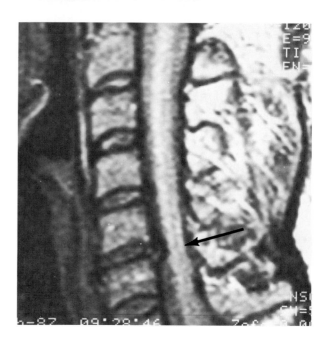

90: C3-4 Disc Herniation   (.6T)

EXAM: MRI of the cervical spine.

CLINICAL INFORMATION: Prior fusions C4-5, C5-6, and C6-7 in a 46-year-old female who now complains of headaches and right-hand numbness.

TECHNIQUE: Sagittal and axial T1- and T2-weighted images were acquired (450/34; 1400/50,100).

FINDINGS: Right-sided extradural defect to the C3-4 level is consistent with disc herniation. The routine double-echo sagittal studies are slightly degraded by motion. However, there is good confirmation on repeat short-sequence sagittal and axial views of the defect.

IMPRESSION: Central and right-sided disc herniation at C3-4.

DISCUSSION: Note first the normal appearance of the three fused levels and the appearance of a disc herniation above this level.

REFERENCE: Modic et al.: *Radiology* **161**:753, 1986.

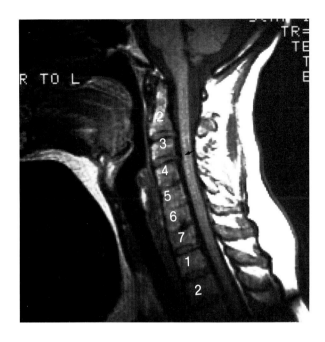

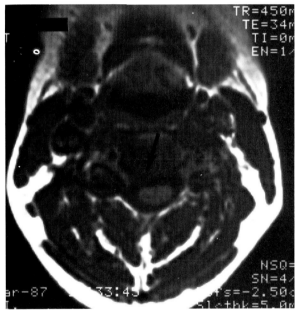

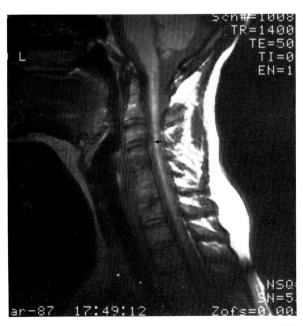

91: Myelomalacia   (.6T)

EXAM: MRI of the cervical spine.

CLINICAL INFORMATION: 40-year-old male with radiculopathy to the right arm.

TECHNIQUE: Surface coil sagittal and axial T1- and T2-weighted images were acquired (2000/34,68; 1000/60).

FINDINGS: A large central and right-sided disc herniation at the C6-7 level is identified. These extend into the central right and neural foraminal canals with displacement of the cord posteriorly and slight flattening of the ventral right aspect of the cord. On the axial images, an area of increased signal from C4 to C7 is seen. The margins are indiscrete, and there is no expansion of the cord parenchyma. The alteration or increase in signal in this region may reflect some cord edema or myelomalacia.

DISCUSSION: The area of nonspecific increased signal is probably, in part, secondary to edema from cord irritation by the large disc herniation at the C6-7 level. These are sometimes difficult to separate from a surface-coil burn artifact because of proximity of the structures to the surface coil. The MR, is, however, useful as well as excluding edema and myelomalacia cysts or other deformities of the cord.

REFERENCE: Quencer et al.: *AJNR* 7:457, May/June, 1986.

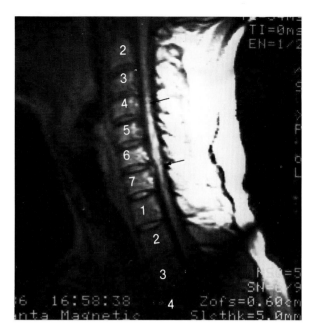

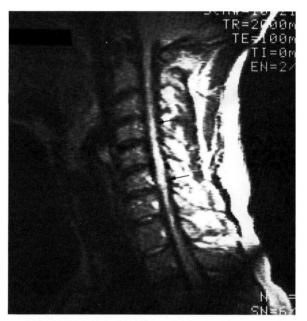

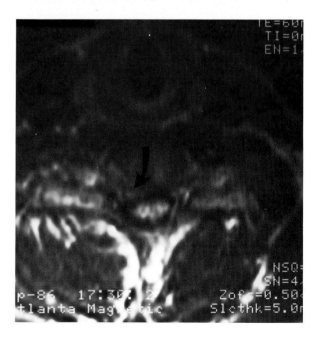

92: Multiple Sclerosis (.6T)

EXAM: MRI of the cervical spine.

CLINICAL INFORMATION: 37-year-old female with numbness in the neck and right arm.

TECHNIQUE: Axial and coronal T1- and T2-weighted images were acquired through the calvarium (2000/34,68; 2000/60,120).

FINDINGS: Numerous white-matter areas of increased signal are seen. These are small, without mass effect, and populated over the roof of the lateral ventricle. In addition, on both coronal and axial views, an area of increased signal in the right superior cervical cord is identified.

IMPRESSION: Findings consistent with multiple sclerosis. Involvement of the upper cervical right hemicord also identified.

REFERENCE: Smoker et al.: *RadioGraphics* **6**:   November, 1986.

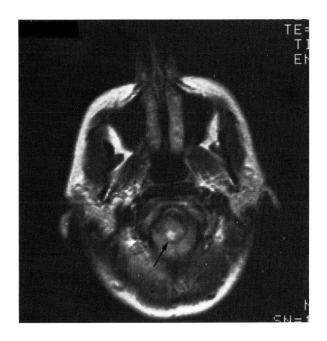

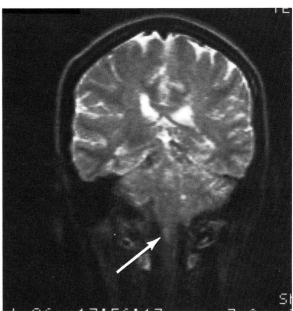

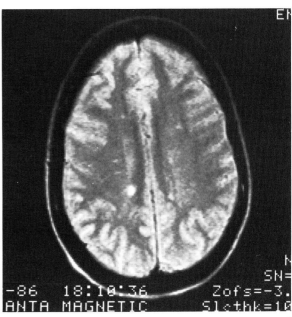

93: Foramen Magnum Meningioma (.6T)

EXAM: MRI of the cervical spine.

CLINICAL INFORMATION: 54-year-old female with left-sided hand and leg problems beginning 3 years before.

TECHNIQUE: Sagittal and axial T1- and T2-weighted images were acquired (2000/40,80; 550/38).

FINDINGS: There is an extramedullary intradural right-sided tumor measuring approximately 4 to 5 cm from the cephalad to caudal dimensions. This measures 2 to 3 cm in transverse dimension. There is marked compression of the upper cervical cord. There is isointensity to the neural structures on the spin density and T1-weighted images and slight increase in signal intensity on the more T2-weighted images. Differential for an extramedullary lesion in this location is between meningioma and neurofibroma.

IMPRESSION: Extramedullary intradural mass felt to represent meningioma.

CONFIRMATION: This patient has been previously diagnosed as having a foramen magnum tumor and was submitted for this evaluation to rule out other cervical disc diseases.

REFERENCE: Smoker et al.: *RadioGraphics* **6**: November, 1986.

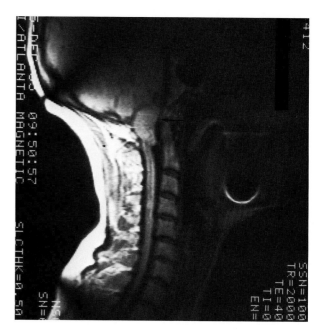

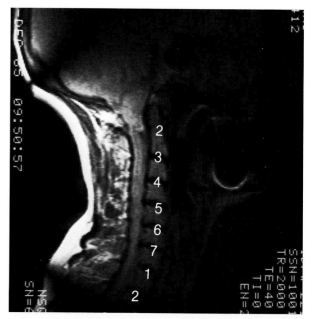

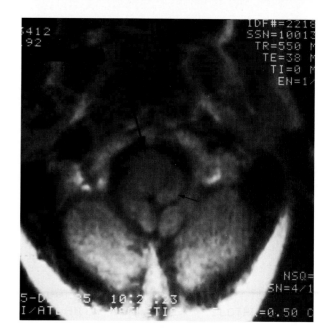

94: Recurrent Dermoid   (.6T)

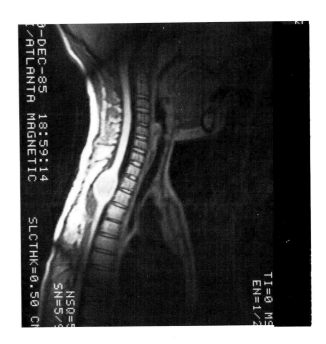

EXAM: MRI of the cervical spine.

CLINICAL INFORMATION: Five-year-old doing well following a prior resection of a dermoid cyst with a prior laminectomy T1 to T4. Now, recurrent gait and clumsiness problem. Rule out recurrence.

TECHNIQUE: Surface coil T1- and T2-weighted images with axial T1-weighted images were obtained (2000/40,80; 600/38).

FINDINGS: There is a focal intramedullary tumor enlarging the cord at the T2 level. The margins of the tumor are discrete, and the tumor shows hyposignal intensity compared to the neural structures. The surrounding neural tissue on the T1- and spin-density-weighted images. This occurs at the site of prior resection.

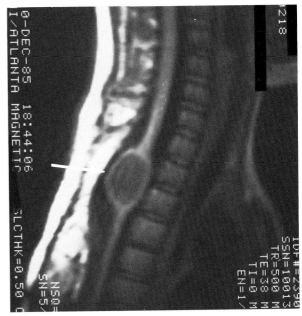

IMPRESSION: Findings consistent with a recurrent intramedullary tumor. By history, prior tumor was dermoid. An ependymoma or a glioma cannot be excluded.

DISCUSSION: This case shows excellent differential sometimes seen between tumor and surrounding normal neural tissue. This is useful in planning an approach to a cord tumor allowing an entry site with minimal disruption of normal tissues.

CONFIRMATION: Recurrent dermoid was removed at surgery shortly after this imaging session.

REFERENCE: Smoker et al.: *RadioGraphics* **6**:   November, 1986.

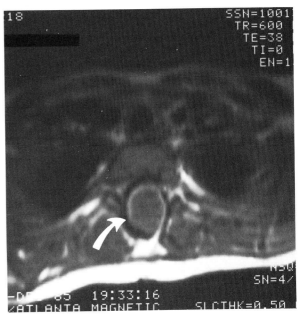

95: Multiple Myeloma (1.5T)

EXAM: MRI of the cervical spine.

CLINICAL INFORMATION: 35-year-old male with neck pain and increasing lower extremity weakness.

TECHNIQUE: Sagittal and axial T1- and T2-weighted images were acquired (2000/25,90; 1000/25).

FINDINGS: Destructive lesion of the seventh cervical vertebral body with tumor extending both anteriorly and posteriorly to the vertebral body and through the right neural foraminal canal at the C6-7 level. There is a high degree of canal obstruction secondary to the extent of tumor.

IMPRESSION: Neoplastic destruction of the seventh cervical vertebra with marked canal destruction secondary to diffuse extension of a neoplastic process.

CONFIRMATION: Aspirate demonstrated myeloma tissue. Also note the characteristic permeated involvement of the skull.

REFERENCE: Lee et al.: *AJNR* **6**:209, March/April, 1985.

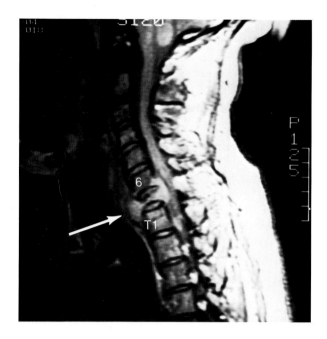

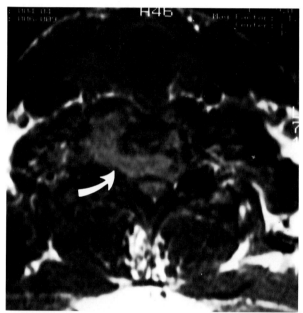

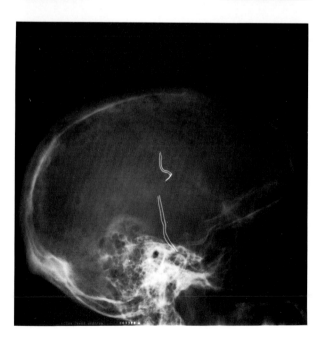

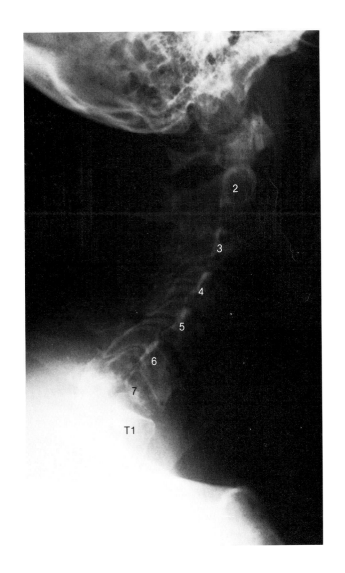

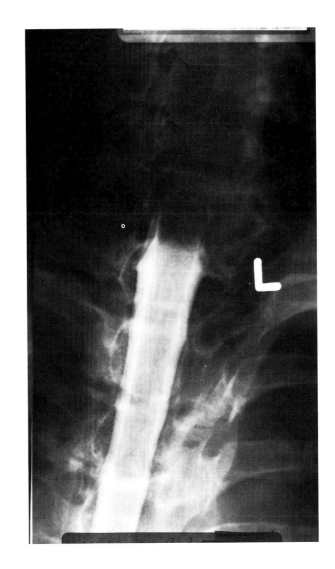

96: C5-6 Disc Herniation (1.5T)

EXAM: MRI of the cervical spine.

CLINICAL INFORMATION: 45-year-old male, with right-sided symptoms and neck pain.

TECHNIQUE: Sagittal and axial T1- and T2-weighted images were acquired (2000/30; 1500/30,60).

FINDINGS: There is evidence for a large extradural defect at the C5-6 disc level. This is identified on both sagittal and axial views. This is consistent with a disc herniation with associated moderate cord deformity at this level. Myelogram done approximately 1 month earlier (Image 3) did not suggest a defect at that time.

IMPRESSION: C5-6 right-sided disc herniation.

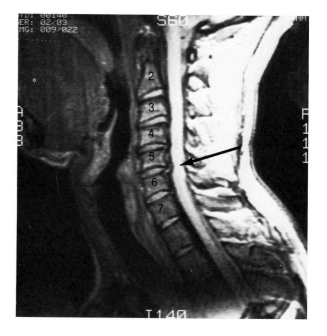

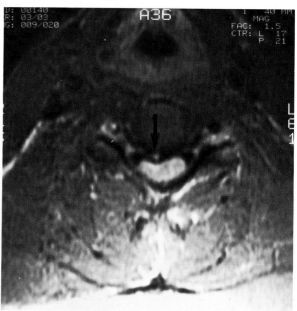

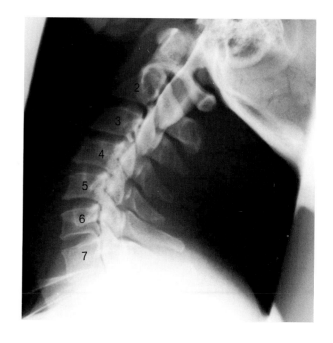

97: Anterior C5-6 Disc Herniation (.6T)

EXAM: MRI of the cervical spine.

CLINICAL INFORMATION: 62-year-old with previous cervical decompression and continued spastic paraparesis.

TECHNIQUE: Sagittal region was studied with a T1-weighted image acquisition in a head series (other images not shown) (500/38).

FINDINGS: A C5-6 anterior disc herniation is identified. There is mild posterior subluxation of C5 in relation to C6. This extends into the posterior canal but does not appear to cause significant canal compression or deform the cord through this region.

IMPRESSION: C5-6 anterior disc herniation.

DISCUSSION: The presence of a disc herniation anteriorly, although not of clinical importance in itself, does indicate significant disease within the disc material and annulus and, on questionable posterior disc herniation, the presence of an anteriorly herniated disc at the same level can act as a confirmation to suspected posterior disc herniation.

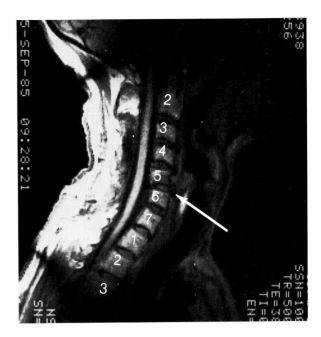

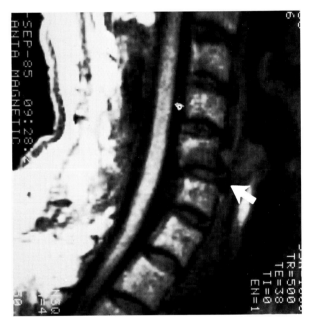

98: Two-Level Fusion (Pre and Postop Study)   (1.5T)

EXAM: MRI of the cervical spine.

CLINICAL INFORMATION: This is a 39-year-old male with two separate studies. The first study followed a C5-6 fusion. The second study follows a C6-7 fusion.

TECHNIQUE: Surface coil sagittal imaging was obtained using T1- and T2-weighting (2000/40,80; 1500/25,90).

FINDINGS: Characteristic loss of signal at the C5-6 level on the first study with central area of increased signal is identified. No epidural defect or abnormality within the canal is identified. Findings are typical for that of a postoperative cervical fusion. The second study shows again similar changes of postoperative fusion.

IMPRESSION: The two studies demonstrate first at C5-6 and then at C6-7, postop fusion.

DISCUSSION: There can be a slight range in the appearance of a postoperative disc. Predominantly, loss of signal and distortion of endplate anatomy is seen. There may be a metal-type artifact identified in the sites. Recent literature suggest that this may be secondary to deposit of small amounts of metal flake from the surgeons' operating instruments.

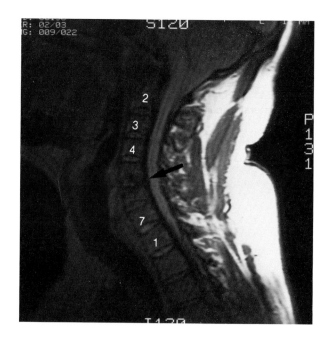

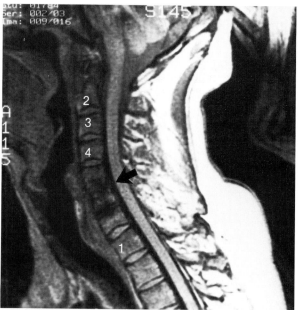

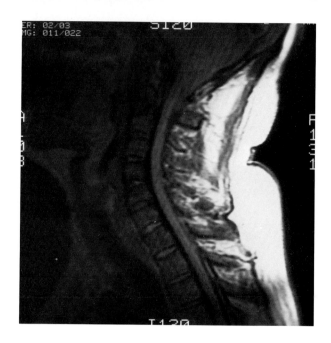

99: Chiari I with Syrinx   (1.5T)

EXAM: MRI of the cervical spine.

CLINICAL INFORMATION: The patient is a 44-year-old female with bilateral upper-extremity difficulty.

TECHNIQUE: Sagittal T1-weighted images were acquired (600/25).

FINDINGS: A prominent Chiari I with large cerebellar peg or protrusion downward of the cerebellar tonsils is identified. This is associated with a large syrinx extending from the C2 to the T9-10 levels.

IMPRESSION: Chiari I with associated syrinx extending from C2 to T8-9.

DISCUSSION: The Chiari I is a form of hindbrain dysgenesis which includes downward placement of cerebellar tonsils. The cutoff suggested in recent literature of the lowermost extent of normal tonsil from the foraminal ring is 4 mm. The size and amount of cerebellar tonsil protrusion can vary. These are felt by various investigators to provide blockage to the normal CSF, and the obstruction caused by the tonsils allows development of a syrinx. These are different from the Chiari II in that the medullary segment is not also herniated, and the Chiari II malformation is always associated with the spinal dysraphic syndrome.

REFERENCE: Bradley et al.: *Radiology* **152**:695, 1984.

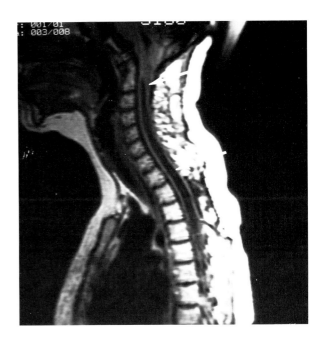

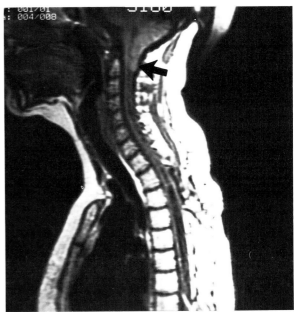

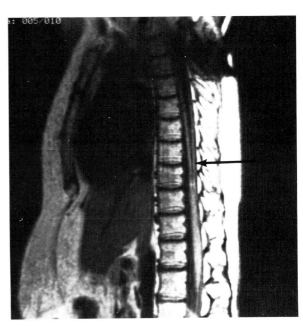

100: Chiari I   (1.5T)

EXAM: MRI of the cervical spine.

CLINICAL INFORMATION: 28-year-old female to rule out C5-6 disease.

TECHNIQUE: Sagittal T1-weighted images were acquired.

FINDINGS: The cerebellar tonsils protrude below the foramen magnum lip. This is consistent with a Chiari I malformation. No syrinx or other abnormality is identified.

IMPRESSION: Chiari I malformation.

REFERENCE: Smoker et al.: *RadioGraphics* **6**: November, 1986.

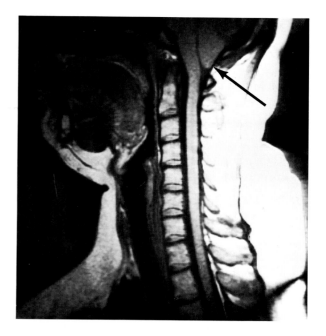

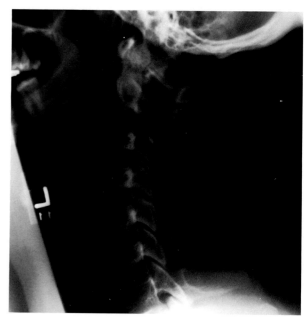

101: Rheumatoid Arthritis with Subluxation (.6T)

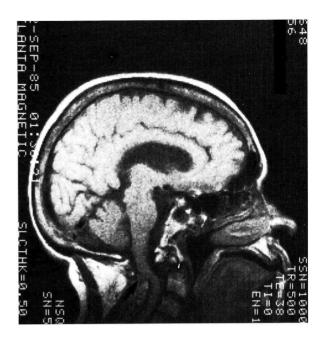

EXAM: MRI of the cervical spine.

CLINICAL INFORMATION: 75-year-old female with hand numbness for the past several years. Patient with proven rheumatoid arthritis.

TECHNIQUE: Surface coil sagittal T1-weighted images were obtained (500/38).

FINDINGS: There is marked kinking of the upper cervical cord in the C1-2 level, secondary to anterior subluxation of the C2 body in relation to the C1 ring. The dens has been eroded and migrated superiorly. This forms an os odentium. The dens is now wedged between the posterior superior aspect of the anterior C1 arch and the inferior aspect of the clivus. There is marked kinking of the cervical cord as it passes through this area.

IMPRESSION: Marked abnormality of the cranial vertebral junction to include erosion and migration of the os and forward subluxation of the C2 body in relation to the C1 bony ring. Marked kinking and compression of the cervical cord at this level. These findings are consistent with changes seen with rheumatoid arthritis.

REFERENCE: Smoker et al.: *RadioGraphics* **6**: November, 1986.

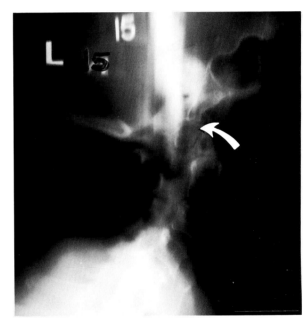

102: Severe Cord Compression Secondary to Pseudomass of Rheumatoid Arthritis (1.5T)

EXAM: MRI of the cervical spine.

CLINICAL INFORMATION: 6-year-old female with known rheumatoid arthritis and numerous neurologic complaints.

TECHNIQUE: Sagittal T1- and T2-weighted images were obtained (1000/30,60).

FINDINGS: There is a marked widening between the anterior arch of C1 and the dens. The dens is irregular and shows an intermediate, rather than high signal of the bone marrow seen in the other cervical vertebral bodies. In addition, surrounding the anterior arch and anterior to the dens, there is an area of large soft tissue mass. This is consistent with a pannus or pseudomass. The resultant subluxation shows marked compression of the cord with slight increase in signal at the level of the dens within the cord material, probably representing edema.

IMPRESSION: C1-2 subluxation with large pseudomass or inflammatory tissue surrounding the C1 arch and dens. Findings are consistent with rheumatoid arthritis. There is severe cord compression at this level.

DISCUSSION: Note that the associated flexion and extension views show the lack of restraint of the dens in regard to the anterior arch of C1. The inflammatory changes have destroyed the integrity of the transatlanto ligament.

   The dens can show a slight decrease in signal intensity in the normal cervical spine; this is, however, advanced beyond that and, with the associated inflammatory mass surrounding it, are consistent with severe involvement from rheumatoid arthritis.

REFERENCES: Smoker et al.: *RadioGraphics* **6**: November, 1986. Sze et al.: *Radiology* **161**:391, 1986.

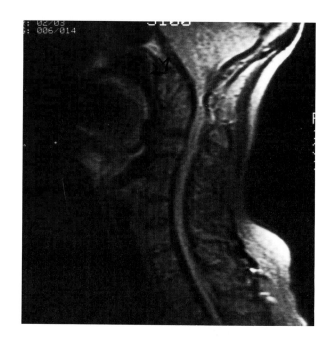

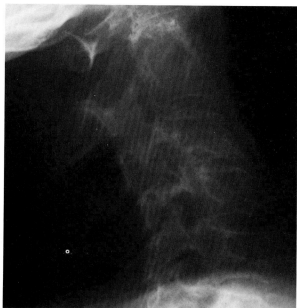

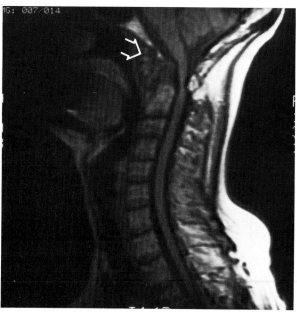

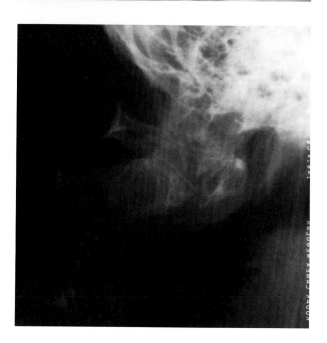

103: Foramen Magnum Colloid Cyst (.6T)

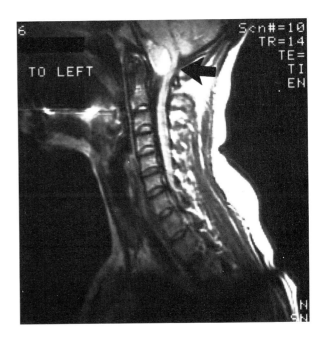

EXAM: MRI of the cervical spine.

CLINICAL INFORMATION: 29-year-old professional dancer with headache and neck pain following a fall 4 months before.

TECHNIQUE: Surface coil sagittal, axial, and coronal views were obtained (900/35; 2000/50,00; 1400/50,100).

FINDINGS: An extradural mass anterior to the medullo-cervical junction is identified with marked posterior displacement and compression of the lower brainstem upper cervical cord. There is an apparent fluid level within this mass. The mass measures approximately 4 cm in overall length and is well-rounded with good borders. This is clearly separated from the cord and upper brainstem. Differential consideration would be that of a dermoid or a subarachnoid cyst, possibly with hemorrhagic content. A large aneurysm from the proximal origin of PICA is felt to be less likely. Neurofibroma or meningioma felt to be less likely, given the presence of a fluid fluid interface.

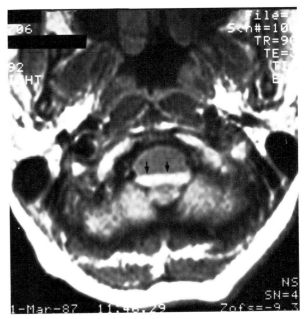

IMPRESSION: Intradural extramedullary mass at the foramen magnum with marked displacement and compression of the medullo-cervical junction. Diagnostic considerations listed above.

CONFIRMATION: At surgery a large colloid cyst was removed. The patient's symptoms were absent following surgery.

REFERENCE: Smoker et al.: *RadioGraphics* **6**:   November, 1986.

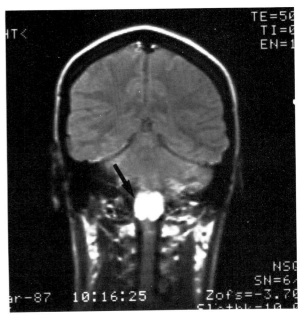

104: Old Compression Fractures   (.6T)

EXAM: MRI of the cervical spine.

CLINICAL INFORMATION: Rule out syrinx in 52-year-old with numbness in the arms, hands, and feet. Severe cervical injuries 18 years before. The patient now also has increasing gait problems.

TECHNIQUE: Surface coil sagittal imaging was acquired (1800/34,100).

FINDINGS: Large posterior osteophytes at C3-4 and C4-5 levels are identified. In addition, deformity consistent with an old compression fracture at C7 is identified. The posterior superior portion of the C7 body protrudes into the posterior canal with some mild effacement for deformity on the ventral aspect of the cord.

IMPRESSION: Large osteophytes at C3-4 and C4-5, with C7 change consistent with old compression-type fracture.

REFERENCE: Penning et al.: *AJR* **146**:793, April, 1986.

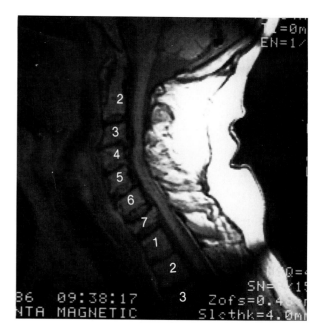

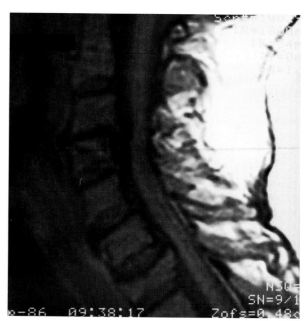

105: Status Post-C5-6 Fusion (1.5T)

EXAM: MRI of the cervical spine.

CLINICAL INFORMATION: 24-year-old female, status post-C5-6 surgery, now has some recurrent symptomatology. Rule out disc herniation.

FINDINGS: The alignment of C1 through C7 is normal. There is absence and total fusion of the C5-6 space. There is no evidence of any epidural extension or defect. The fusion appears to be solid.

IMPRESSION: Status post-C5-6 fusion. Note abnormal discogram obtained preoperatively.

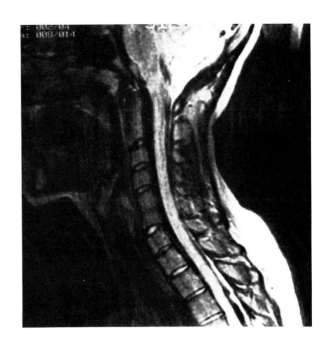

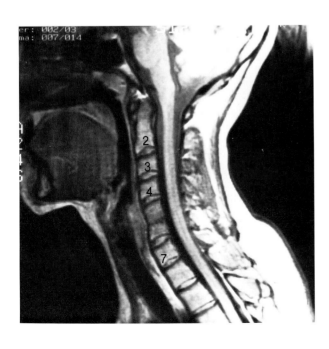

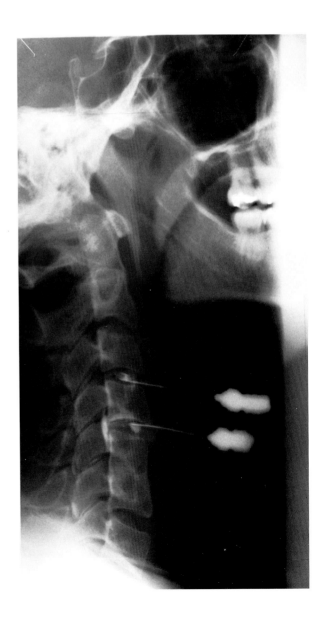

106: C6-7 Fracture
Subluxation (1.5T)

EXAM: MRI of the cervical spine.

CLINICAL INFORMATION: 18-year-old male involved in a severe motor vehicle accident.

TECHNIQUE: Spin density sagittal images were obtained (600/25).

FINDINGS: There is anterior subluxation of the C6 vertebral body in relation to C7. There is a small amount of material posterior to this which may represent a traumatic disc herniation. The intraspinous processes are widened. This is consistent with a marked flexion injury and disruption of the intraspinous processes and posterior longitudinal ligament. In addition, on the right lateral sagittal cut (Image 2), there is evidence of a fracture extending through the facet on the left. There is marked anterior subluxation of the C6 superior facet in relation to C7, suggesting disruption of the ligamentous capsule. The facet has not extended enough anteriorly to become locked.

IMPRESSION: Fracture subluxation C6-7 with abnormal subluxation of the left C6 in relation to C7 and fracture through the C6 facet right side.

DISCUSSION: Unusually good detail of the bony structures is identified and the complicated facet relationships are simplified on the available parasagittal views. The use of MR as an imaging tool in the acutely injured patient is growing. The need to move the patient only once is a definite advantage. The need for monitoring devices and life-support equipment is a major disadvantage to most multitrauma patients with severe or suspected cord and cervical spinal canal problems.

REFERENCE: Gebarski et al.: *Radiology* **157**:379, 1985.

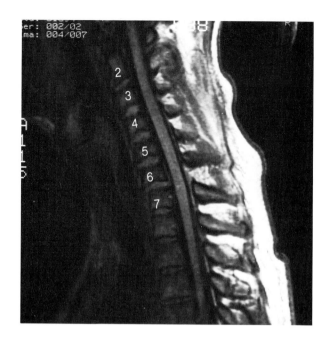

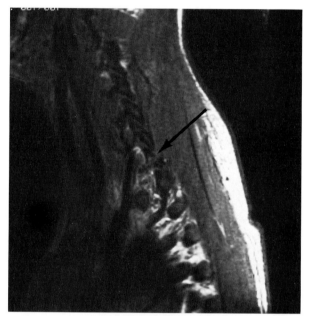

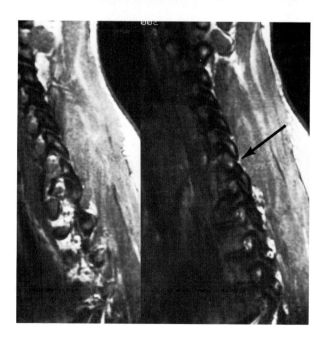

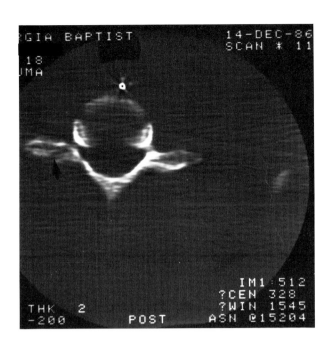

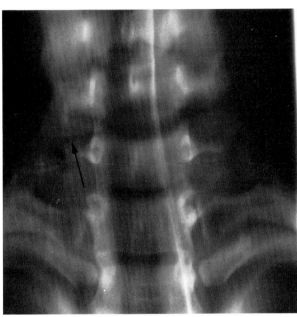

107: Severe Myelomalacia (.6T)

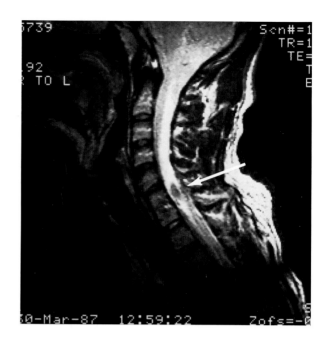

EXAM: MRI of the cervical spine.

CLINICAL INFORMATION: 26-year-old male involved in a motor vehicle accident with prior cervical fracture has had severe headache, left arm, and hand radiculopathy since motor vehicle accident.

TECHNIQUE: Surface coil sagittal axial T1- and T2-weighted images were obtained (1400/50,100; 450/34).

FINDINGS: There is a CSF irregular cystic structure centered at the C6 level. This mildly expands the cord at this level. Superior to this is a small eccentric syrinx extending up to the C4 level. The cord superior to this to the foramen magnum is diffusely small. The cord inferior to the C6 cystic area is markedly atrophied. The entire cervical cord shows increased signal on the more T2-weighted images.

IMPRESSION: Severe myelomalacia involving the cervical cord with moderate atrophy of the upper cervical cord and more severe generalized atrophy inferior to the cystic myelomalacia.

REFERENCE: Chakeres et al.: *AJNR* 8:5, January/February, 1987.

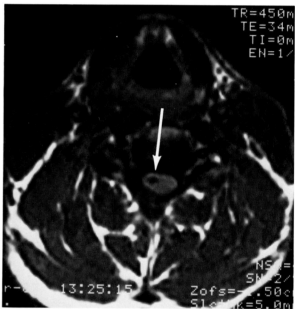

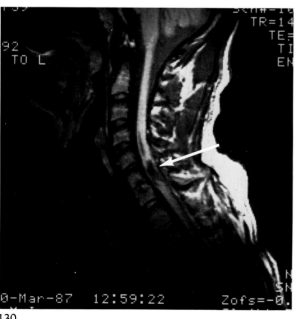

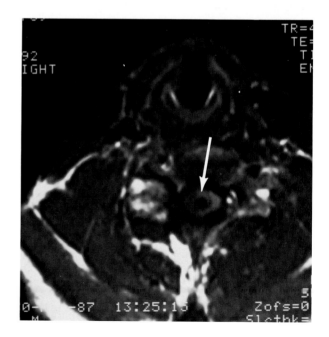

108: Dislodged Fusion Mass (.6T)

EXAM: MRI of the cervical spine.

CLINICAL INFORMATION: 47-year-old female. Recent C5-6 fusion with good results and elevation of symptomatology. Patient is now, however, compliant with several postoperative restrictions and returns with some focal neck pain.

TECHNIQUE: Sagittal T1- and T2-weighted images were obtained (1800/45,90).

FINDINGS: The fusion mass has been dislodged and is located anterior to the vertebral body. High-signal focus is seen in the fossa of the fusion mass, representing collection of fluid and old hemorrhage.

IMPRESSION: Dislodged fusion body at the C5-6 level.

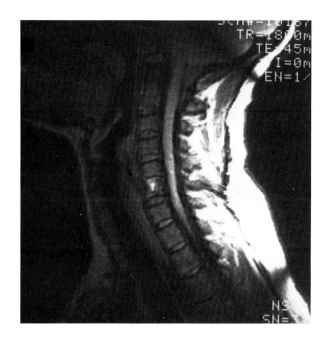

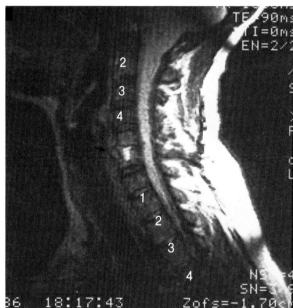

109: Cystic Myelomalacia (.6T)

EXAM: MRI of the lower thoracic and upper lumbar region.

CLINICAL INFORMATION: 31-year-old male who fell from a tree several years earlier.

TECHNIQUE: Surface coil T1- and T2-weighting were acquired (2000/40,80; 500/30).

FINDINGS: Marked compression of the L1 vertebral body and comminuted fracture identified. There is retropulsion of a portion of the posterior L1 body into the canal. The terminal spinal cord at this level shows evidence of compression and increased signal reflecting myelomalacia. In addition, there is a suggestion centrally of posttraumatic cyst or syrinx development (small arrows).

DISCUSSION: Excellent evaluation of the location of the bony fragments and underlying neural tissue damage is offered in this sagittal case.

REFERENCE: McArdle et al.: *AJNR* 7:885, September/October, 1986.

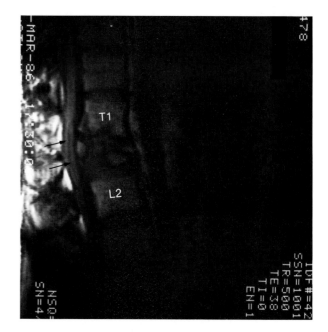

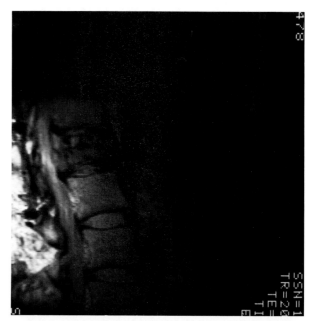

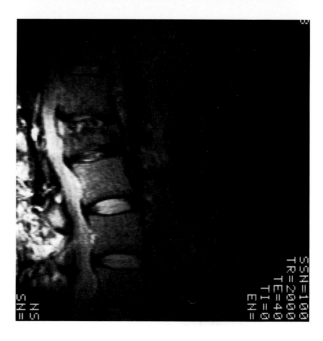

110: Compression Fracture with Canal Compromise (1.5T)

EXAM: MRI of the thoracic spine.

CLINICAL INFORMATION: Patient is a 20-year-old female involved in a motor vehicle accident with severe trauma to the vertebral column.

TECHNIQUE: Surface coil sagittal imaging was acquired through the thoracic and upper lumbar region (1500/25, 70).

FINDINGS: There is marked retrolisthesis of L1 in reference to T12 with compression fracture through the L1 vertebral body. The anterior portion of the L1 vertebral body remains aligned to the T12 inferior endplate. This marked subluxation results in severe compromise of the canal with retrolisthesis of the L1 vertebral body severely compromising the canal. Severe compression of the terminal cord at this level is also identified.

IMPRESSION: Marked retrolisthesis of L1 in reference to T12 with marked loss of canal dimension.

DISCUSSION: All studies were dramatic in demonstrating this severe injury and malalignment with regard to the bony structures. The MR adds significant information in demonstrating the relationship of the neural structures to the associated bony injuries. Image 4 is a three-dimensional reformation of thin axial CT cuts acquired through the level of injury.

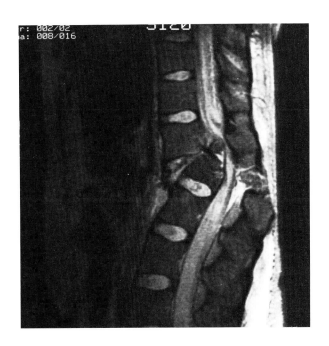

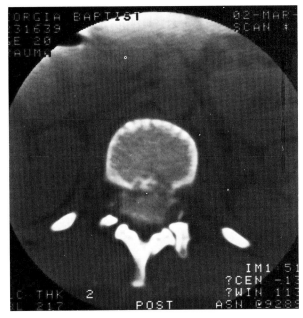

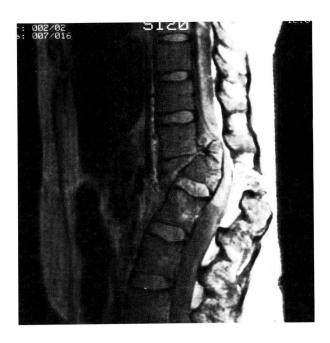

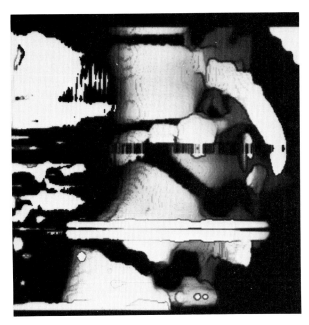

111: Cystic Myelomalacia (1.5T)

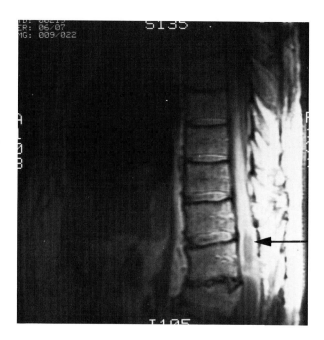

EXAM: MRI of the thoracic spine.

CLINICAL INFORMATION: 56-year-old male with history of prior severe trauma to the vertebral column.

TECHNIQUE: Surface coil sagittal and axial T1- and T2-weighted images were acquired (2000/30,90; 1000/25).

FINDINGS: Large, predominantly cystic, expansion of the terminal cord, beginning at approximately the T11-12 level and continuing into the conus, is identified on both the sagittal and axial images. The remnant neural tissue surrounds the large cystic space. The sagittal and axial images correlate nicely to myelography showing diffuse expansion of the terminal portion of the cord.

IMPRESSION: Cystic myelomalacia.

DISCUSSION: The presence of cord cysts or cystic myelomalacia following trauma to the cord can be well-demonstrated with MR. The large size of our case can be well-evaluated prior to any attempt at decompression for progressive neural loss in such patients. Note also the excellent evaluation of the remnant neural tissue.

REFERENCE: Quencer et al.: *AJR* **147**:125, July, 1986.

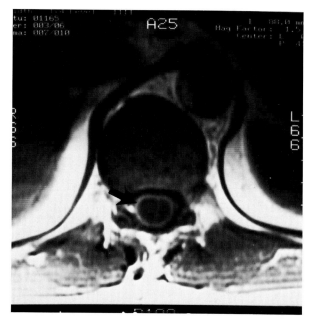

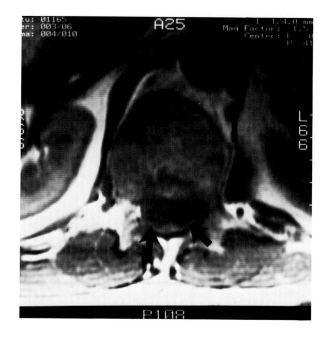

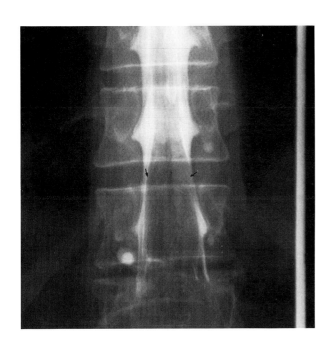

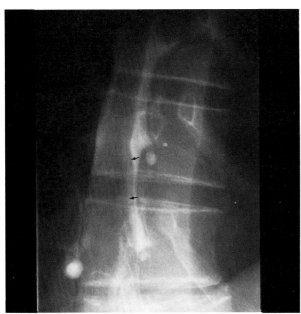

112: Metastatic Disease (.6T)

EXAM: MRI of the thoracic spine.

CLINICAL INFORMATION: 76-year-old male with a known pancoast tumor of the lung. Now with a nonspecific spinal level. Increasing loss of strength in the lower extremities.

TECHNIQUE: Surface coil and body coil T1-weighted images were obtained (450/34; 350/26).

FINDINGS: Large metastatic deposit is seen extending from the T1 to T3 levels. This invades and destroys the posterior spinous processes in these levels. This also extends into and completely surrounds the cord in this region. Maximal cord compression is seen at the T2-3 level.

IMPRESSION: Large amount of metastatic disease with significant soft tissue component posterior to the canal. Evidence for cord compression from the T1 to T3 levels with marked involvement of the vertebral bodies.

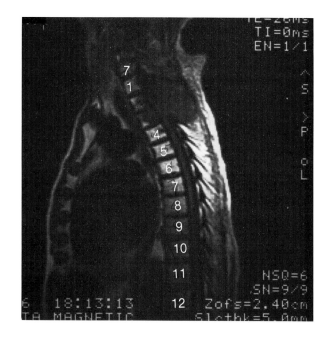

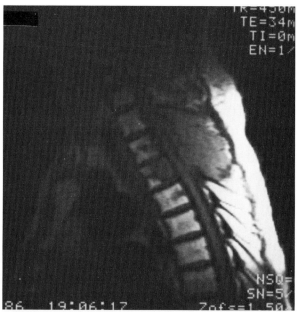

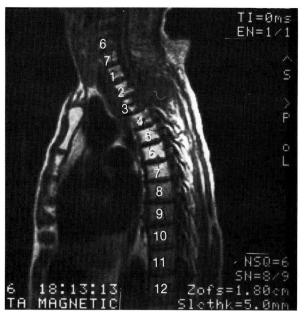

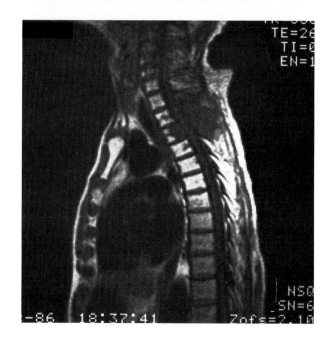

113: Intramedullary Tumor (.6T)

EXAM: MRI of the thoracic cord.

CLINICAL HISTORY: 28-year-old female. Numb from the waist down with recent loss of bladder control.

TECHNIQUE: Surface coil sagittal and axial T1- and T2-weighted images were acquired (2000/45,90).

FINDINGS: There is extension and expansion of the cord from the T7 to T9 levels. This has the appearance of an intramedullary tumor. Along the superior aspect are several rounded areas of signal void. These may represent small cysts or focal areas of calcification. No vascular structures are suggested on the contiguous images. The findings are most consistent with a primary glioma of the thoracic cord. The presence of cysts in the cord can be associated with a glioma, such as an astrocytoma or a hemangioblastoma.

IMPRESSION: Intramedullary tumor, probably a glioma.

DISCUSSION: Even retrospectively, the myelogram done at the same time shows little suggestion of enlargement of the cord through this area of interest.

CONFIRMATION: Glioblastoma biopsied at surgery.

REFERENCE: Bradley et al.: *Radiology* **152**:695, 1984.

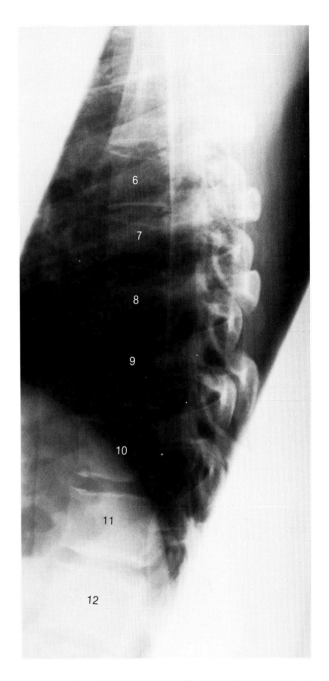

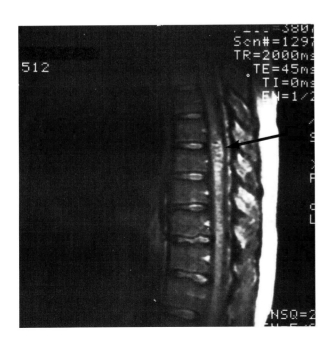

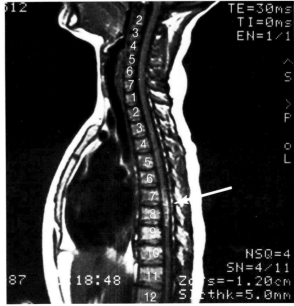

114: Metastatic Breast Cancer (1.5T)

EXAM: MRI of the thoracic spine.

CLINICAL INFORMATION: 62-year-old female with known breast CA and nonspecific back pain.

TECHNIQUE: Surface coil sagittal T1- and T2-weighted images were acquired through the mid- and lower-thoracic and lumbar spine (1500/25,70).

FINDINGS: The bone marrow shows marked alteration and decrease in normal signal intensity. There are several focal rounded areas of increased signal intensity on the more T2-weighted images, representing focal islands of fat within the bone marrow. The other areas of decreased signal are most consistent with that of diffuse metastatic involvement through the bone marrow containing portions of the vertebral bodies.

IMPRESSION: Widespread metastatic change secondary to diffuse breast metastasis. Note made also of several rounded areas of increased signal representing islands of bone-marrow fat.

REFERENCE: Porter: *Diagnostic Imaging* February, 1987.

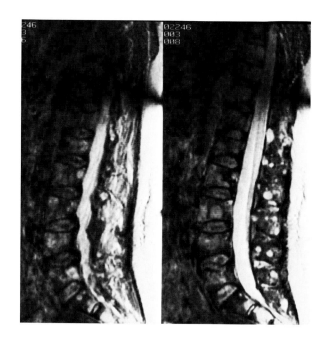

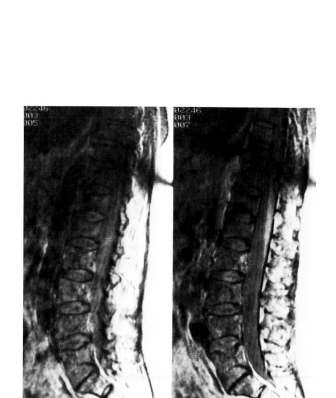

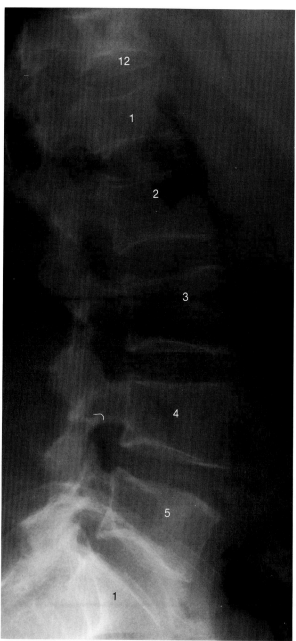

115: Metastatic Lung Disease   (1.5T)

EXAM: MRI of the thoracic spine.

CLINICAL INFORMATION: 75-year-old female with resected lung cancer.

TECHNIQUE: Surface coil sagittal and axial T1- and T2-weighted images were acquired (1200/25,90; 500/25).

FINDINGS: The T9 vertebral body shows marked decrease in signal intensity with some compressive change. In addition, an epidural soft tissue mass fills into the right portion of the canal and deviates the cord to the left side. Changes suggest cord compression at this level. Extension of tumor into the lamina and posterior epidural space is also identified.

IMPRESSION: Metastatic disease involving the T9, T10, and T11 vertebral bodies, with evidence on sagittal and axial scans to suggest extension of metastatic disease into the epidural space with cord compression.

REFERENCE: Porter: *Diagnostic Imaging* February, 1987.

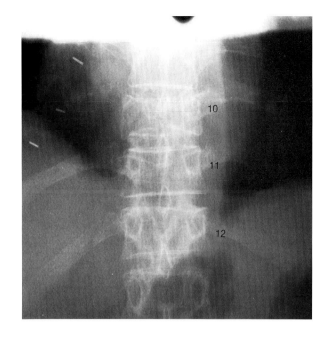

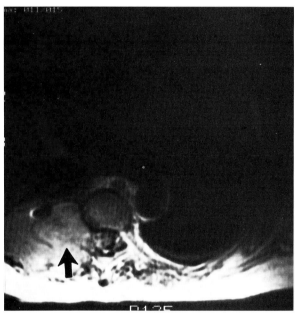

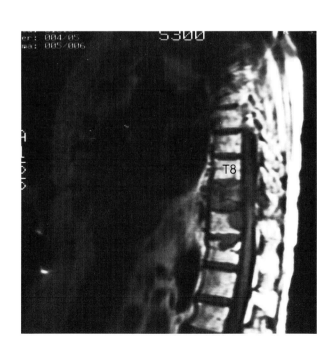

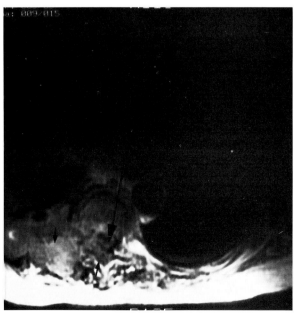

116: Widespread Metastases (1.5T)

EXAM: MRI of the thoracic spine.

CLINICAL INFORMATION: 69-year-old female complaining of diffuse back pain. Rule out cord compression. The patient has a known primary malignancy.

TECHNIQUE: Surface coil sagittal T1- and T2-weighted images were acquired from the lumbar and thoracic region (800/25,60). TR was reduced because of patient discomfort and inability to remain still for long periods of time.

FINDINGS: Diffuse replacement of the normal bone-marrow signal throughout the entire bone-marrow spaces of the vertebral columns. Disc maintains normal signal intensity. There is a slight scoliosis; however, the canal and cord show no evidence of compromise.

IMPRESSION: Widespread decrease in bone marrow of the vertebral bodies consistent with widespread metastatic disease. No cord compression was identified.

REFERENCE: Porter: *Diagnostic Imaging* February, 1987.

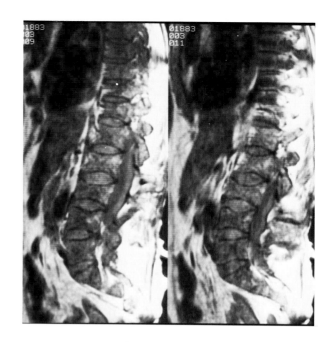

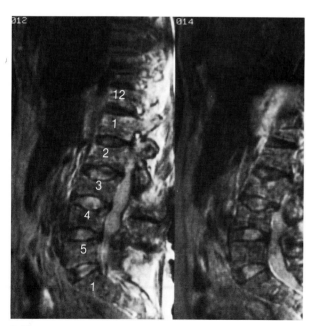

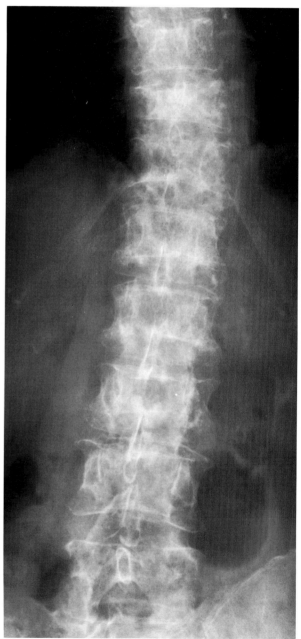

117: Compression Fractures (1.5T)

EXAM: MRI of the thoracic spine.

CLINICAL INFORMATION: 59-year-old female with diffuse back pain.

TECHNIQUE: Sagittal and coronal T1- and T2-weighted images were acquired (500/25; 800/25).

FINDINGS: Numerous vertebral bodies show both compression and replacement of bone marrow with low-signal intensity. The disc material appears to be spared. There is some mild lipping of the endplates in the canal, but no significant cord compression is identified.

IMPRESSION: Numerous metastatic areas of involvement with compression fractures. No evidence of cord compression.

DISCUSSION: MR offers excellent evaluation of the entire vertebral column for exclusion of cord compression and involvement of the vertebral bodies by metastatic disease. This is highly preferable, particularly in widespread metastases, rather than total spinal column myelography, which is uncomfortable for the patient and time-consuming for the radiologist.

REFERENCE: Beltran et al.: *Radiology* **162**: 565, 1987.

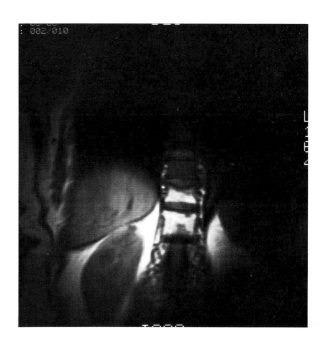

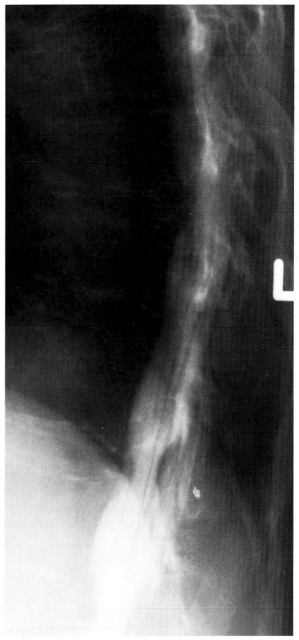

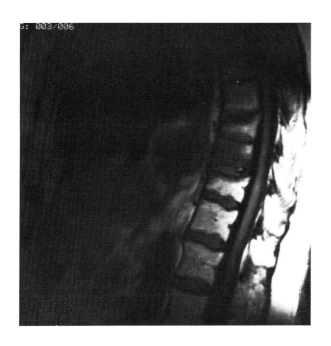

118: Metastatic Breast Cancer (1.5T)

EXAM: MRI of the thoracic spine.

CLINICAL INFORMATION: Rule out spinal cord compression in patient with known primary disease (breast CA).

TECHNIQUE: Sagittal images through the cervical and thoracic spine were obtained with T1- and T2-weighting (1200/20,90; 500/20).

FINDINGS: Marked decrease in signal intensity of the T2-3 vertebral body which shows epidural extension into the posterior column with compression of the cord. This is consistent with widespread metastatic disease and high-grade obstruction.

IMPRESSION: Bony metastatic change involving T2-3 with extension into the posterior epidural space of metastatic disease with high-grade cord compression.

DISCUSSION: Excellent delineation is offered of the metastatic disease and extension into the epidural space with graphic demonstration of the cord compression. In addition, note the excellent evaluation of the upper cervical cord. A case with this quality of detail obviates the need for myelography. This also excludes the presence of any more cephalad metastasis, not recognized on myelography, thus obviating the need for a cervical puncture and myelogram.

REFERENCE: Panshter et al.: *Applied Radiology*: 61, November/December, 1984.

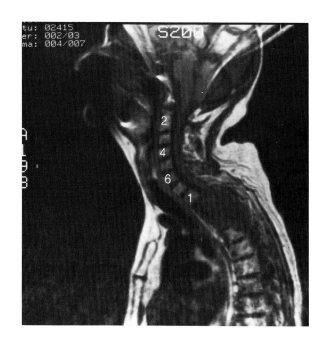

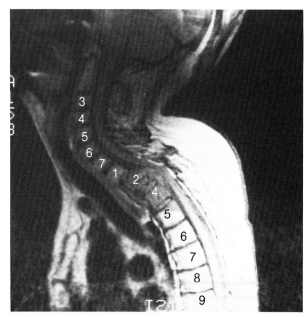

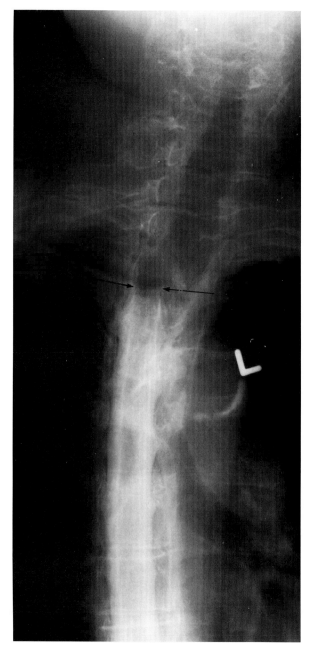

119: T9-10 Disc Herniation (.6T)

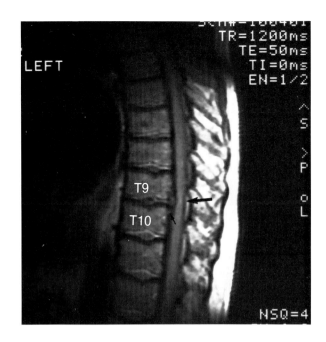

EXAM: MRI of the thoracic spine.

CLINICAL INFORMATION: Rule out transverse myelitis in a 57-year-old male, beginning with tingling and numbness in the feet. Also sensation of extremities falling asleep, more left-sided.

TECHNIQUE: Surface coil T1- and T2-weighting images were obtained (1200/50,100).

FINDINGS: Extradural defect centered at the T9-10 level is seen protruding into the central canal. This shows moderate compression of the cord with slight increase in cord signal through this area. A portion of this defect is probably also secondary to osteophyte extending off the posterior superior endplate of T10 (small arrow).

IMPRESSION: Herniation T9-10.

DISCUSSION: The disc herniation can be well-demonstrated. In addition, there is a wealth of information about the degree of identified cord compression that is particularly well-demonstrated in this case (large arrow). In addition examination of the compressed cord for slight increase in signal may reveal the presence of some edema or early changes of myelomalacia. Several excellent papers on myelopathy secondary to trauma have been presented. Mechanisms of encroachment upon the cord of a chronic nature, such as from a disc herniation, osteophyte, or spinal canal stenosis, can be well imaged such as seen here.

REFERENCE: Gebarski et al.: *Radiology* **157**:379, 1985.

120: T8-9 Disc Herniation (.6T)

EXAM: MRI of the thoracic spine.

CLINICAL INFORMATION: Persistent midback pain. No evidence of radiculopathy.

TECHNIQUE: Surface coil sagittal and axial T1- and T2-weighted images were acquired (1400/50,100; 500/34).

FINDINGS: There is an extradural defect centered at the T8-9 level, protruding into the central spinal canal and slightly to the right of midline. This deviates the cord slightly. There is no underlying cord deformity. The extradural mass is confluent with a similar signal intensity to that of the disc material at T8-9. Findings most consistent with a central and right-sided disc herniation at T8-9.

IMPRESSION: T8-9 central and right-sided disc herniation.

DISCUSSION: The sagittal view adds a dramatic portrayal of disc herniation which can be seen as well on the submitted axial images on the CT (Image 1). Note, in addition, at T11-12, the well-developed osteophyte and anterior disc herniation.

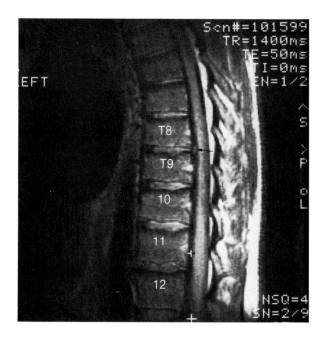

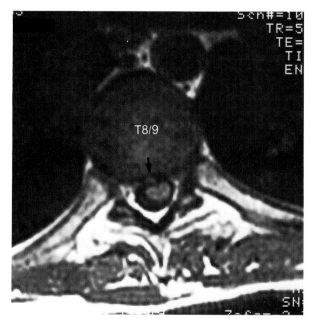

121: Posttraumatic Syrinx   (.6T)

EXAM: MRI of the thoracic spine.

CLINICAL INFORMATION: 43-year-old male with right-sided numbness and problems with ambulation. In 1963, he suffered a broken back from a fall.

TECHNIQUE: Surface coil sagittal imaging with T1-weighting was acquired from the occiput to the sacrum.

FINDINGS: There is a marked compression fracture and accentuated thoracic kyphosis centered at the T8 level. There is also a large syrinx extending from the C3 to the T12 levels. Marked narrowing of the canal at the thoracic kyphotic apex is identified (Image 1).

IMPRESSION: Syrinx extending from C3 to the T12 interspace with suggestion of canal stenosis at the T8 level. Marked compression and kyphotic angulation at the T8 level.

DISCUSSION: The full extent of the posttraumatic syrinx can be identified, as well as assessment of the cavity following decompression with a tube. Note the metal artifact from placements of a drainage tube and Harrington rods for stability. Small arrows also delineate the syrinx cavity.

REFERENCE: Barski et al.: *Radiology* **157**:379, 1985.

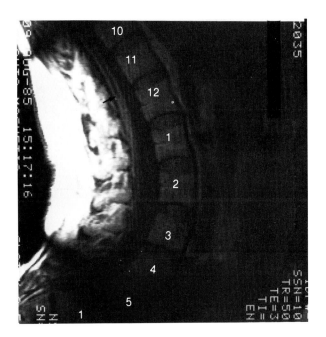

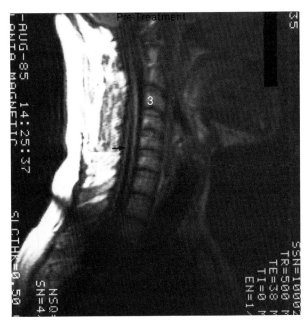

Pre-Treatment

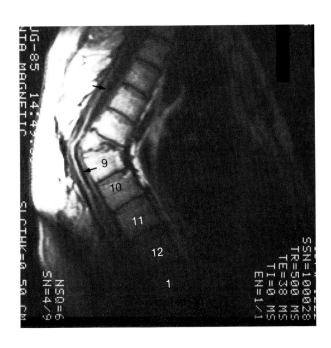

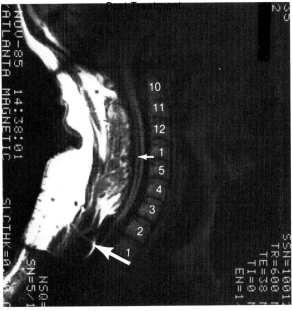

Post-Treatment

122: T11-12 Discitis   (.6T)

EXAM: MRI of the thoracic cord.

CLINICAL INFORMATION: This is a 14-year-old female with low back and bilateral leg pain.

TECHNIQUE: Surface coil sagittal T1- and T2-weighting was acquired through the thoracic spine (2000/40,80).

FINDINGS: Decreased signal in the disc space at the T11-12 levels is identified on the T1-weighted images, and there is persistent decrease on the more T2-weighted images. In addition, the anterior portions of the superior T12 and inferior T11 endplate are distorted and show decreased signal compared to the normally higher bone-marrow signal intensity in the remainder of the bodies. The involvement of the endplates and depression of signal in the disc is most consistent with discitis, with extension into the vertebral bodies consistent with osteomyelitis.

IMPRESSION: T11-12 discitis with associated osteomyelitis at the T11 and 12 vertebral bodies.

DISCUSSION: As per our reference article, loss of differentiation of the endplates and vertebral disc space is a good indicator of an inflammatory, rather than metastatic, involvement of vertebral bodies. This may be more of a differential problem in which the disc is not involved to exclude early neoplastic disease. Severe degenerative changes can cause alteration of both the disc material and surrounding endplates as well. This can usually be separated out by the history. Comparing our case with that of the reference article, we did not, however, experience increased signal in the disc at this time. Perhaps this is because of earlier imaging of our case than was seen in the reference article. Note also the good exclusion on the axial images of any epidural or subdural extension of the infectious process.

REFERENCE: Modic et al.: *Radiology* **157**:157, 1987.

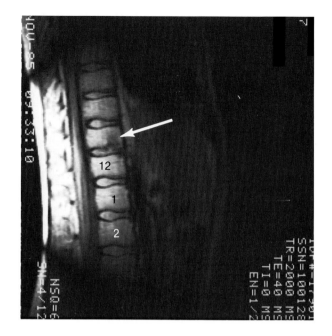

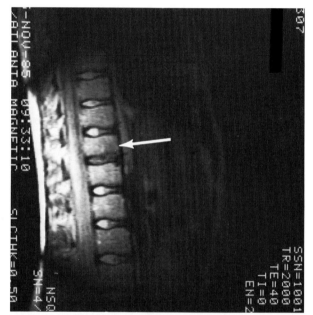

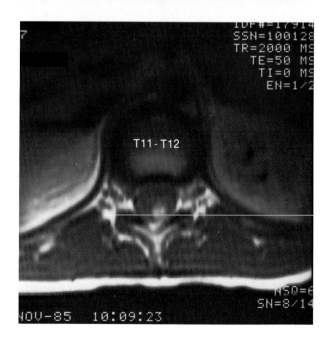

146

123: Multiple Sclerosis   (.6T)

EXAM: MRI of the thoracic spine.

CLINICAL INFORMATION: 35-year-old male with numbness from the waist down.

TECHNIQUE: Surface coil sagittal and axial T1- and T2-weighted images were obtained (1400/45,90; 1000/60).

FINDINGS: There is a flame-shaped area of increased signal at the T7-8 level seen on both the sagittal and axial images. There may be some minimal expansion or swelling of the cord at this level. This, in conjunction with MS demonstrated on the cranial study, is most consistent with a thoracic cord area of demyelination.

IMPRESSION: MS involving the cord at the T7-8 level.

DISCUSSION: Flame-shaped nonspecific area which may slightly enlarge the cord during active demyelination, but without any other features of a mass, can be seen in approximately 5 percent of multiple sclerosis patients.

REFERENCE: Hyman et al.: *AJNR* **6**:229, 1985.

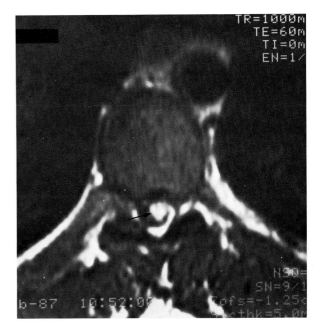

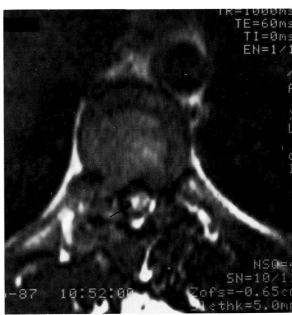

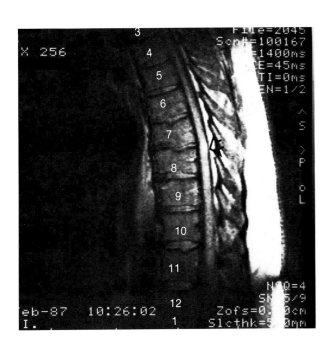

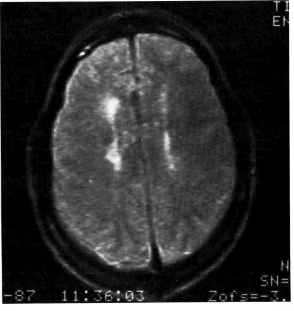

124: Multiple Sclerosis (1.5T)

EXAM: MRI of the thoracic spine.

CLINICAL INFORMATION: 21-year-old female. Rule out upper thoracic myelopathy.

TECHNIQUE: Surface coil T1- and T2-weighted images were acquired (1500/25,70).

FINDINGS: The flame-shaped area of increased signal intensity is identified at the T5 level. This does not expand the cord. In association with findings consistent with intracranial MS, this is most consistent with a plaque of multiple sclerosis.

IMPRESSION: Thoracic cord plaque of demyelination.

REFERENCE: Maravilla et al.: *AJR* **144**:381, February, 1985.

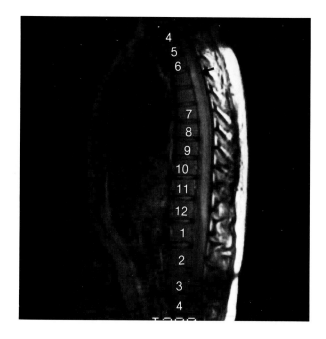

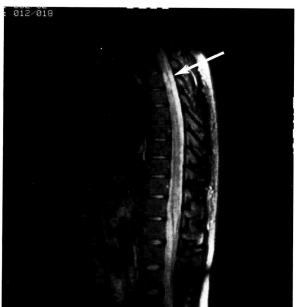

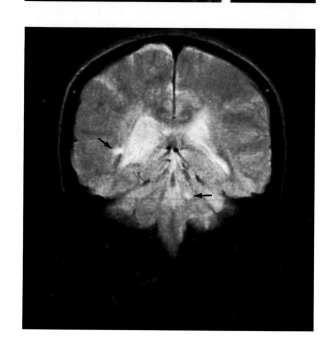

125: Arteriovenous Malformation (.6T)

EXAM: MRI of the thoracic spine.

CLINICAL INFORMATION: 70-year-old male with insulin-dependent diabetes now presents with acute onset of paraplegia.

TECHNIQUE: Surface coil T1- and T2-weighted images were acquired (1200/50,100).

FINDINGS: Characteristic tubular worm-shaped structures surrounding the conus at the T12-L1 level are identified. The cord is not expanded. No altered signal seen within the cord. The prominence of these tubular low-signal areas suggests large draining veins. The presence of large draining veins in this area without associated distortion of the cord raises the possibility of an AVM.

IMPRESSION: Thoracic AVM.

DISCUSSION: This was confirmed on myelography and arteriography. The excellence of MR noninvasive modality for cord evaluation for evidence of AVM is well-demonstrated in this case. MR usually allows visualization and localization of the AVM's nidus. Arteriography is usually necessary as a preoperative staging but, as a radiographic method of investigation, it has a high risk of complication, is time-consuming, and is somewhat tedious.

REFERENCE: Di Chiro et al.: *Radiology* **156**:689, 1985.

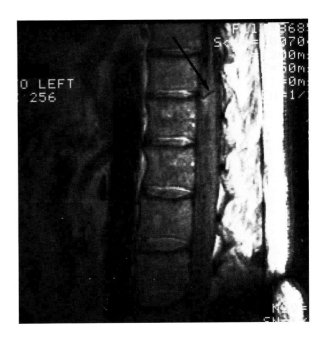

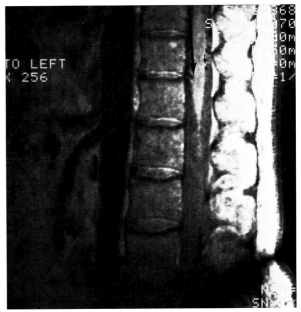

126: Grade I Spondylolisthesis (.6T)

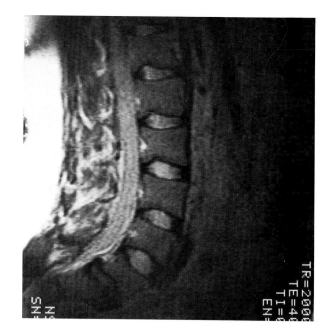

EXAM: MRI of the lumbar spine.

CLINICAL INFORMATION: Rule out disc herniation in 34-year-old male with low back pain.

TECHNIQUE: Surface coil sagittal imaging was obtained (2000/40,80).

FINDINGS: There is a Grade I spondylolisthesis or slippage anteriorly of L5 in relation to the S1 vertebral body. There is a mild degenerative loss of signal within the disc material at L5-S1. There is a pseudobulging or prominence of the disc material posteriorly at the L5-S1 level.

IMPRESSION: Grade I spondylolisthesis with mild degenerative changes within the disc.

DISCUSSION: Pseudobulging is a characteristic of the spondylolisthesis. The annulus is distorted secondary to slippage of the superior vertebral body and presents itself as a wide bulging disc. MR adds further to the appreciation of this phenomenon, demonstrating both the disc and vertebral body in the sagittal plane. Most of the pseudobulging discs encountered at our clinic tend to be degenerated in appearance.

REFERENCE: Teplick et al.: *AJNR* 7:479, May/June, 1986.

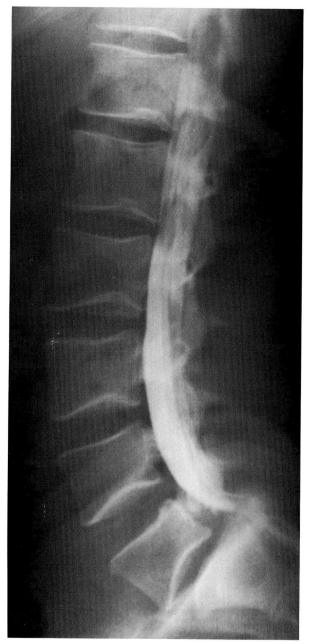

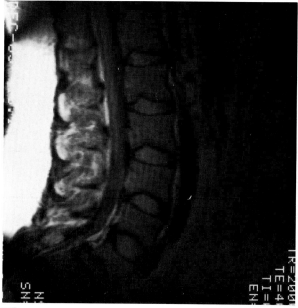

127: Neurofibroma   (.6T)

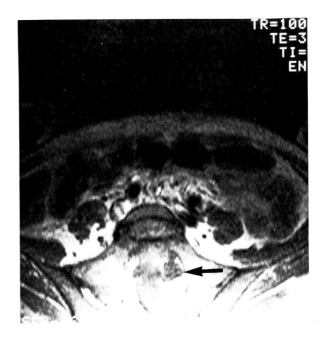

EXAM: MRI of the lumbosacral spine.

CLINICAL INFORMATION: Female with CT scan demonstrating mass in the region of the L5 root. Rule out tumor.

TECHNIQUE: Sagittal, axial, and coronal T1-weighted images were obtained (1000/38; 600/38).

FINDINGS: In the region of the left S2 root, there is a mass with slight angular margins and evidence for expansion of the bony canal. This mass is adjacent to the left S1 root (large arrow). The presence of erosion with fairly well-marginated edges and expansion of the bony canal suggests that this is a slow-growth process. This raises the possibility of a benign nerve sheath tumor, such as a neurofibroma, meningioma, or neurolemmoma.

IMPRESSION: Left S2 nerve sheath neurofibroma.

REFERENCE: Hyman: *AJNR* **6**:229, March/April, 1985.

Courtesy of Al Alexander, Lancaster Magnetic Imaging.

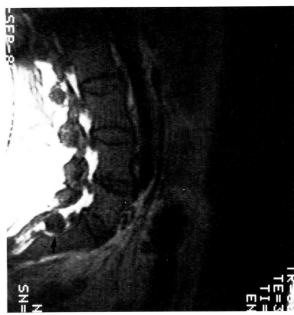

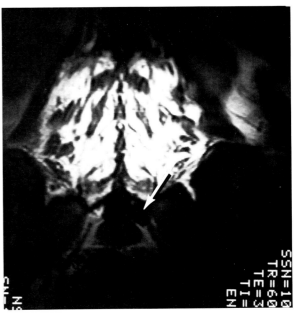

128: Osteoma   (.6T)

EXAM: MRI of the lumbosacral spine.

CLINICAL INFORMATION: A 41-year-old male with low back and left leg pain.

TECHNIQUE: Sagittal and axial T1- and T2-weighted images were acquired (1400/50,00; 500/30).

FINDINGS: The discs showed no evidence of degenerative change; however, there is a focal patch of increased bony density or sclerosis in the left sacrum at the S1 level. This correlates with the focal area of sclerosis on the CT scan. This is left-sided, and there is no evidence of a fracture. No other areas of similar increased bony density are identified on the MR or the CT scan. With the history of associated pain to the S1 root distribution on the left, we suspect that this represents an osteoid-osteoma.

IMPRESSION: Osteoid-osteoma.

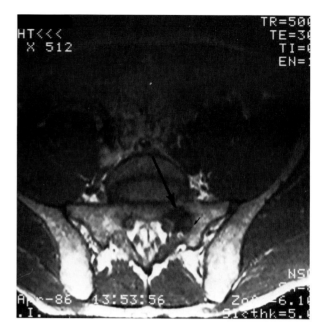

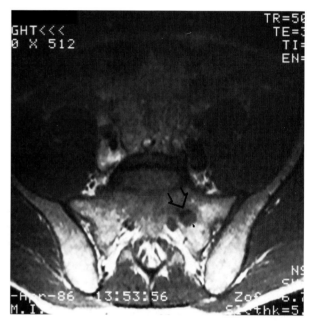

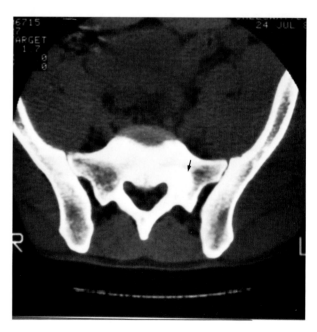

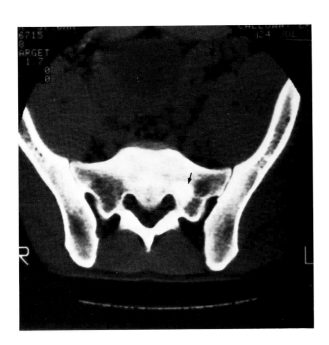

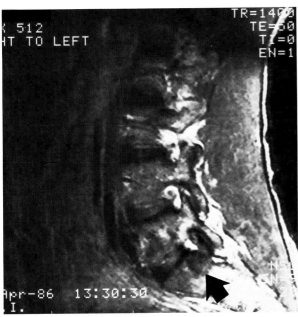

129: Hemangioma (.6T)

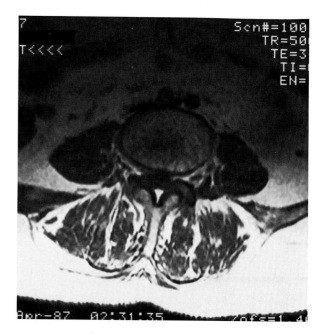

EXAM: MRI of the lumbosacral spine.

CLINICAL INFORMATION: Rule out disc herniation in 71-year-old female.

TECHNIQUE: Surface coil sagittal and axial T1- and T2-weighted images were acquired (1400/50,100; 500/31).

FINDINGS: Heavy degenerative changes identified at the L5-S1 level without evidence of disc herniation. There is also a large posterior bony osteophyte at the L2-3 level.

Incidental note is made of a striated appearance to the L4 vertebral body with slight expansion of its posterior margin into the canal. The striated or celery-stalk appearance and increased signal compared to the other vertebral bodies raise the possibility of a diffuse hemangioma.

IMPRESSION: Hemangioma of the L4 vertebral body. Posterior osteophyte at L2-3 and heavy degenerative change at L5-S1.

DISCUSSION: The speckled appearance on the CT and the celery-stalk appearance on both plain film and MR are characteristic of a hemangioma. Although thought to be benign, the hemangioma can expand the architecture of the vertebral body and can grow into the epidural space, causing canal obstruction. Note the posterior bulging of the vertebral body in our case and the comparative axial views of the speckled pattern on the CT and MR.

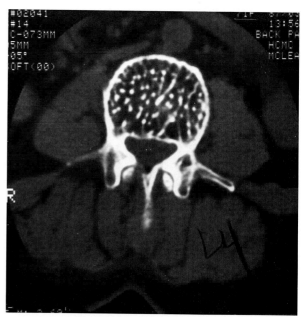

REFERENCES: Paushter et al.: *Applied Radiology*: 61, November/December, 1984. Modic et al.: *Neurosurgery* **15**:483, 1984.

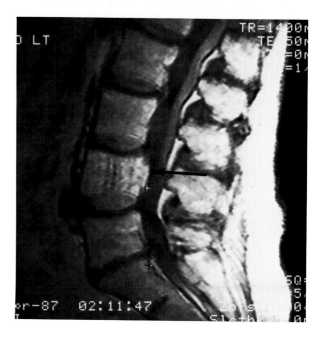

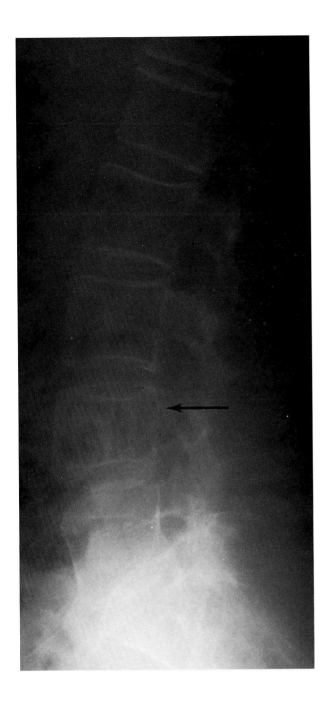

130: Neurofibroma (.6T)

EXAM: MRI of the lumbosacral spine.

CLINICAL INFORMATION: Low back and left-sided radiculopathy. Rule out disc herniation in middle-aged patient.

TECHNIQUE: Sagittal and axial T1- and T2-weighted images were acquired in addition to spin density and T2-weighted sagittal images. (2200/50,100; 1000/35; 600/35).

FINDINGS: There is a large mass replacing and expanding the size of the left psoas muscle and extending in dumbbell fashion through the neural foraminal canal at the L3-4 level. The mass invades the canal and also invaginates or scallops out the posterior portion of the L3 vertebral body. The mass has well-defined borders. Given the dumbbell shape, bony remodeling or scalloping, and the homogeneous signal that was identified, we suspect that this may represent a large neurofibroma.

DISCUSSION: Excellent delineation of the tendency of neurofibroma to extend in dumbbell fashion into the neural foraminal canals, with scalloping or remodeling of bone, can be identified here.

REFERENCE: Burk et al.: *Radiology* **162**:797, 1987.

Courtesy of Dr. Al Alexander/Paul Collura, Lancaster Magnetic Imaging

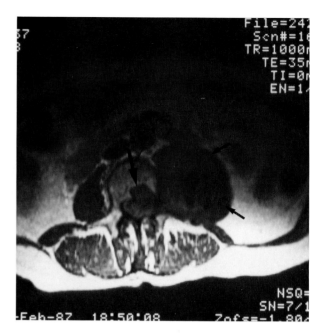

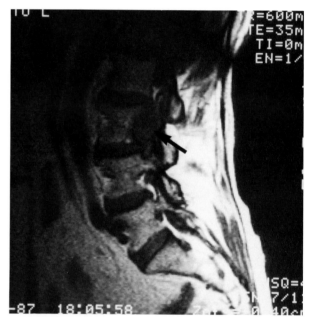

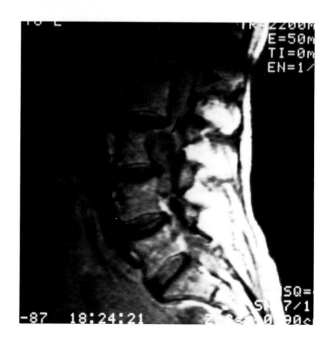

131: Hemangioma   (.6T)

EXAM: MRI of the lumbosacral spine.

CLINICAL INFORMATION: A 34-year-old female with back pain.

TECHNIQUE: Surface coil sagittal and axial T1- and T2-weighted images were acquired (1400/5,100; 600/34).

FINDINGS: There is a rounded area of increased signal intensity on both the T1- and T2-weighted images in both sagittal and axial planes. This does not deform the vertebral body and is located in its left midportion. This does not involve the disc space or encroach into the epidural space. The characteristic high signal can be seen with focal fatty deposit or hemangioma.

IMPRESSION: High-signal focus within the vertebral body is most consistent with a small incidental bone hemangiona.

REFERENCE: Paushter et al.: *Applied Radiology*: 61, November/December, 1984.

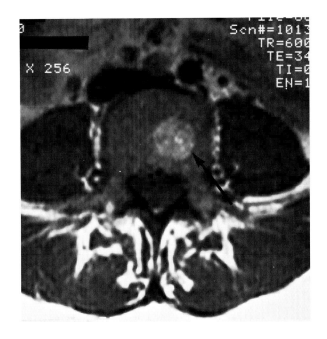

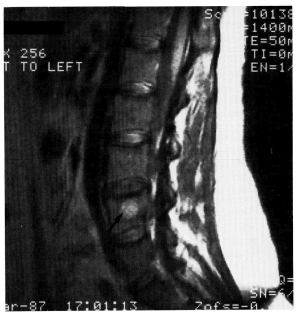

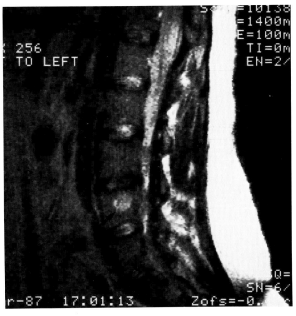

132: Metastatic Breast Disease (1.5T)

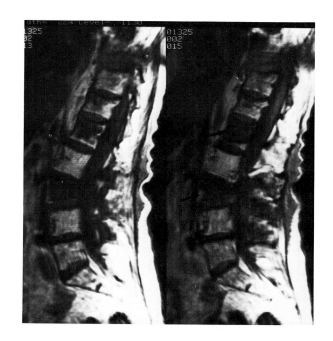

EXAM: MRI of the lumbosacral spine.

CLINICAL INFORMATION: This is a 77-year-old female with metastatic breast CA.

TECHNIQUE: Surface coil sagittal T1- and T2-weighted images were acquired (1800/20,90).

FINDINGS: Areas of decreased signal in the bone marrow are identified on the L1 and L3 vertebral bodies. There is also extension of abnormality into the soft tissues to the left of midline and extending posteriorly at the L3 level. This appears to encase and provide at least a moderate canal stenosis at the L3 level (large arrow, Image 2).

IMPRESSION: Findings consistent with metastatic disease with at least moderate canal stenosis at the L3 level secondary to extension of metastatic change in the epidural space and soft tissues of the canal.

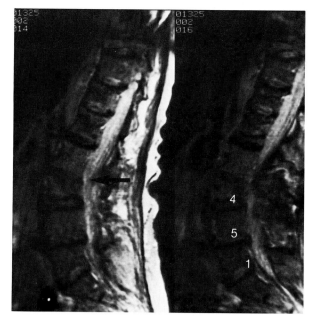

133: Medulloblastoma (Drop-Seed Metastases) (.6T)

Pre-Treatment

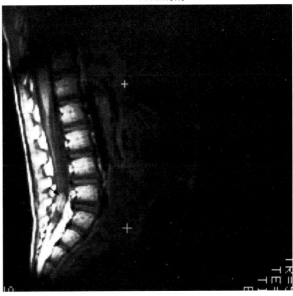

EXAM: MRI of the lumbosacral spine.

CLINICAL INFORMATION: This is a patient with a known medulloblastoma.

TECHNIQUE: Coronal T1-weighted images were obtained on the preliminary study (500/28). In a follow-up study, T1- and T2-weighted images were obtained (1400/50,100).

FINDINGS: There is evidence for a rounded intradural mass at the L5-S1 level consistent with a drop-seed metastasis. On the follow-up scan, following interval chemotherapy, the mass is no longer identified, suggesting resolution of the metastatic deposit.

IMPRESSION: Evidence for a drop-seed metastasis from a medulloblastoma with marked regression to a baseline following chemotherapeutic intervention.

DISCUSSION: Medulloblastoma shown on Image 2 is a tumor with a tendency to metastasize via the CSF pathway. Note that the smaller arrow indicates a suprasellar metastasis.

REFERENCE: Post et al.: *AJNR* **8**:339, March/April, 1987.

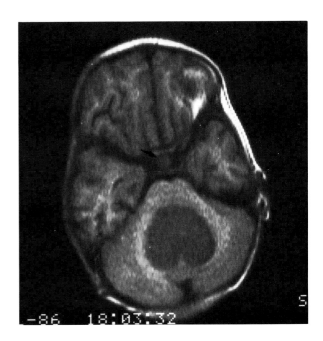

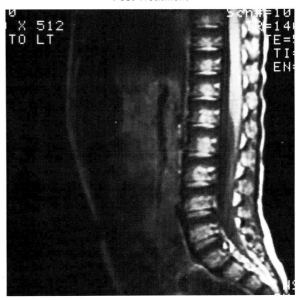
Post-Treatment

159

134: Compression Fractures with Canal Stenosis (1.5T)

EXAM: MRI of the lumbosacral spine.

CLINICAL INFORMATION: A 44-year-old male involved in a recent motor vehicle accident.

TECHNIQUE: Short sagittal acquisition was obtained secondary to claustrophobia; no further imaging could be obtained (400/25).

FINDINGS: L1 shows minimal compressive-type change. L2 is fractured with retropulsion of the posterior portion of the body into the canal with an area of marked canal stenosis.

IMPRESSION: Compression fractures of the L1 and L2 bodies with marked retropulsion of L2 with resultant moderate to severe canal stenosis.

DISCUSSION: Although the cord terminates at the T12-L1 level, the roots of the cauda equina can be compressed (large arrows). Note the smaller rootlets as they course toward their exit under the respective pedicles (small arrows).

REFERENCE: Kulkarni et al.: *Radiology* **164**:834, 1987.

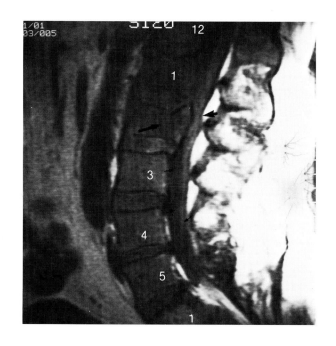

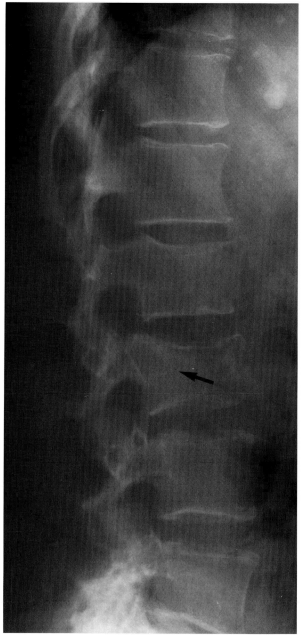

135: Compression Fractures with Canal Stenosis (.6T)

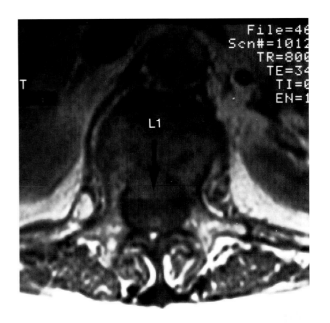

EXAM: MRI of the lumbosacral spine.

CLINICAL INFORMATION: Rule out lumbar abnormality in a 67-year-old with low back pain and left hip pain.

TECHNIQUE: Surface coil and axial imaging were obtained (1500/50,100; 800/34).

FINDINGS: There is a retropulsion of a large fragment of the anterior posterior L1 vertebral body into the canal with resultant moderate canal stenosis. There is a slight increase in signal in the terminal cord and root, suggesting the possibility of some gliosis from edema. There is preservation of the disc. There is, however, some moderate to severe degenerative change from T11 through S1.

IMPRESSION: Compression fracture of L1 with retropulsion of fragment, as described, with at least moderate canal stenosis at this level.

DISCUSSION: Retropulsed vertebral body in relationship to the conus is shown well. Although, on the axial images, a more spacious canal is suggested, the sagittal images clearly show the stenosis (large arrows). Increase in signal in the neural tissues, particularly in the cord, can reflect edema or myelomalacia. Posttraumatic cyst, hemorrhage, and tears are also easily identified within the tissue of the spinal cord. This is a distinct and marked advantage over CT which requires contrast and delayed scans to image the larger cysts and irregularities in a damaged cord.

REFERENCE: Kulkarni et al.: *Radiology* **164**:837, 1987.

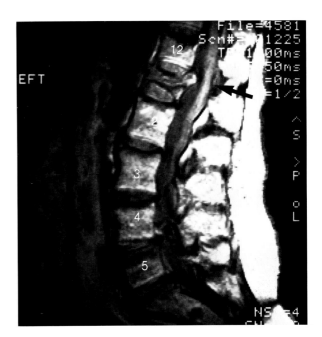

136: L4-5, L5-1 Disc Herniation (.6T)

EXAM: MRI of the lumbosacral spine.

CLINICAL INFORMATION: A 30-year-old, who injured back while lifting at work, is now complaining of low back and left leg pain.

TECHNIQUE: Sagittal and axial T1- and T2-weighted images were acquired (1800/34,68; 1000/60).

FINDINGS: Two midline disc herniations are identified on both the sagittal and axial images as protruding disc material which extends beyond the posterior bony margin of the vertebral discs. The L5-S1 annulus shows a tear or rent on the midline cut.

IMPRESSION: Two-level disc herniation involving L4-5 and L5-S1 disc spaces.

DISCUSSION: Although the annulus appears intact on the sagittal image, the axial image shows the eccentric bulge of a herniated, rather than a diffusely bulging, disc.

REFERENCE: Modic et al.: *AJR* **147**:757, October, 1986.

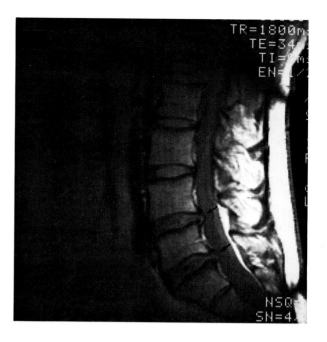

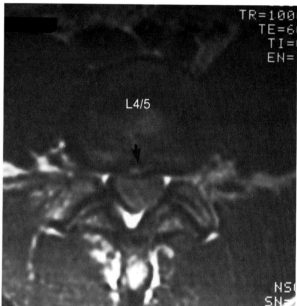

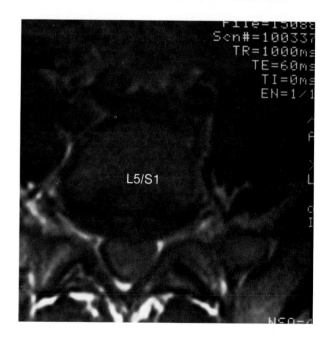

137: L2-3 Disc Herniation   (.6T)

EXAM: MRI of the lumbosacral spine.

CLINICAL INFORMATION: A 53-year-old female with back pain following lifting of heavy object. She is now complaining of back and right leg pain.

TECHNIQUE: Sagittal T1- and T2-weighted images were acquired (2000/45,90).

FINDINGS: There is central and right-sided disc herniation at the L2-3 level, best identified on the sagittal views. This is also loss of signal intensity at the T3, L3-4, and L4-5 levels, reflecting moderate to severe degenerative change within the disc material. There is also moderate to marked disc bulge at the L3-4 level.

IMPRESSION: L2-3 disc herniation with degenerative change.

REFERENCE: Modic et al.: *AJR* **147**:757, October, 1986.

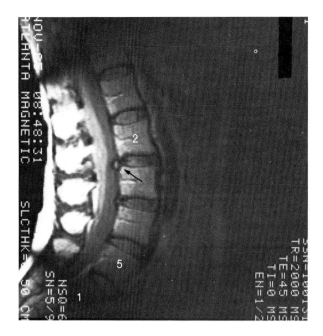

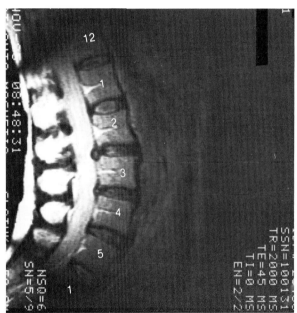

138: Large L5-S1 Disc Herniation with Fragment   (.6T)

EXAM: MRI of the lumbosacral spine.

CLINICAL INFORMATION: A 59-year-old with back and right leg pain. Rule out disc herniation.

TECHNIQUE: Sagittal and axial T1- and T2-weighted images were acquired through the lumbar spine (1800/45,90; 1000/60).

FINDINGS: The alignment of the vertebral bodies is maintained. There is a large central and right-sided extradural defect which shows slightly increased signal intensity compared to the CSF in the thecal sac and in the disc material at the L5-S1 level. The L5-S1 disc shows decreased signal consistent with degenerative change, as well as narrowing of the intervertebral space. The axial images showed the extruded free fragment extending down along the posterior right portion of the S1 vertebral body, displacing the S1 root on the right laterally and deforming the ventral aspect of the thecal sac.

IMPRESSION: Large L5-S1 herniated disc fragment.

DISCUSSION: As in our reference article, we have encountered several free fragments which show increased signal compared to the disc space. The associated presence of narrowing and degenerative change within the disc space, as well as the evidence of mass effect, further supports, the diagnosis of herniation with a free fragment.

REFERENCE: Modic et al.: *AJNR* 7:709, July/August, 1986.

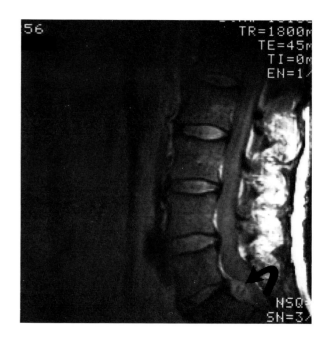

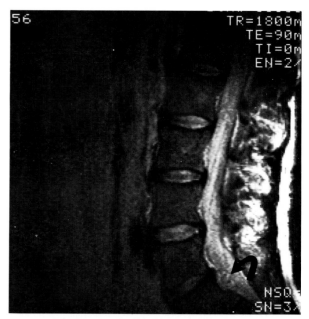

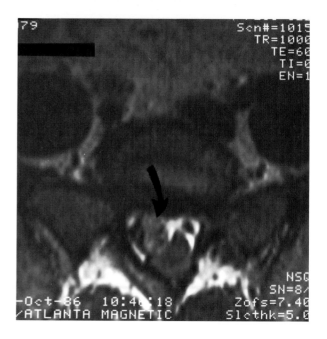

139: Large L4-5 Disc Herniation (.6T)

EXAM: MRI of the lumbosacral spine.

CLINICAL INFORMATION: A 37-year-old male with back and leg pain. Rule out disc herniation.

TECHNIQUE: Sagittal and axial T1- and T2-weighted images were acquired (1200/45,90; 1000/60).

FINDINGS: The alignment of the vertebral bodies is maintained. There is moderate to severe loss of signal in the L4-5 and L5-S1 discs. There is a large central and left-sided extradural defect extending from the disc space. This elevates the ventral thecal sac and markedly deforms it on the sagittal views. There is at least a moderate to severe canal stenosis secondary to a large mount of disc material herniated into the canal.

IMPRESSION: Large L4-5 disc herniation.

REFERENCE: Maravilla et al.: *AJNR* **6**:237, March/April, 1985.

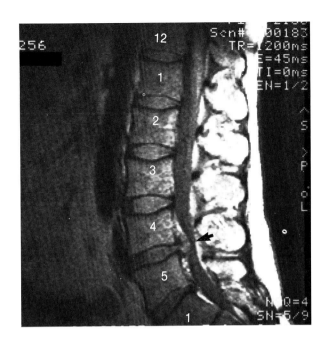

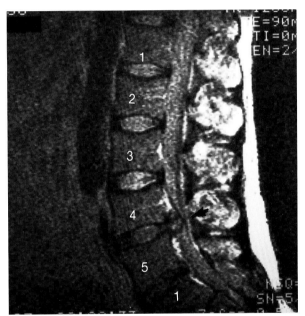

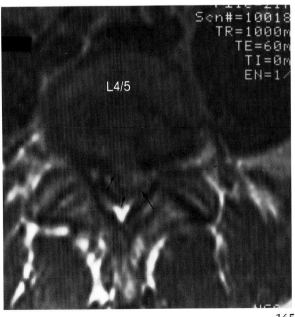

140: Pars Intraarticularis Defects (.6T)

EXAM: MRI of the lumbosacral spine.

CLINICAL INFORMATION: A 37-year-old with back pain beginning 2 weeks before.

TECHNIQUE: Surface coil sagittal and axial T1- and T2-weighted images were acquired (1800/34,85; 1000/60).

FINDINGS: Grade I spondylolisthesis or slippage of the L5 body in relation to S1 is noted with marked narrowing and degenerative change and almost total absence of disc material at the L5-S1 level. In addition, bilateral bony defects are seen through the region of the pars intraarticularis.

IMPRESSION: Changes of Grade I spondylolisthesis with bilateral bony pars defects are demonstrated on both sagittal and axial views.

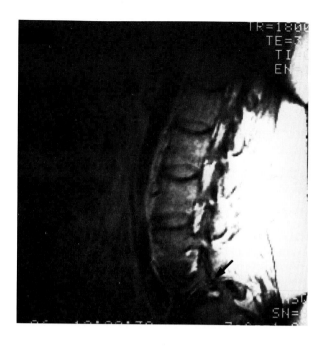

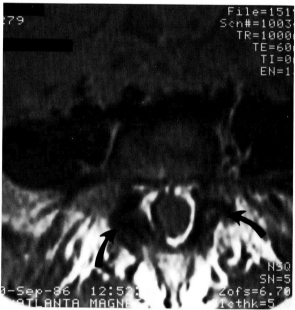

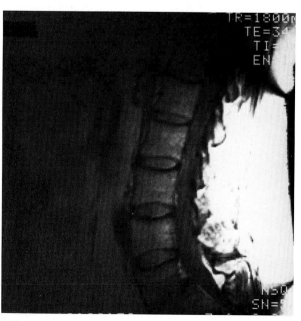

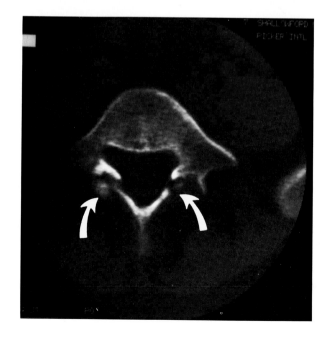

141: Normal Spine (1.5T)

EXAM: MRI of the lumbar spine.

CLINICAL INFORMATION: A 52-year-old female with back and leg pain.

TECHNIQUE: Surface coil sagittal and axial images were obtained (1500/20,70).

FINDINGS: The alignment of the vertebral bodies and disc spaces is normal. No evidence of disc herniation is identified.

IMPRESSION: Normal MRI.

DISCUSSION: Note the high signal of normal healthy disc as well as the high signal in midvertebral bodies representing the entry site of vertebral basilar venous complex. Note correlation between another patient's extensive multilevel discography and the information available on sagittal MR. Sensitivity to internal disc morphology suggests that all information other than that of provocative symptomatology is available on the MR scan.

REFERENCE: Reicher et al.: *AJR* **147**:891, November, 1986.

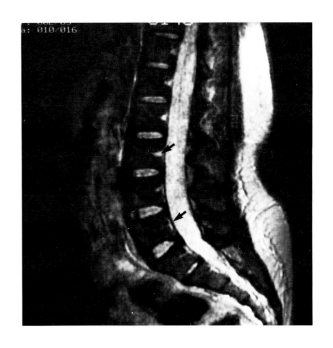

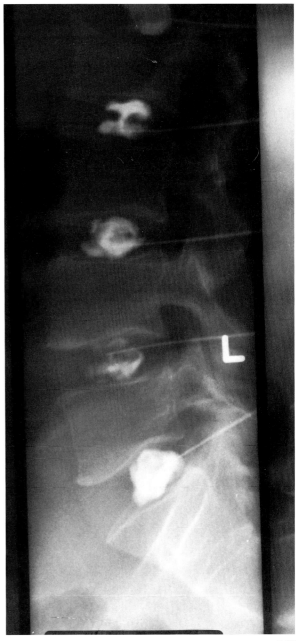

142: Metastases (Medulloblastoma) (.6T)

EXAM: MRI of the lumbar spine.

CLINICAL INFORMATION: An 8-year-old with a medulloblastoma with severe right hip pain.

TECHNIQUE: Sagittal and axial T1-weighted images were acquired (600/34).

FINDINGS: A large right paraspinal mass is seen invading into the thecal sac and extending from the L2 to the L3 superior endplates. There is extensive epidural spread as well as a large amount of soft tissue invasion and tumor to the right of the canal in the paraspinal musculature. This is consistent with a metastatic involvement from known medulloblastoma.

IMPRESSION: Intrathecal extension of a large right paraspinal metastasis with evidence for canal obstruction.

DISCUSSION: This is an excellent example of the ability to image the total tumor volume, which is also displayed on the axial CT but perhaps somewhat less dramatically. Medulloblastoma can have drop-seed metastasis, and the ability of MR to image the neural axis can obviate the need for myelography, extensive CT scan, and, hence, radiation in the pediatric age-group patient.

REFERENCE: Siegel et al.: *JCAT* **10**:593, July/August, 1986.

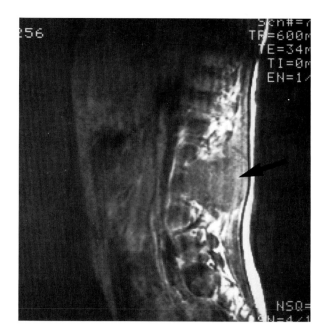

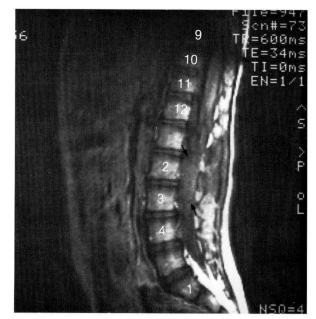

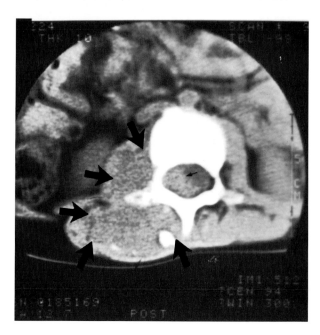

143: Metastases (Poorly Differentiated Adenocarcinoma) (1.5T)

EXAM: MRI of the lumbar spine.

CLINICAL INFORMATION: A 40-year-old male with proven metastatic, poorly differentiated adenocarcinoma to the left abdominal wall.

TECHNIQUE: Surface coil sagittal T1-weighted images were acquired (500/25).

FINDINGS: No evidence of vertebral body collapse or canal compromise is identified; however, there is marked signal loss in the L2 vertebral body, as well as in the L4-5 and L5-S1 vertebral bodies. This is consistent with diffuse metastatic involvement. There is increased signal in the L3 vertebral body. This may be an unusual manifestation of metastases or may represent hemorrhage in a metastatic region.

IMPRESSION: Metastatic involvement of lumbar vertebral bodies without canal compromise.

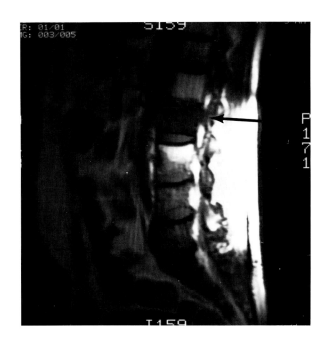

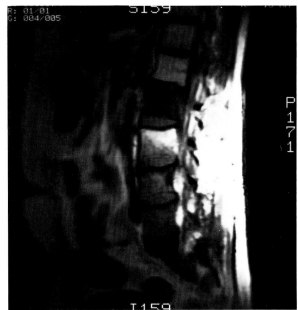

144: Progression of an L5-S1 Disc Herniation   (1.5T)

EXAM: MRI of the lumbar spine.

CLINICAL INFORMATION: A 36-year-old male, with studies approximately 4 months apart. The symptoms of numbness in left leg had accelerated to include loss of sensation.

TECHNIQUE: Surface coil sagittal and axial T1- and T2-weighted images were acquired (1000/50,100; 1000/25).

FINDINGS: On the first study, there is definite disc herniation with effacement of the normal epidural fat in the central and left side with no deviation of the S1 root. There is also marked degenerative loss of signal. In the second study, there is gross extrusion of disc material into the epidural space, and a marked deformity is also appreciated on the axial scans.

IMPRESSION: Progression of an L5-S1 disc herniation in central and left side as seen in two studies separated by several months.

REFERENCE: Modic et al.: *AJR* **147**:757, October, 1986.

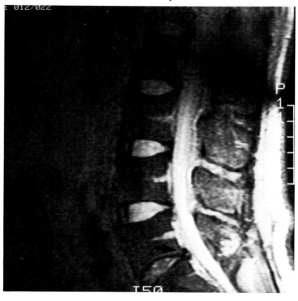

First Study

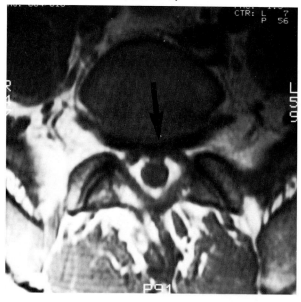

First Study

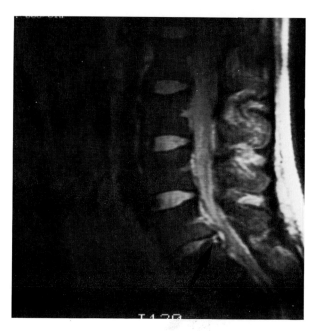

First Study

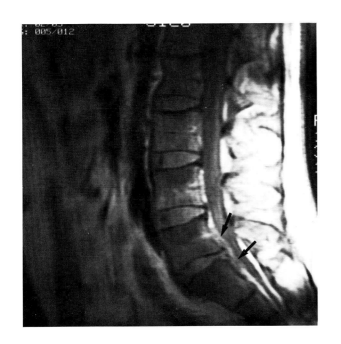

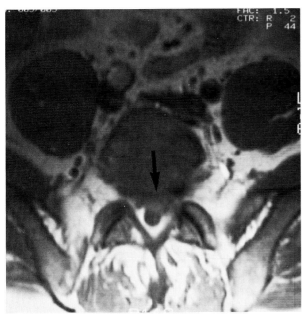

145: L4-5, L5-S1 Disc Herniation with Discogram Correlation   (1.5T)

EXAM: MRI of the lumbar spine.

CLINICAL INFORMATION: A 42-year-old male with predominant complaint of low back pain.

TECHNIQUE: Surface coil sagittal and axial images were obtained (1000/20,90; 1000/40).

FINDINGS: There is a decrease in signal intensity at the L4-5 and L5-S1 levels with associated narrowing and large central and right-sided disc herniation at the L5-S1 level. L4-5 herniation is central and slightly more to the left of midline.

IMPRESSION: L4-5, L5-S1 disc herniation.

DISCUSSION: Correlation with an old exam is available in this case. Note the similar information available both on the sagittal MR and the discography at both levels.

REFERENCE: Ramsey: *Diagnostic Imaging* June, 1987.

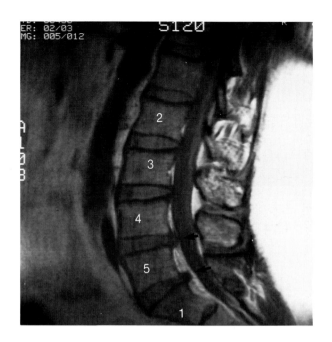

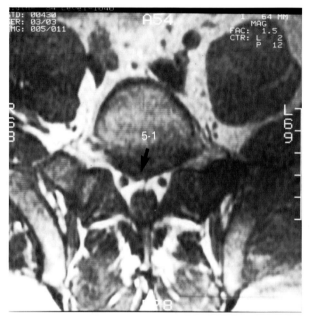

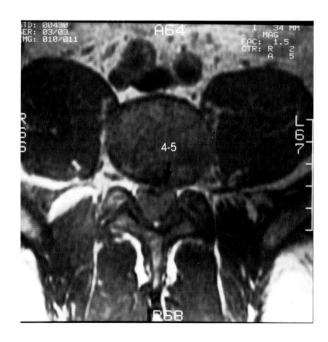

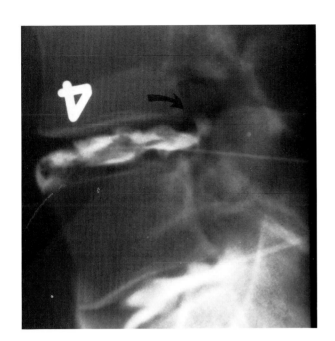

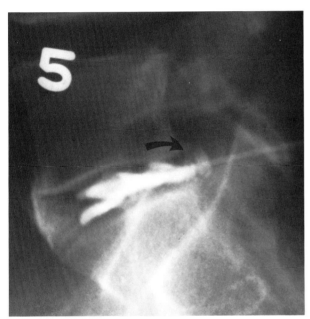

146: Three-Level Disc Herniation (1.5T)

EXAM: MRI of the lumbar sacral spine.

CLINICAL INFORMATION: The patient is a 58-year-old male with a predominant complaint of back pain.

TECHNIQUE: (1500/25; 1000/20,70).

FINDINGS: Three-level disc herniation is identified. L5-S1 is central and large. L4-5 is diffusely herniated, but more so on the right. L3-4 is central.

IMPRESSION: Three-level disc herniation involving the L3-4, L4-5, and L5-S1 levels.

REFERENCE: Ramsey: *Diagnostic Imaging* June, 1987.

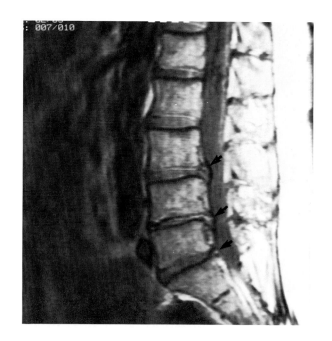

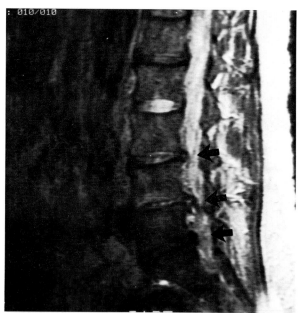

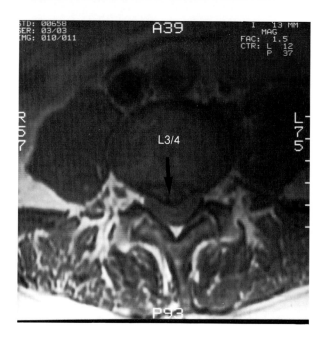

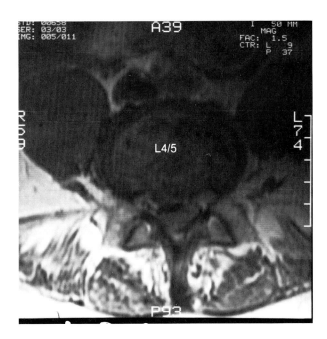

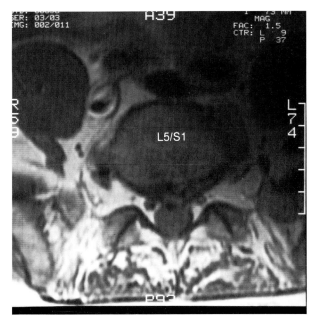

175

147: Canal Stenosis Secondary to Disc Bulge and Ligamentous Hypertrophy (.6T)

EXAM: MRI of the lumbar spine.

CLINICAL INFORMATION: A 70-year-old male with pain and burning in feet bilaterally.

TECHNIQUE: Surface coil sagittal and axial images with T1- and T2-weighting were acquired (1400/50,100).

FINDINGS: There is marked disc bulge and degenerative change at the L4-5 level. This diffuse disc bulge and extradural defect combined with marked posterior-element hypertrophy results in a marked canal stenosis at the L4-5 level. Heavy degenerative changes in all lumbar discs are noted. Retrolisthesis of L5 on S1 with diffuse bulging is noted also.

IMPRESSION: Severe canal stenosis at the L4-5 level secondary to marked diffuse disc bulge and hypertrophy of the posterior elements.

REFERENCE: Han et al.: *AJR* **141**:1137, 1983.

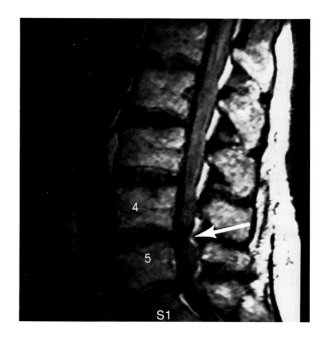

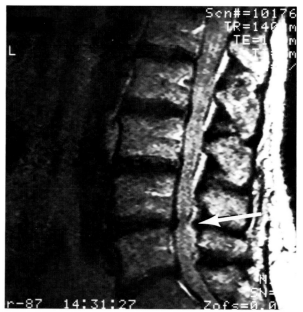

148: L4-5 Herniation   <small>(1.5T)</small>

EXAM: MRI of the lumbar sacral spine.

CLINICAL INFORMATION: A 45-year-old male with L4 radiculopathy, left.

TECHNIQUE: Surface coil sagittal and axial images were acquired (1600/25,90; 1000/25).

FINDINGS: There is a focal disc herniation involving the L4-5 neuroforaminal and left central canals. This is well-identified on both axial and sagittal images.

IMPRESSION: Left central and neuroforaminal canal disc herniation, L4-5.

DISCUSSION: We maintain that MRI is more sensitive to disc disease because of its ability to image in several planes. We are reluctant on a routine schedule to omit axial exams, unless, under careful scrutiny, the sagittal images, including good cuts through the neuroforaminal canals, are deemed normal. Such a case is included here where a sagittal study may omit explanation of left-sided radiculopathy.

REFERENCE: Modic et al.: *AJR* **147**:757, October, 1986.

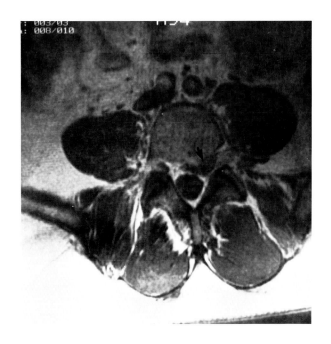

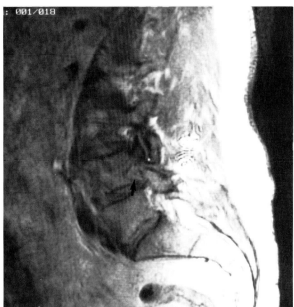

149: Large L5-S1 Disc Herniation (1.5T)

EXAM: MRI of the lumbar sacral spine.

CLINICAL INFORMATION: Rule out disc herniation in a 41-year-old male with left-sided symptoms.

TECHNIQUE: Surface coil axial and sagittal images were acquired (2000/40,80; 1000/25).

FINDINGS: There is an obvious large disc herniation at the L5-S1 level. Marked extrusion into the canal markedly effaces the thecal sac. There is some sparing or deviation of the remaining sac to the right of midline.

IMPRESSION: Large L5-S1 disc herniation.

DISCUSSION: Although the large disc herniation is apparent on CT, its most posterior extent is not fully appreciated or could erroneously be underestimated as a volume artifact.

REFERENCE: Modic et al.: *AJR* **147**:757, October, 1986.

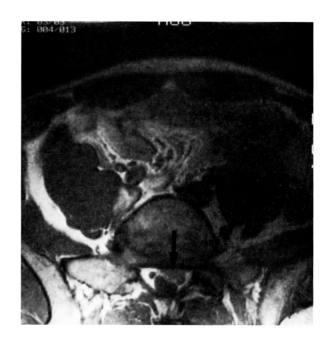

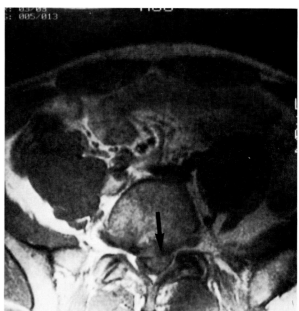

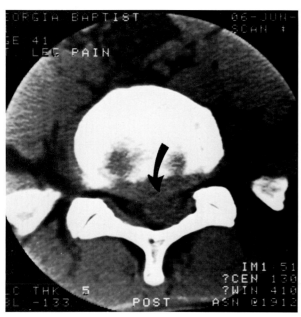

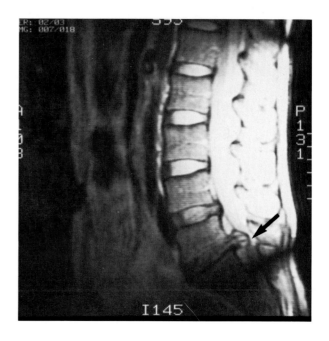

150: Postsurgical Meningocele (1.5T)

EXAM: MRI of the lumbar spine.

CLINICAL INFORMATION: Patient is a 34-year-old female with prior disc surgery at the L4-5 and L5-S1 levels.

TECHNIQUE: T1- and T2-weighted images were acquired (1500/20,70; 1000/25).

FINDINGS: L4-5 and L5-S1 discs show decrease in disc signal intensity on T2-weighted images, as well as narrowing of the intervertebral disc space. This is secondary to a combination of degenerative and postsurgical change. In addition, the posterior bony processes have been removed at both levels. There is a posterior enlargement of the thecal sac in this region consistent with a pseudomeningocele. No evidence of disc herniation is identified, and upper levels are normal.

IMPRESSION: Postsurgical meningocele.

REFERENCE: Ross et al.: *Radiology* **164**:851, 1987.

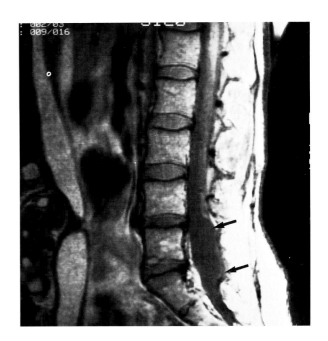

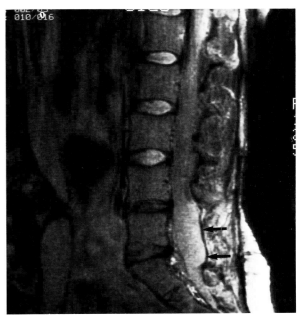

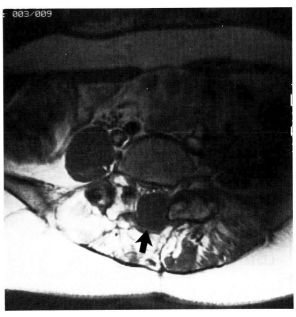

151: Metastatic Breast CA   (.6T)

EXAM: MRI of the thoracic and lumbar spine.

CLINICAL INFORMATION: A 44-year-old female with known breast CA.

TECHNIQUE: Surface coil sagittal and axial T1- and T2-weighted images were obtained (1800/40,80) (450/26; 100/60).

FINDINGS: Numerous areas of decreased signal intensity in all of the vertebral bodies of the midthoracic through the sacral region are identified. No cord compression is seen. The vertebral discs are uninvolved. No evidence of cord compression is identified. The widespread loss of signal located within the vertebral bodies is most consistent with metastatic disease.

IMPRESSION: Multifocal lesions compatible with metastatic disease.

DISCUSSION: The evaluation of the canal demonstrates no evidence of cord compression on contiguous images (some not shown). The fairly specific involvement of the vertebral bodies with decreased signal intensity identifies numerous levels of involvement. These correlate with metastatic involvement.

REFERENCE: Ramsey: *Diagnostic Imaging* August, 1986.

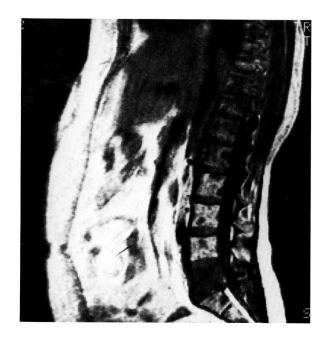

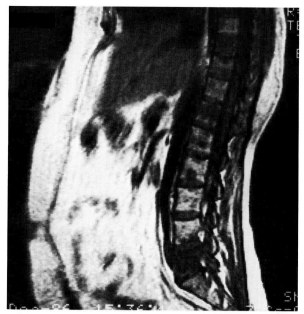

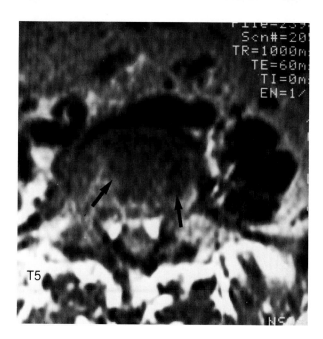

152: Bilateral Avascular Necrosis (1.5T)

EXAM: MRI of the hips.

CLINICAL INFORMATION: A 49-year-old male with bilateral hip pain.

TECHNIQUE: Spin-density-weighted images were obtained in the coronal and axial views (1500/20).

FINDINGS: Bilateral altered signal is identified in the femoral heads. On the right, a bright cystic-type deformity is seen in the weight-bearing surface. On the left, there is altered, markedly decreased signal as well as evidence of flattening of the femoral head.

IMPRESSION: Findings consistent with bilateral avascular necrosis.

DISCUSSION: Avascular necrosis can have several different patterns, two of which are included here.

CONFIRMATION: Pathologic specimen following left hip prosthesis.

REFERENCE: Markisz et al.: *Radiology* **162**:717, 1987.

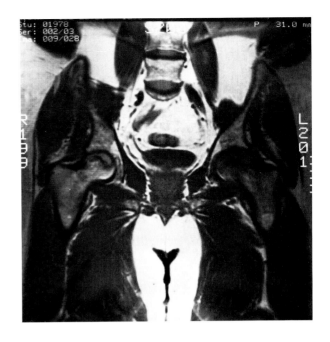

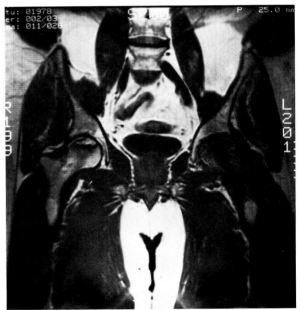

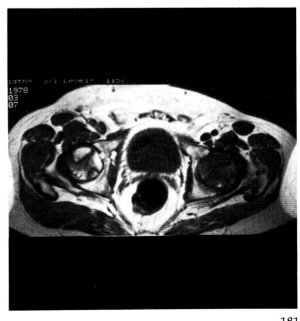

153: Avulsion Injury   (.6T)

EXAM: MRI of the hips.

CLINICAL INFORMATION: A 27-year-old male with low back and right hip pain, which occurred while lifting a heavy object.

TECHNIQUE: Body coil axial and sagittal T1-weighted images were acquired (800/30).

FINDINGS: The coronal images demonstrate discontinuity of the normal low signal of the capsule and cortex along the inferior aspect of the femoral head and neck. There is a slight overall increase in signal intensity, reflecting some localized edema and fluid at this level. This signal is in the region of the attachment of the ilio-femoral ligament and obturator externis and, possibly, the adductor magnus muscle to the capsule and femoral lesser trochanter.

IMPRESSION: Asymmetry in the right hip probably represents avulsion from the capsule and lesser trochanter insertion of muscles in the femur. Note made of a small amount of surrounding inflammatory fluid.

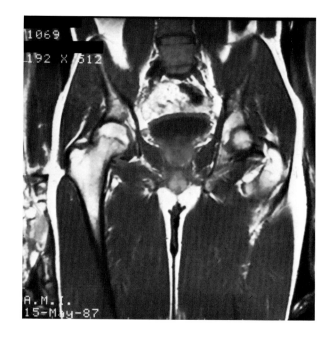

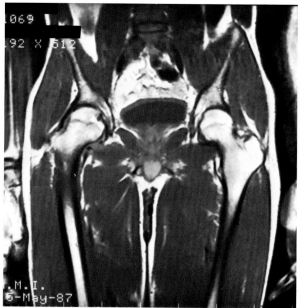

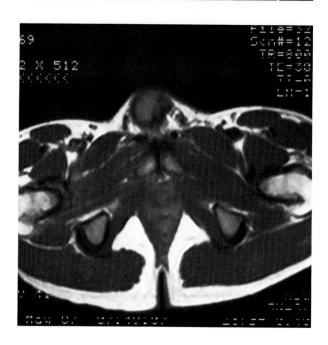

154: Diffuse Atrophy   (1.5T)

EXAM: MRI of the thigh musculature.

CLINICAL INFORMATION: A 69-year-old female with marked muscle atrophy secondary to hip and knee fracture and secondary changes of disuse.

TECHNIQUE: Coronal and axial T1- and T2-weighted images were acquired through the thigh musculature (700/25).

FINDINGS: There is marked asymmetry of the vastus medialis, lateralis and intermedias muscle on the left thigh versus the normal right side. This is a nonspecific atrophy of disuse. No underlying bone tumor or abnormalities are identified.

IMPRESSION: Generalized atrophy of the vastus musculature secondary to disuse.

REFERENCE: Murphy et al.: *AJR* **146**:565, March, 1986.

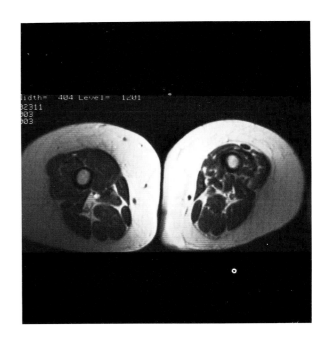

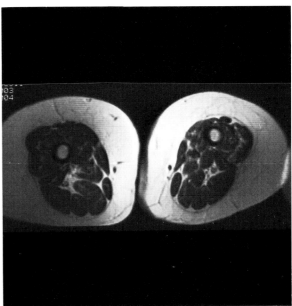

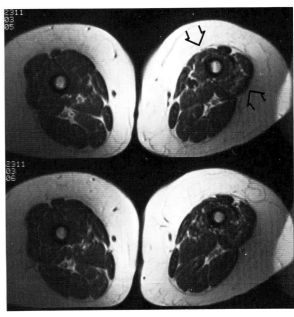

155: Popliteal Cyst   (.6T)

EXAM: MRI of the knee.

TECHNIQUE: Coronal T1- and T2-weighted images were acquired (2500/38/900/38).

FINDINGS: There is a rounded cystic lesion posterior to the knee which exhibits short T1 and prolonged T2 characteristics. This is consistent with simple cystic structures, such as a popliteal cyst.

IMPRESSION: Popliteal cyst.

CONFIRMATION: Confirmed at surgery.

REFERENCE: Beltron et al.: *Radiology* **158**:133, 1986.

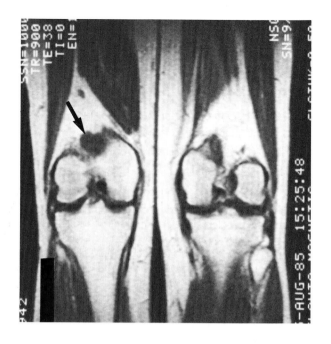

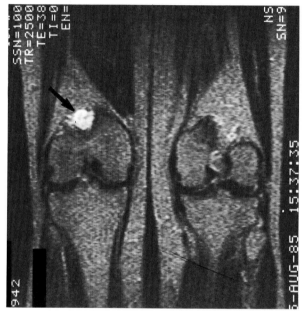

156: Fracture and Avascular Necrosis (.6T)

EXAM: MRI of the feet.

CLINICAL INFORMATION: A 24-year-old male, with severe injury to the talar bones from a fall 6 months before. Rule out avascular necrosis.

TECHNIQUE: Coronal and sagittal T1-weighted images were obtained (800/32).

FINDINGS: A fracture through the midportion of the talus is identified with sclerosis of the margins of the left foot. The signals in both the anterior and posterior segments of the talus are, however, normal. In the right foot, there is an area along the weight-bearing surface of wedged-shaped, decreased signal consistent with avascular necrosis.

IMPRESSION: (1) Fracture through the midtalus, left foot, and (2) avascular necrosis talus, right foot.

REFERENCE: Gillespy et al.: *Radiology Clinics of North America* **24**:193, 1986.

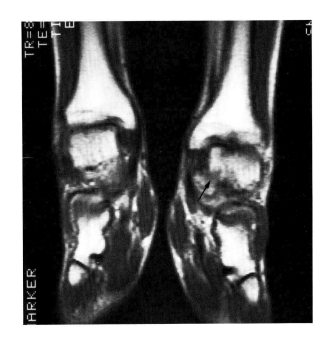

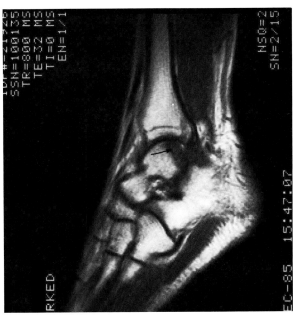

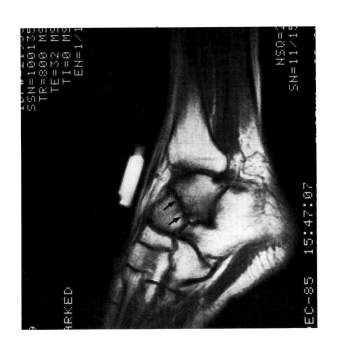

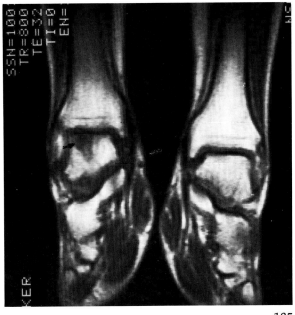

157: Neurofibroma of the Sciatic Nerve (.6T)

EXAM: MRI of the pelvis.

CLINICAL INFORMATION: 14-year-old male with reduced motion of the right foot for over 2 years with flatfootedness and lack of flexion and extension. No pain.

TECHNIQUE: Axial and coronal T1-weighted images were acquired (700/32).

FINDINGS: There is asymmetry of the right sciatic nerve which is enlarged along its course from the level of the greater trochanter by approximately 3 cm caudally. It enlarges up to 1½ cm in greatest dimension.

IMPRESSION: Asymmetric right sciatic nerve most compatible with a focal neurofibroma.

DISCUSSION: The ease of visualizing the distal sciatic nerves and subcutaneous tissue, as well as the pelvis, is a rewarding additional imaging maneuver when the conventional spine-imaging modalities fail to demonstrate a cause for radiculopathy.

REFERENCE: Cohen et al.: *AJNR* 7:337, March/April, 1986.

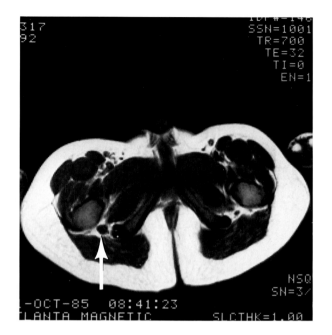

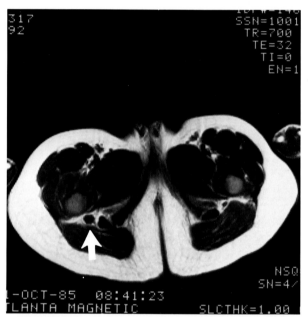

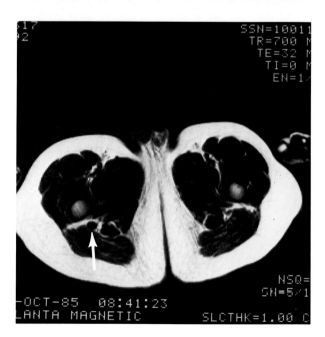

158: Desmoid of the Calf   (.6T)

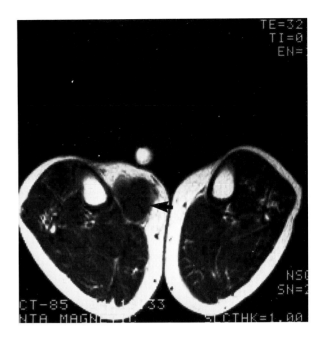

EXAM: MRI of the subcutaneous tissues of the calf.

CLINICAL INFORMATION: A 59-year-old female with a growth noted in the left leg. The patient noticed a recent increase in size.

TECHNIQUE: Sagittal and axial T1-weighted images were obtained (700/32).

FINDINGS: Located within the subcutaneous fat overlying the anterior portion of the tibia is a rounded, discrete low-signal-intensity mass. This abuts, but does not appear to invade, the musculature or cortex of the tibial shaft. This has a rounded configuration and measures approximately 4 cm in greatest extent. The homogeneous character with good margins and lack of any evidence of invasion of the muscle or bone suggest that this is a benign tumor, such as a fibroma.

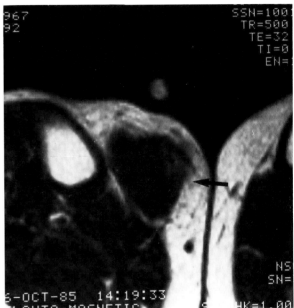

DISCUSSION: The axial scans through soft tissue tumors are comparable to CT. However, our experience has been that there is far more detail secondary to the inherent contrast of fat on MRI. The coronal and sagittal orientations also add a wealth of information. There seems to be, in most cases, enough vascular information available to obviate the need for angiography. The attachment to associated muscle and bone is also obvious as demonstrated here.

CONFIRMATION: Desmoid tumor was removed at surgery.

REFERENCE: Murphy et al.: *Radiology* **160**:135, 1986.

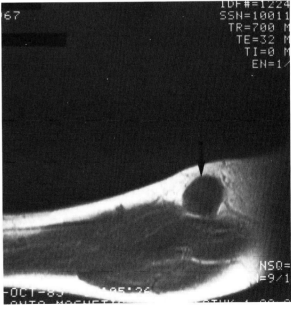

159: Ischial Fracture (.6T)

EXAM: MRI of the pelvic bones.

CLINICAL INFORMATION: Nonathletic, slightly overweight 12-year-old male fell while running in physical education class, fracturing both the scapula and left ischium.

TECHNIQUE: Axial and coronal body coil images were obtained with T1- and T2-weighting (1000/25; 2000/40,80).

FINDINGS: High-signal intensity seen to displace the obturator internis muscle adjacent to the ischium and the inner aspect of the pubic bone. This high-signal area is felt to represent acute hematoma.

IMPRESSION: Hematoma and edema surrounding the ischial fracture. The actual fracture is not seen by MRI. The remainder of the MR images included suggested no evidence of an infiltrative lesion or abnormality within the bone marrow.

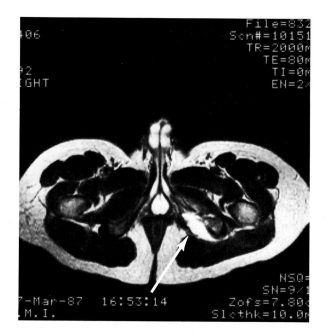

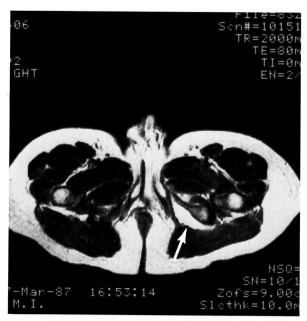

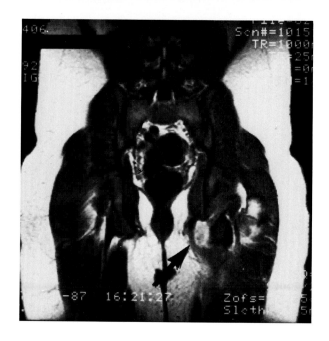

160: Ewing's Sarcoma (.6T)

EXAM: MRI of the pelvis.

CLINICAL INFORMATION: A 7-year-old female with known Ewing's sarcoma, now on chemotherapy. MRI for evaluation of total tumor extent prior to block resection.

TECHNIQUE: Coronal and axial T1 images were obtained (400/21).

FINDINGS: There is expansion of the right superior pubic ramus with periosteal reaction and an enlargement of the overall bony shaft. There is replacement of the normal bright-signal bone marrow of the bone with iso- to hyposignal intensity when compared to the soft tissue structures such as muscle. The area of abnormal change appears to be limited to the pubic bone. This does not cross the symphysis and does not extend into the acetabulum or iliac bone.

IMPRESSION: Ewing's Sarcoma of the pubic bone.

DISCUSSION: Plain film and CT remain the preferred modality for evaluating calcified change; however, MRI demonstrates elegantly the replacement of the normal bone marrow and the relationship of bone tumor to the surrounding structures such as muscle and vascular structures. The evaluation of the joint and adjacent bony structures is also well-portrayed. Note on the coronal views the suggestion of an onion-skinning or periosteal reaction (arrow).

REFERENCES: Boyko et al.: *AJR* **148**:317, February, 1987. Zimmer et al.: *Radiology* **155**:709, 1985.

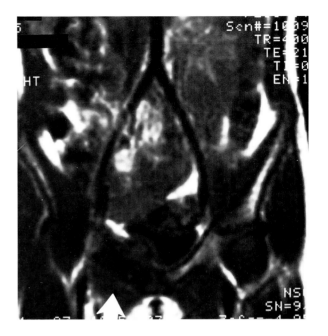

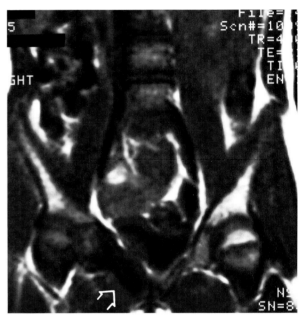

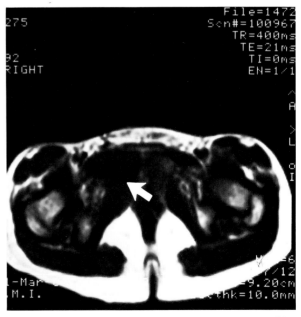

161: Changes of Biopsy   (1.5T)

EXAM: MRI of the thigh.

CLINICAL INFORMATION: A 49-year-old female with a small squamous cell CA that was removed in an office visit inspection of a skin mass. This was associated with a small sinus tract.

TECHNIQUE: Coronal and axial T1- and T2-weighted images were obtained (400/24; 2000/40,80).

FINDINGS: An irregular area of signal is seen superficial and medial to the medial musculature of the thigh. This shows increased signal on the more T2-weighted images. This is quite nonspecific and may represent inflammatory edema and hemorrhage. The coronal views are more bothersome in indicating a possible focal mass but, when correlated with the axial images, no definite mass can be identified.

IMPRESSION: An area of abnormal signal in the subcutaneous tissues lateral to the thigh musculature. This most likely represents edema and hemorrhage. No definite mass is identified.

CONFIRMATION: A more thorough excision through the sinus tract area following the initial biopsy failed to produce any additional malignant tissue, and all changes were attributed to trauma from the local biopsy site.

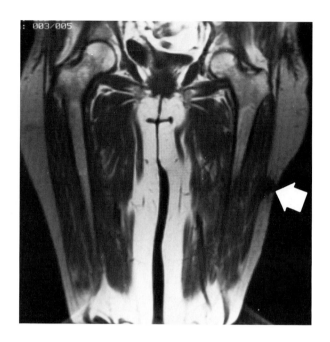

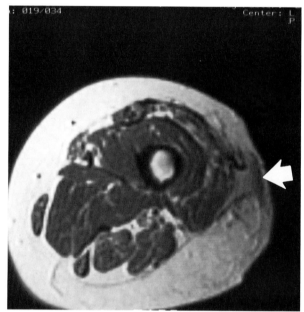

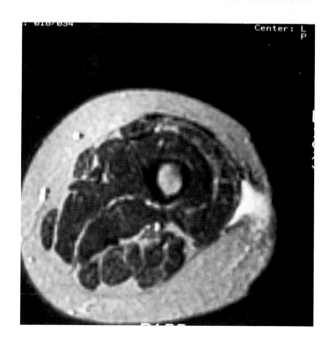

162: Hematoma (.6T)

EXAM: MRI of the right leg.

CLINICAL INFORMATION: Swelling in the right posterior leg following an injury 5 weeks before.

TECHNIQUE: Sagittal and axial T1- and T2-weighted images were acquired (1800/40,80; 650/21).

FINDINGS: A discrete high-signal intensity lesion is identified, which is contained within the medial gastrocnemius muscle on the right. The high-signal characteristics on both the T1- and T2-weighted images suggest that this is consistent with a hematoma.

DISCUSSION: Hematoma.

Courtesy of Al Alexander and Perry Miller of Lancaster Magnetic Imaging.

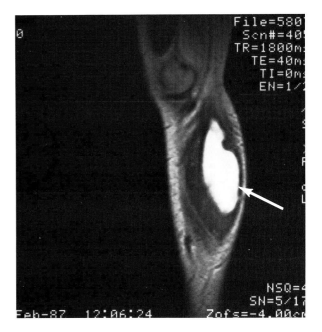

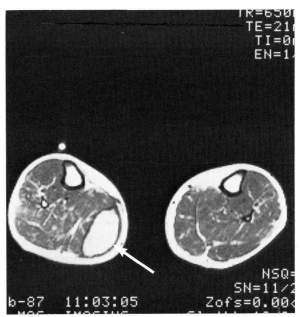

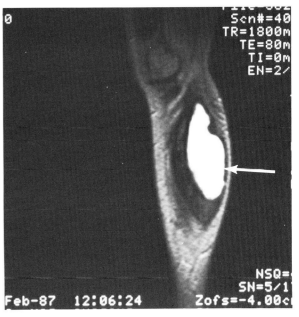

163: Sinus Tract   (1.5T)

EXAM: MRI of the pelvis.

CLINICAL INFORMATION: A 63-year-old male with radiation osteonecrosis of the sacrum and enlarged soft tissue mass in the left inguinal region.

TECHNIQUE: Coronal T1-weighted images were obtained (2000/25).

FINDINGS: Soft tissue collection arising from the area of the radiation-destroyed sacro-iliac joint is seen extending along the course of the psoas muscle. This may be within the parenchyma of the psoas muscle out into the inguinal region. It is consistent with a sinus tract. Infection of the fluid cannot be excluded.

DISCUSSION: Note the good correlation between the coronally demonstrated sinus tract and fluid on the MR and the fistulogram done following the MR.

REFERENCE: Gillespy et al.: *Radiology Clinics of North America* **24**:193, 1986.

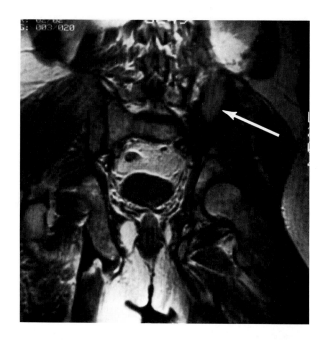

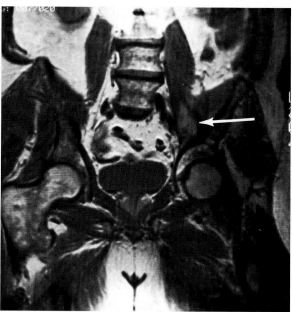

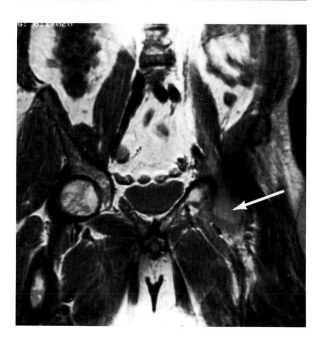

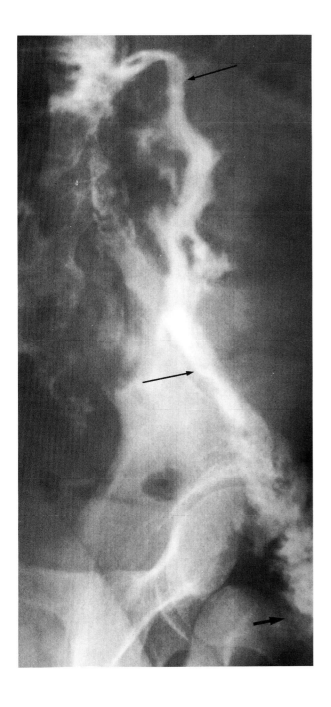

164: Radiation Osteonecrosis (1.5T)

EXAM: MRI of the pelvis.

CLINICAL INFORMATION: This is a 63-year-old male with prior radiation, now with an enlarging mass in the inguinal region on the left side.

TECHNIQUE: Coronal and axial T1- and T2-weighted images were acquired (2000/25,90).

FINDINGS: There is marked distortion and very low signal surrounding the left half of the sacrum and S-I joint, suggesting marked loss. There is an overall impression of loss of bone anatomy rather than a mass. With the history of prior significant radiation, we suspect that this all represents old radiation osteonecrosis.

IMPRESSION: Radiation osteonecrosis.

REFERENCE: Gillespy et al.: *Radiology Clinics of North America* **24**:193, 1986.

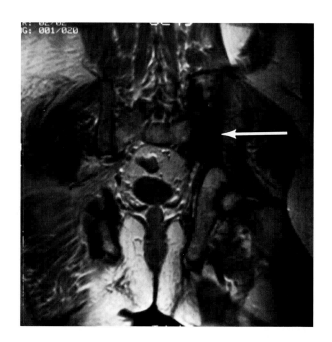

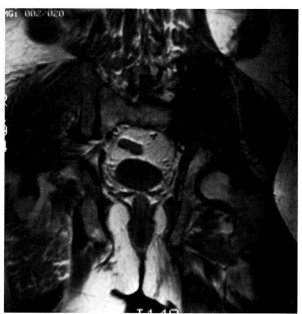

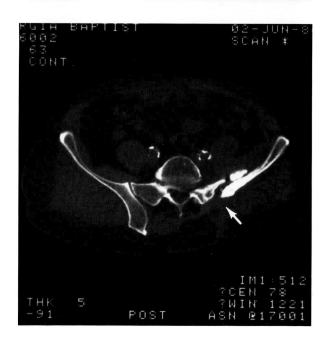

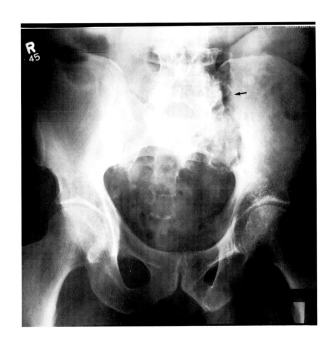

165: Lymphangioma   (.6T)

EXAM: MRI of the left lower extremity.

CLINICAL INFORMATION: This is a 14-year-old with marked asymmetry of the extremities with diffuse enlargement of the left extremity and clinical diagnosis of a lymphangioma.

TECHNIQUE: Coronal and axial cuts were obtained from the lower abdomen to the level of the knee with spin density images (850/30).

FINDINGS: Marked asymmetry of the subcutaneous tissue is identified. The left side is abnormal. There are various areas of intermediate soft-tissue-type signal extending through the subcutaneous fat. There are several large rounded structures seen extending along the lateral subcutaneous tissue representing vascular structures. Smaller strandlike areas are also seen infiltrating up into the subcutaneous tissues of the lower abdominal wall. The underlying muscles show no loss of mass. There is an increase in the fascial planes. There appears to be no direct invasion into the muscle or bony structures.

IMPRESSION: Diffuse lymphangioma involving soft tissues from the lower abdominal wall through the entire left leg.

DISCUSSION: This is a particularly graphic demonstration of the asymmetry of the subcutaneous tissue as well as a demonstration of the diffuse profound involvement of the leg with lymphangioma.

REFERENCE: Cohen et al.: *Radiology* **158**:475, 1986.

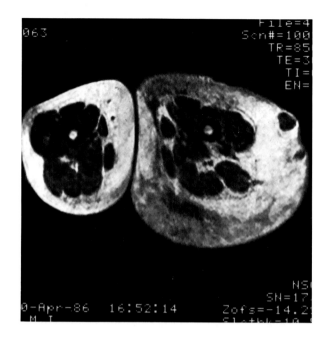

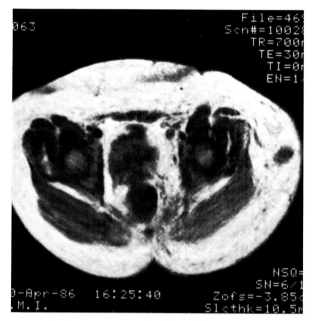

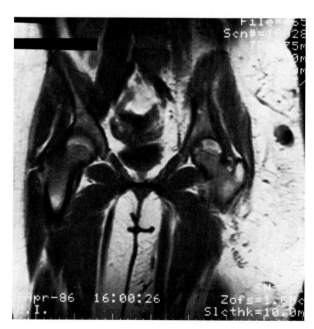

166: Calcific Tendonitis   (1.5T)

EXAM: MRI of the foot.

CLINICAL INFORMATION: Right posterior foot pain and perception of a small lump in a 34-year-old male.

TECHNIQUE: Spin density images in the sagittal, coronal, and axial planes were obtained through the mid- and hindfoot (1000/20).

FINDINGS: A nonspecific area of intermediate signal adjacent to, but not apparently invading, the musculature and tendon of the calcaneus is identified. Differential concern for a periosteal sarcoma or a small tumor arising from the tendon or muscle was raised.

IMPRESSION: Question a small periosteal sarcoma. There is, however, no evidence of cortical invasion. Also question a benign chondroma.

DISCUSSION: Of particular concern to the clinician, prior to resecting this area, was the relationship of this abnormality to the tendon and muscle in the foot. The advantage of the numerous planes of orientation for acquiring information allows good demonstration of all the associated tendon, muscle, and bone structures of the foot and ankle.

CONFIRMATION: At surgery, nonspecific focus of calcification was obtained and diagnosed as a nonspecific myositis ossificans or calcific tendonitis possibly from old trauma. No malignant tissue was identified.

REFERENCE: Beltran et al.: *Radiology* **162**:735, 1987.

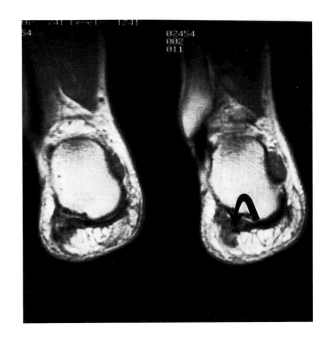

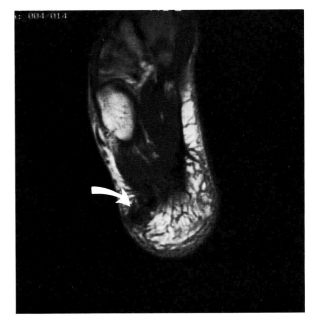

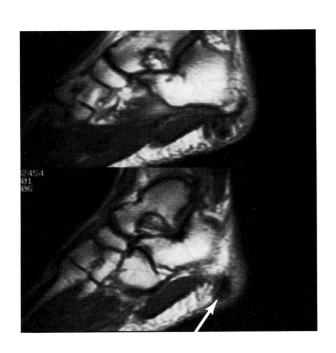

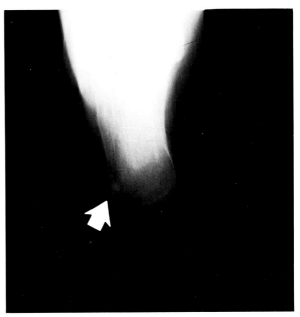

167: Rhabdomyosarcoma (.6T)

EXAM: MRI of the neck.

CLINICAL HISTORY: A 15-year-old female, who, 7 months earlier, had noticed some bumps on her left neck. These have enlarged with patient now having difficulty turning head and being unable to sleep. Arm feels "strange" and occasionally goes to sleep.

TECHNIQUE: Axial spin density and double-echo techniques were employed in the coronal and axial orientation (725/35; 1400/40,80).

FINDINGS: Soft tissue mass in the left neck measuring 7 cm in depth, 9 cm in greatest transverse diameter, and approximately 9 cm in distance. This begins at approximately the level of the tip of the epiglottis and extends into the anterior superior left pleural space. No evidence of direct lung parenchyma invasion is seen. There is displacement of the sternocleidomastoid muscle, and the signal of the tumorous mass occupies the right longus coli muscle as well as totally replaces the scalenus medias and posterior muscle. The mass has fairly well-marginated edges and shows an increased signal intensity to that of muscle on both the more T1- and T2-weighted sequences. There is no evidence of direct extension into the neural foraminal canal; however, the mass sits right in the region of the brachial plexus and exiting roots.

IMPRESSION: A hemangioma was considered; however, clinically, this mass is quite firm and hard and does not reduce or increase with positional maneuvers. The differential is between that of an adherent group of lymph nodes from lymphoma versus a rhabdomyosarcoma. The nonvisualization of several of the strap muscles in the neck supports the diagnosis of rhabdomyosarcoma.

REFERENCE: Stork et al.: *Radiology* 150:455, 1984.

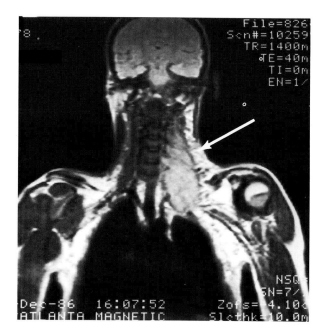

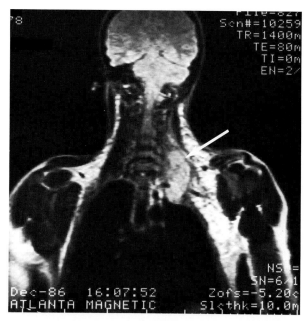

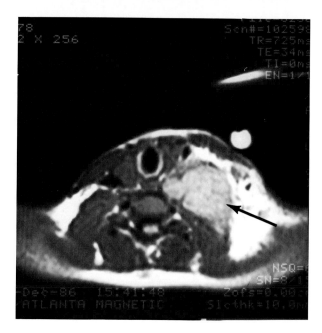

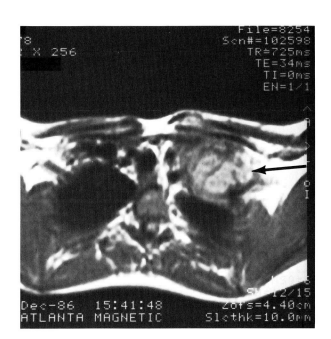

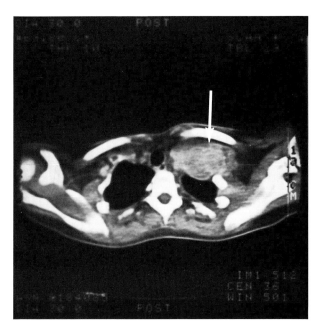

168: Osteogenic Sarcoma (.6T)

EXAM: MRI of the pelvis.

CLINICAL INFORMATION: A patient with known osteogenic sarcoma, leg and hip pain on left.

TECHNIQUE: Axial and coronal T1- and T2-weighted images were obtained (1500/21,42).

FINDINGS: There is decreased signal in the bone marrow of the left iliac. This does not appear to cross into the ischial bone or into the hip capsule. The sacrum also maintains normal signal. There is evidence for periosteal reaction or elevation with mild deviation of the associated musculature away from the cortex.

IMPRESSION: Abnormal left iliac bone showing decreased signal within the bone marrow and periosteal reaction. This is compatible with osteogenic sarcoma.

DISCUSSION: MR offers good visualization of the entire extent of primary bone tumor. Evaluation of the total amount of bone marrow in addition to the tumor's relationship to the surrounding musculature, viscera, and vascular structures. Like the authors of our reference article, we too feel that this is an excellent primary imaging modality for evaluation of bone tumor and should be a useful modality for follow-up to check response to chemical and surgical intervention.

REFERENCE: Boyko et al.: *AJR* **148**:317, February, 1987.

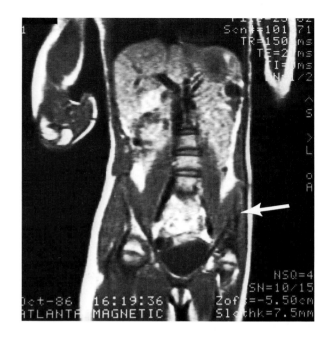

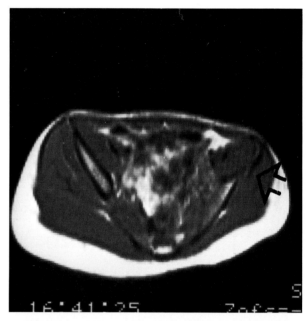

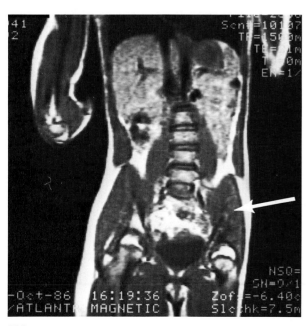

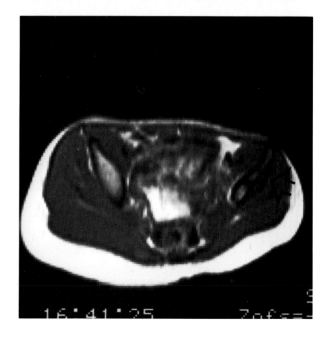

169: Sarcoma of the Scapular Muscles (.6T)

EXAM: MRI of the shoulder.

CLINICAL INFORMATION: A 69-year-old female with painful left shoulder.

TECHNIQUE: Body coil spin density and T2-weighted images were acquired (1500/45,90).

FINDINGS: Soft tissue mass arising from the medial or inner aspect of the scapular body is identified. This shows increased signal on the T2-weighted images. The mass measures approximately 11 cm in cranial caudad dimension and 6.7 cm in transverse and posterior dimension. There is evidence of scalloping of the inner table of the scapula, but we suspect the mass is arising directly from the muscles of the scapula. The margins of the mass are discrete, and there is no evidence of invasion into the chest wall.

IMPRESSION: Sarcoma of the scapular muscles.

DISCUSSION: Offering the most exact information of the tumor volume and its relation to the adjacent structures, MR is a useful primary modality in evaluation of bone and soft tissue tumors. This is particularly useful in patients who would be candidates for block resection of malignant tumors. The involvement of bone marrow, soft tissue extension, joint involvement, and relation to any vascular structures are the largest strong points of MR over CT. Plain film and CT remain the more definitive investigational tools for evaluation of cortical destruction.

REFERENCE: Bloem et al.: *RadioGraphics* 5:853, November, 1985.

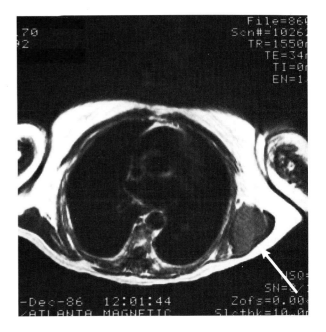

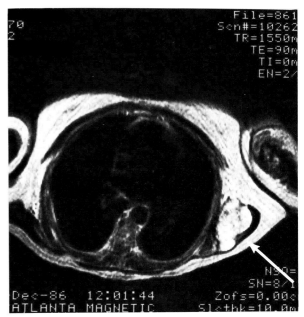

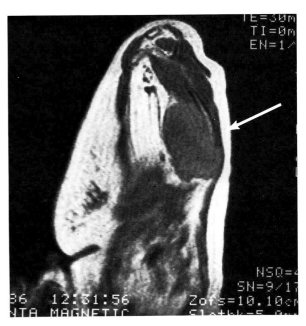

170: Polio (.6T)

EXAM: MRI of the left leg.

CLINICAL INFORMATION: Left leg mass in a 35-year-old female complaining predominantly of lower back pain, but also question slight increase in size of the left leg, possibly a mass, in the past several months.

TECHNIQUE: Coronal and sagittal T1- and T2-weighted images were acquired (1500/40,80; 500/21).

FINDINGS: There is a slight asymmetry with fatty replacement in the left gastrocnemius muscle head. No mass is identified.

IMPRESSION: Focal fatty infiltration of medial head of the left gastrocnemius muscle. Question of a local trauma or possibly an old viral inflammation to explain changes.

CONFIRMATION: The patient relates a history of polio from childhood.

REFERENCE: Murphy et al.: *AJR* **146**:565, 1986.

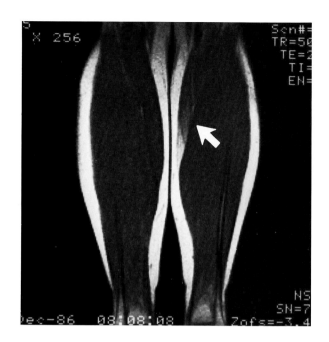

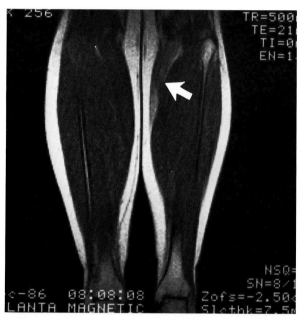

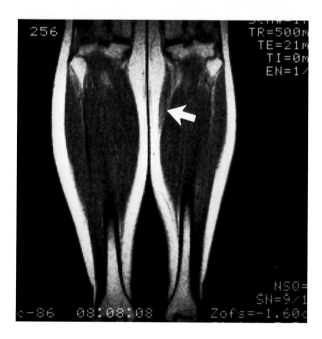

171: Bilateral Avascular Necrosis (.6T)

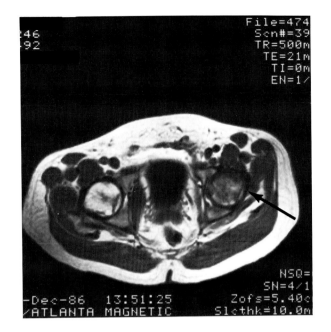

EXAM: MRI of the hip.

CLINICAL INFORMATION: A 41-year-old male with left hip pain.

TECHNIQUE: Axial and coronal T1-weighted images were obtained (500/21).

FINDINGS: Irregular low signal seen on the weight-bearing surface of the left hip, which is also flattened in its contour. In addition, on the right side, there is a well-circumscribed area of increased signal consistent with early cystic change of avascular necrosis.

IMPRESSION: Bilateral avascular necrosis, left side more advanced with femoral head flattening. The right side shows earlier cystic-type change.

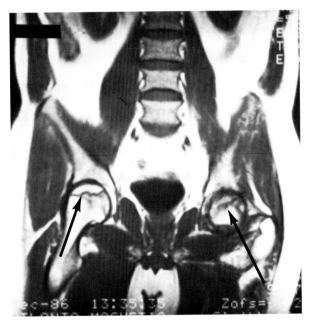

DISCUSSION: Conversion of the hematopoietic substance to fatty marrow is known to correlate with the physiologic decrease in intramedullary blood flow. Early conversion of this marrow within the intratrochanteric marrow has been seen with patients with AVN. This alteration to fat may be an early sign for patients at risk for AVN.

The distribution of the hematopoietic marrow correlates with the marrow's blood supply. In patients of all ages, there is some fatty marrow within the femoral epiphysis. Ischemic necrosis of the bone has been noted to occur almost exclusively within the fatty marrow of the femoral head and neck.

REFERENCE: Mitchell et al.: *Radiology* **161**:739, 1986.

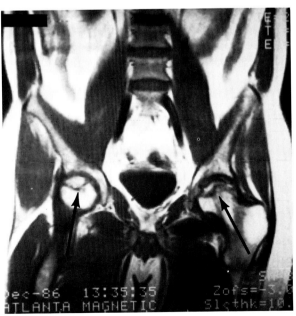

172: Avascular Necrosis   (.6T)

EXAM: MRI of the hip.

CLINICAL HISTORY: A 35-year-old with painful left hip. Rule out AVN.

TECHNIQUE: Coronal and axial spin density images were obtained (825/30).

FINDINGS: There is marked signal loss involving the large portion of the left femoral head and neck extending down into the shaft below the intratrochanteric line. In addition, an area of intermediate signal outside of the low-signal bone cortex is identified, representing fluid within the capsule.

IMPRESSION: This is a typical case of avascular necrosis showing the characteristic low signal associated with the interruption of blood flow to the femoral head and neck as contrasted to the normal bone marrow signal seen on the right side. The amount of signal loss is extensive and is seen to extend below the intratrochanteric line.

DISCUSSION: A gross appraisal of any femoral head flattening can be offered with MR. This is an important diagnostic feature for the orthopedic surgeon. Small amounts of fluid can be seen in the avascular necrotic hip. Fluid can occur just prior to the avascular necrosis but is seen in greatest amounts in the femoral heads that have already been slightly flattened. Note the capsular fluid (small arrows).

REFERENCE: Mitchell et al.: *AJR* **146**:1215, June, 1986.

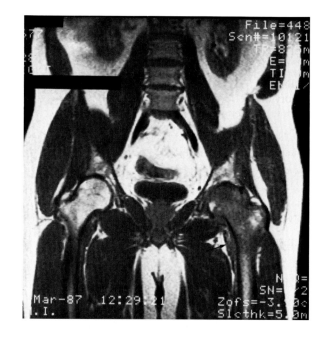

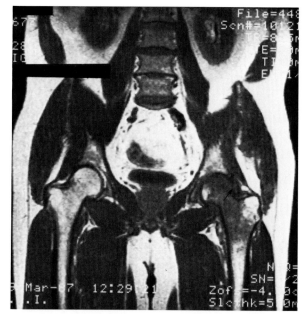

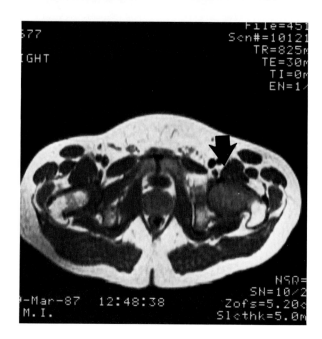

173: Medial Meniscal Tear   (.6T)

EXAM: MRI of the right knee.

CLINICAL HISTORY: A 31-year-old female with a two-year history of knee pain. No history of injury: the knee intermittently become swollen.

TECHNIQUE: Coronal and sagittal spin density images were obtained (900/34; 1050/34).

FINDINGS: An area of increased signal in the posterior horn of the medial meniscus is identified. The meniscus otherwise appears intact. This finding is consistent with horizontal tear and chronic mixed degeneration within the meniscus.

IMPRESSION: Horizontal tear in the posterior horn, medial meniscus.

DISCUSSION: The horizontal tear is secondary to chronic shearing forces on the meniscus. These normally occur in older individuals. This contrasts to the acute, linear meniscal tear injuries in the athletic young adult. This is one form of injury (mixoid degeneration) in which the outer capsule of the meniscus may remain intact and be missed, even upon direct arthroscopic examination.

REFERENCE: Reicher et al.: *Radiology* **162**:547, 1987.

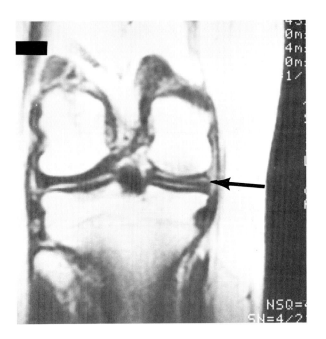

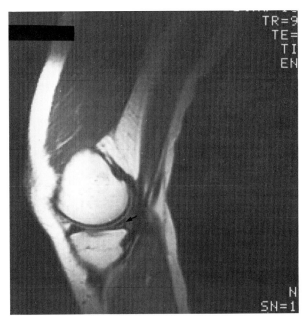

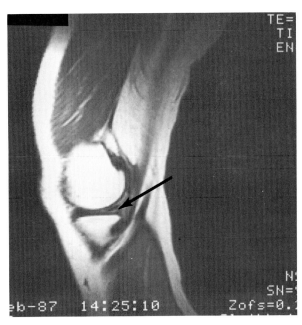

174: Anterior Cruciate Damage/ Joint Effusion   (.6T)

EXAM: MRI of the knee.

CLINICAL INFORMATION: A 31-year-old with prior reconstruction of the anterior cruciate ligament. Question retear of the cruciate.

TECHNIQUE: Coronal and sagittal spin density images were obtained (750/35).

IMPRESSION: The posterior cruciate is unremarkable. The collateral ligaments and the menisci are intact. Note is made of a small amount of joint effusion tracking into the suprapatella bursa.

The anterior cruciate ligament is well-attached to both its femoral and tibial attachments. There is, however, a zone of intermediate signal surrounding the cruciate suggestive of some diffuse enlargement of the ligament, possibly from some hemorrhage or edema.

IMPRESSION: Anterior cruciate remains intact. There is, however, suggestion of some inflammatory change throughout the cruciate ligament. Joint effusion.

DISCUSSION: We favor a technique of imaging the routine knee in the sagittal and coronal views with a T1- or spin-density-weighted image. Although some authors advocate the use of a longer TR sequence to convert the normal joint fluid into an arthrographic effect, we feel that the normal contrast between the joint fluid and the very low signal menisci and ligaments is in itself satisfactory. Note the appearance of the normal posterior cruciate and the presence of joint effusion.

REFERENCE: Li et al.: *JCAT* 8:1147, 1984.

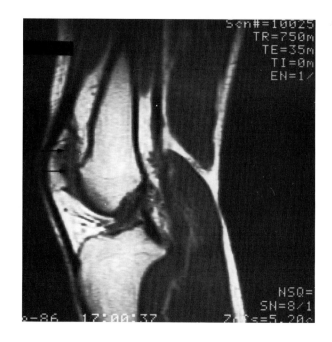

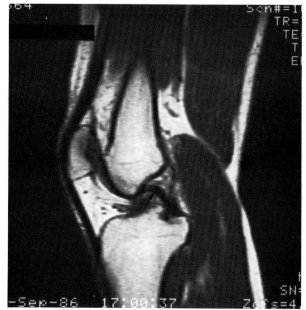

175: Cystic Tumor of the Calcaneus   (.6T)

EXAM: MRI of the foot.

CLINICAL INFORMATION: A 37-year-old female with persistent pain in the heel.

TECHNIQUE: Coronal T1- and spin-density-weighted images were acquired (735/34; 1250/43).

FINDINGS: Well-marginated cystic lesion in the body of the calcaneus is identified. Within the central portion is a low-signal-intensity area, probably representing a free-floating bone fragment. The bone marrow signal of the remainder of the calcaneus is normal, and the edges of this lesion are quite discrete.

IMPRESSION: Cystic bubbly-type lesion of the right calcaneus. Suspect most compatible with a simple bone cyst with fractured and free-floating fragment. Aneurysmal bone cyst and giant cell tumors cannot be excluded.

DISCUSSION: The bone tumors are well-displayed. The relationship to the cortical margin, bone marrow, tendon and muscle is also well-displayed. The ability to view these in more than one dimension adds immensely to the appreciation of the total volume. As a general rule, with MRI most malignant tumors tend to alter or show decreased signal within the bone in addition to the malignant features well known to plain radiography.

REFERENCE: Beltran et al.: *Radiology* **158**:689, 1986.

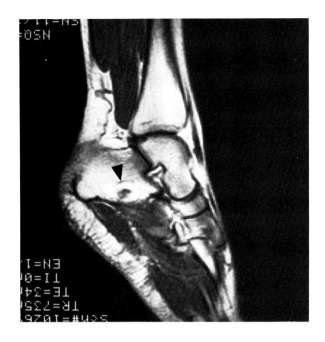

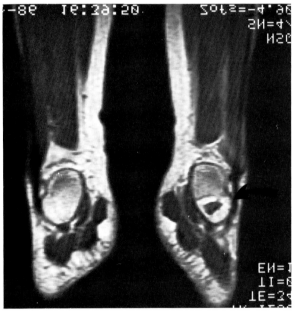

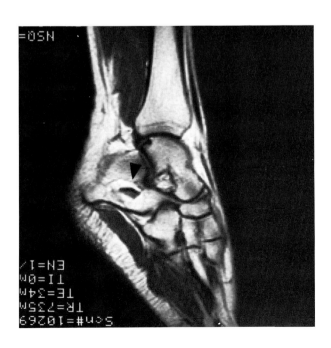

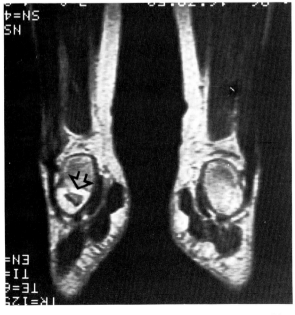

176: Septic Arthritis (.6T)

EXAM: MRI of the knee.

CLINICAL INFORMATION: A 51-year-old male fell approximately 1 year prior to this examination. An open sinus tract draining fluid has developed with a fullness or mass in the posterior calf.

TECHNIQUE: Surface coil coronal and sagittal spin echo and double-echo axial exams were obtained through the knees (900/34; 1500/24,48).

FINDINGS: There is marked narrowing, irregularity, and destruction of the knee joint with a loss of almost all the normal features, including marked irregularity of the tibial and femoral articular surfaces. The posterior cruciate ligament is just barely identified (Image 1, small arrows). There is a large amount of fluid throughout the knee as well as an extensive amount of fluid tracking posterior to it and down overlying the calf musculature (Image 2, arrows). A marked amount of destruction and history of a draining sinus are most consistent with severe septic arthritis and development of large

IMPRESSION: Severe arthritic change secondary to trauma and superimposed sepsis. All findings are consistent with that of septic arthritis.

DISCUSSION: This dramatic demonstration of septic arthritis with tracking fluid or abscess into the calf demonstrates nicely the ability of MRI to reveal the total extent of infected fluid as well as appeciation for the loss of normal knee anatomy from trauma or inflammation.

REFERENCE: Beltran et al.: *Radiology* 158:133, 1986.

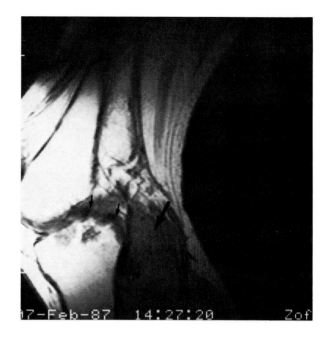

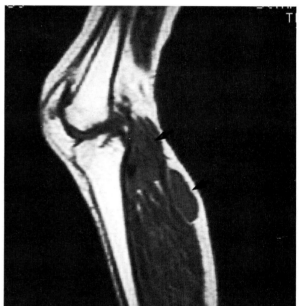

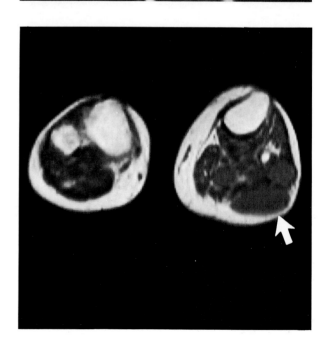

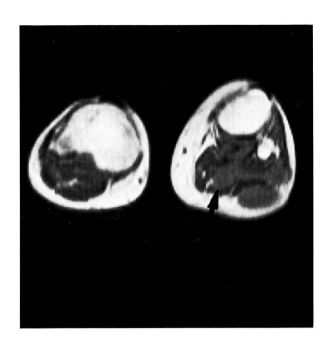

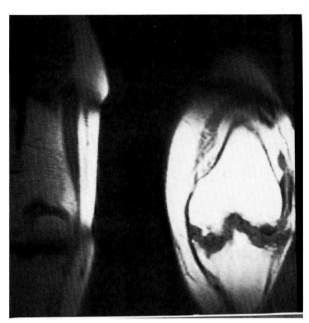

177: Lateral Meniscal Tear (1.5T)

EXAM: MRI of the knee.

CLINICAL INFORMATION: This is a 65-year-old female with an acute twisting injury and right compartment knee pain. Rule out meniscal tear.

TECHNIQUE: Coronal and sagittal spin density images were obtained (1000/20).

FINDINGS: A linear area of increased signal is seen extending through the midportion of the lateral meniscus of the right knee.

IMPRESSION: Lateral meniscus tear.

DISCUSSION: Normal meniscus appears as a black-wafer-like structure. Two types of tears are identified. An acute linear or cephalad-directed tear can be identified as well as a chronic or recurrent injury tear, referred to as a horizontal tear. This is seen as an anterior-to-posterior tear through the meniscus.

REFERENCE: Beltran et al.: *Radiology* **159**:747, 1986.

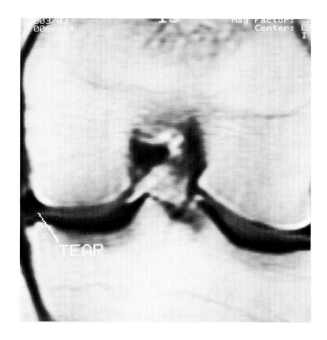

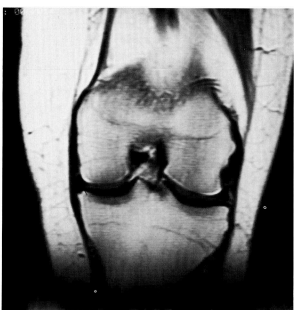

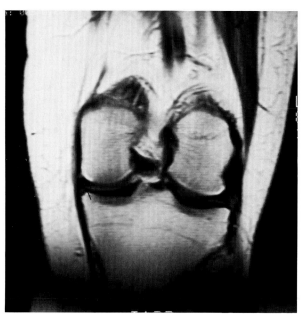

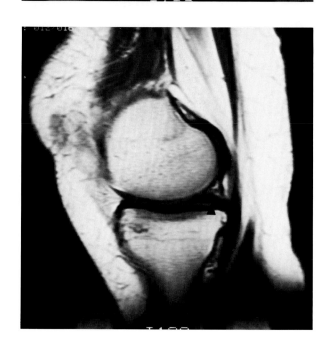

178: Multiple Tears of the Lateral Meniscus with Joint Effusion (.6T)

EXAM: MRI of the knee.

CLINICAL INFORMATION: Patient with long history of right knee pain.

TECHNIQUE: Spin-density-weighted images were obtained in coronal and sagittal plane (900/34; 800/34).

FINDINGS: There is joint effusion present represented by the intermediate signal in the capsule tracking into the suprapatella bursa. In addition, only small fragments of a low-signal area representing portions of the severely damaged lateral meniscus are identified.

IMPRESSION: Extensive damage to the right lateral meniscus including numerous tears and detachment of the meniscus from the capsule. Joint effusion.

DISCUSSION: The details of the menisci and collateral and cruciate ligaments offered by MRI in such a sensitive fashion make the need for arthrography almost nonexistent. The presence of effusion in the acute or chronically injured knee is easily demonstrated as seen in our case.

REFERENCE: Gallimore & Harms: *Radiology* **160**:457, 1986.

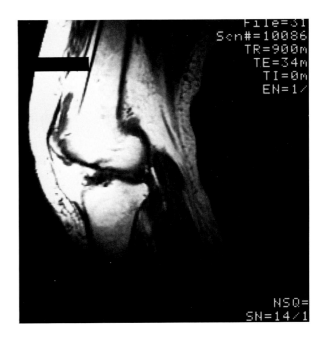

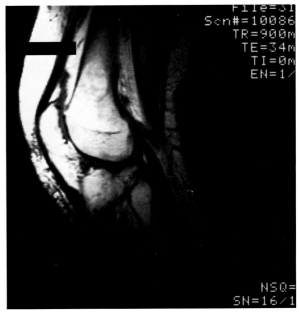

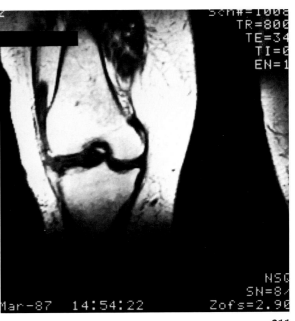

179: Collateral Ligament Damage (.6T)

EXAM: MRI of the knee.

CLINICAL INFORMATION: A 40-year-old male. Rule out torn meniscus.

TECHNIQUE: Coronal and sagittal spin density images were obtained (800/33).

FINDINGS: An area of altered irregular intermediate signal is seen tracking along the lateral aspect of the lateral meniscus and the lateral collateral ligament. The collateral ligament remains attached. There is a question of a possible tear through the lateral aspect of the lateral meniscus attachment to the capsule.

IMPRESSION: Evidence of some inflammatory change along the lateral meniscus and collateral ligament. Evidence of disruption consistent with acute injury to the collateral ligament and possibly to the lateral meniscus.

DISCUSSION: The normal appearance of the collaterals is that of very low signal intensity similar to that of the meniscus or the anterior and posterior cruciates. The alteration or increase of signal reflects surrounding edema or hemorrhage around the site of injury. At times, a direct visualization of a torn collateral ligament can be identified. The authors of our review article consider a ligament to be torn if the high-intensity signal in and around the collateral ligament can be identified. The evaluation of the collateral ligaments is an area often silent to both arthrogram and arthroscopic investigation.

REFERENCE: Turner et al.: *Radiology* **154**:717, 1985.

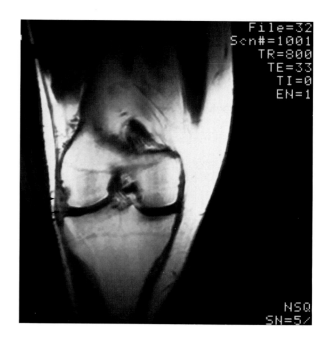

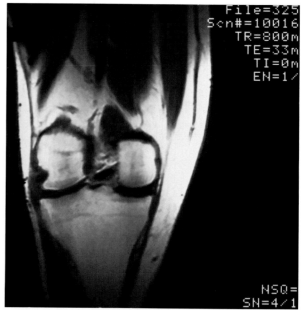

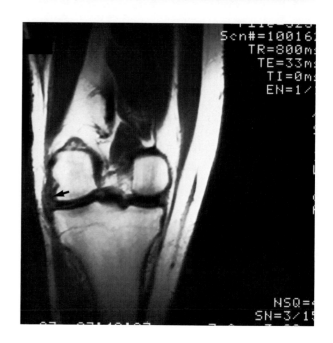

180: Bilateral Avascular Necrosis   (.6T)

EXAM: MRI of the hip.

CLINICAL INFORMATION: AVN confirmed by prior studies in the right hip. CT done recently of left hip is negative. Minimal cortisone treatment in the past. Rule out AVN now on the left.

TECHNIQUE: T1-weighted images were acquired in the coronal and axial planes (700/32).

FINDINGS: There is definite avascular necrosis identified in the right hip with similar loss of signal and bright cystic-type change seen in the left hip.

IMPRESSION: Findings consistent with AVN in both hips.

DISCUSSION: Our reference authors have divided the different morphologic presentations of AVN into Classes A through D which correlate with early to late AVN. Class A, or early AVN, is consistent with a signal similar to that of fat. Class B has a blood or subacute hemorrhage isointensity. Class C, a later stage including fibrosis and sclerosis, becomes less signal intense. The final Class D, or late stage, is the sclerotic bony reaction, with marked decreased signal intensity.

REFERENCE: Mitchell et al.: *Radiology* **162**:709, 1987.

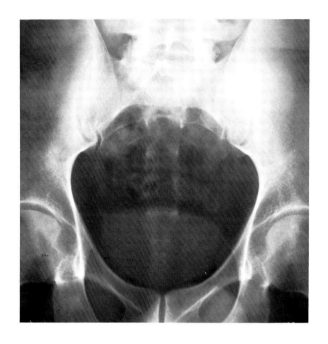

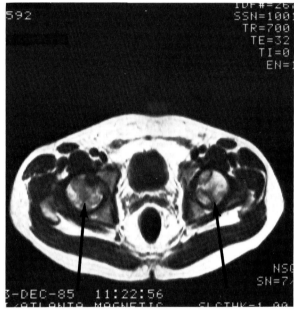

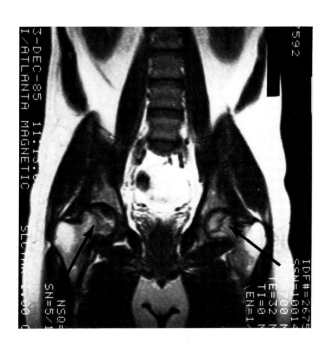

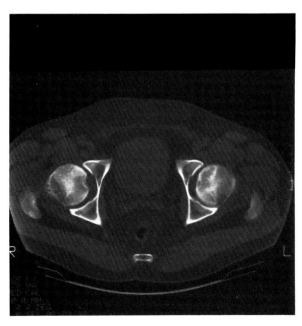

181: Septic Joint Effusion   (.6T)

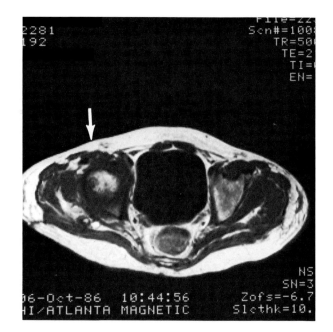

EXAM: MRI of the hip.

CLINICAL INFORMATION: Osteomyelitis of the right femoral head, proven by biopsy to be positive for salmonella. Continued pain in the right hip and leg. Patient is a 44-year-old male.

TECHNIQUE: Axial and coronal T1-weighted images were obtained (500/20).

FINDINGS: There is decreased signal in the acetabular head and femoral neck. The femoral head has normal signal on sequential cuts (not shown). There is also a large amount of fluid within the right hip capsule.

IMPRESSION: Findings consistent with a hip joint effusion, probably septic, given history.

DISCUSSION: Correlates of CT and nuclear medicine scans are included. Without history, it would be difficult to exclude an arthritis or an AVN due to large amount of fluid here.

REFERENCE: Mitchell et al.: *AJR* **147**:67, July, 1986.

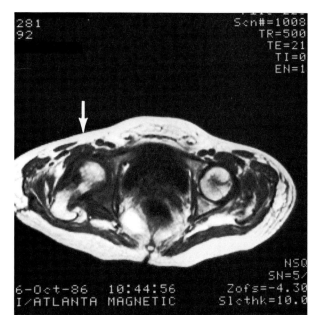

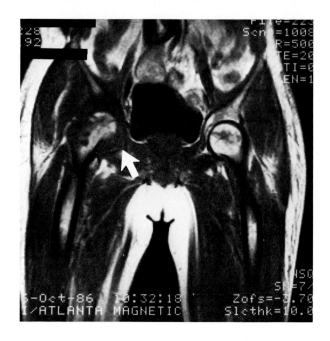

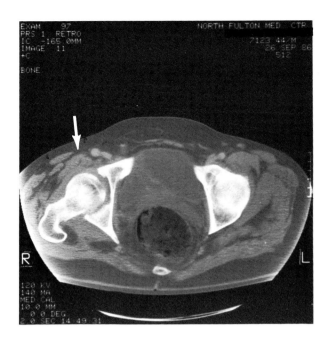

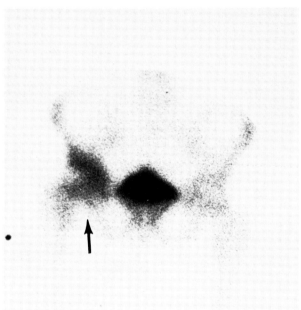

215

182: Alveolar Soft Part Sarcoma (1.5T)

EXAM: MRI of the right thigh.

CLINICAL INFORMATION: A 9-year-old female with noticable, mildly painful thigh mass.

TECHNIQUE: Axial and coronal T1- and T2-weighted images were acquired (800/25, 1600/40).

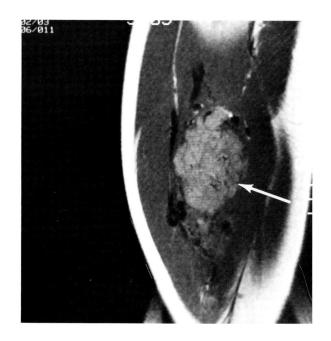

FINDINGS: A markedly vascular mass is identified. This arises between the cleft of the vastus lateralis and media. This abuts, but does not appear to invade or distort, the bony cortex. The edges of this mass are poorly defined, and the mass shows increased signal intensity in both T1- and T2-weighted images, suggesting either a large fatty content or possibly blood content from vascular channels.

DISCUSSION: The MR shows dramatically the full extent of the tumor area, as well as the vascularity obviating the need for angiography in this case. Excellent delineation of the location of the tumor in relation to the muscle bundles and the bony cortex is offered. The bone marrow can also be well-evaluated and, in this particular case, shows no evidence of involvement. The marked vascularity and indiscrete borders suggest a malignant potential. Sarcomas and rhabdomyosarcomas were considered.

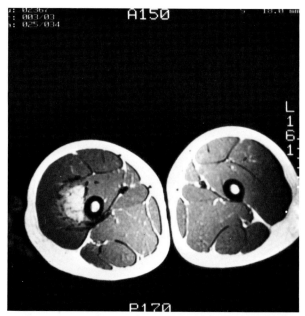

IMPRESSION: This tumor was excised with an apparent capsule at surgery. There was a marked amount of bleeding. Final pathologic diagnosis was alveolar soft part sarcoma.

REFERENCE: Aisen et al.: *AJR* **146**:749, April, 1986.

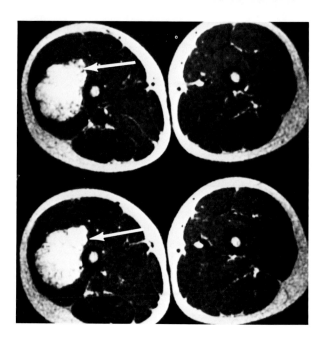

183: Anterior and Posterior Cruciate Ligament Tears (.6T)

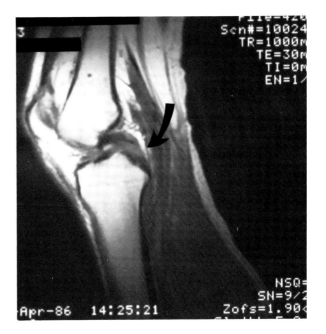

EXAM: MRI of the knee.

CLINICAL INFORMATION: These are two patients in their forties with recent athletic trauma to and pain in the knee. Rule out cruciate ligament damage.

TECHNIQUE: Sagittal T1-weighted images were obtained (1000/30).

FINDINGS: Image 1 demonstrates a cleft or tear through the posterior cruciate ligament. Image 2 demonstrates a defect through the midsubstance of the anterior cruciate ligament. These findings are consistent with tears. The attachment of the cruciate ligaments to the bone remains intact.

IMPRESSION: Example of both anterior (Image 2) and posterior (Image 1) cruciate ligament tears.

REFERENCE: Gallimode et al.: *Radiology* 160:457, 1986.

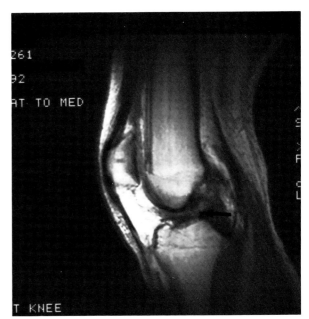

184: Thymoma   (.35T)

EXAM: MRI of the mediastinum.

CLINICAL INFORMATION: This is an 86-year-old female with clinical findings of myasthenia gravis.

TECHNIQUE: Cardiac-gaited T1-weighted scans were obtained in the axial plane through the mediastinum (500/30).

FINDINGS: A discrete well-marginated lesion measuring 3.75 cm is identified in the left anterior mediastinum. The edges are well-demarcated. No adenopathy or parenchymal lesions are detected.

IMPRESSION: Anterior mediastinal mass most consistent with a thymoma due to the clinical information of myasthenia gravis.

DISCUSSION: The anterior mediastinal differential favors thymoma in the presence of myasthenia gravis. The surgical removal of a thymoma may improve the clinical state of myasthenia gravis. Presurgical localization and identification of the mass is of help to the surgeon and the features of invasiveness or noninvasiveness can be evaluated with MRI. Our reference article provides two additional examples of thymoma.

REFERENCE: Batra et al.: *AJR* **148**:515, March, 1987.

Courtesy of Dr. Dan Boon and Pasadena Magnetic Imaging.

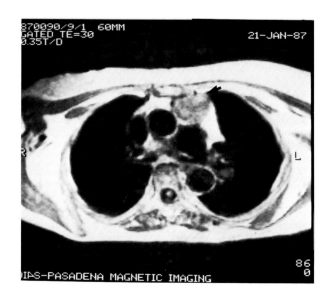

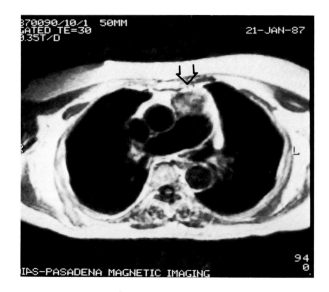

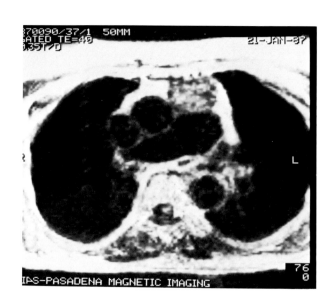

185: Right Upper Lobe Abscess (1.5T)

EXAM: MRI of the chest.

CLINICAL INFORMATION: This is a 46-year-old male with numerous intrathoracic operations and persistence of a right upper lobe mass.

TECHNIQUE: Gaited coronal and axial scans were obtained through the mediastinum (1091/25; 2180/35,70).

FINDINGS: A cavity or air fluid level is identified in the medial portion of the right upper lobe. There is some retraction of the hilar elements. There was no evidence of adenopathy or other areas of abnormality.

IMPRESSION: Right upper lobe abscess.

DISCUSSION: Percutaneous drain was placed via CT guidance, and a mixed flora was cultured including both gram-positive and gram-negative organisms. The cavity initially did well, with both drainage and localized injection of antibiotics into the drainage catheter.

As per our reference article, there is little in the way of signal characteristics to allow for a clear differential between infectious and neoplastic causes of parenchymal infiltrates and masses or cavities as seen here. There is, however, good morphologic delineation of the abscess cavity and the inflammatory fluid and contents. There is also good orientation of the normal mediastinal and hilar structures to the abscess. The ability to image the process in more than one plane allows for increased understanding of the exact location, volume, and extent of this proven inflammatory mass.

REFERENCE: Moore et al.: *AJR* **146**:1123, June, 1986.

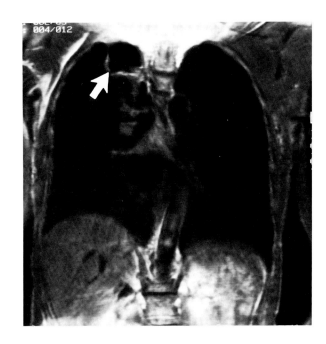

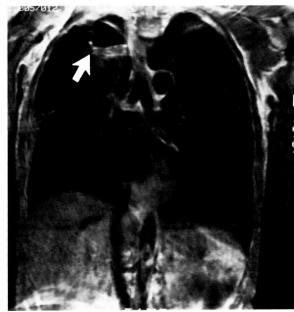

186: Adenobronchial Lesion with Distal Atelectasis Metastases—Right Hepatic Lobe (.6T)

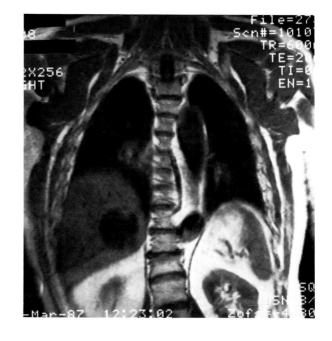

EXAM: MRI of the chest.

CLINICAL INFORMATION: A 75-year-old with mass identified on screening x-ray.

TECHNIQUE: Nongaited axial and coronal images were obtained (1500/30,60; 600/20).

FINDINGS: Soft tissue mass was identified radiating from the inferior posterior hilar region on the right side. This is associated with intermediate signal replacing the hilar structures immediately adjacent to this mass. This is of concern for a possible endobronchial lesion and adenopathy with some distal atelectasis and retained secretions. Note is made of an apparently metastatic lesion in the posterior right hepatic lobe.

IMPRESSION: Endobronchial lesion with adenopathy and distal atelectasis associated with metastatic deposit in the right hepatic lobe.

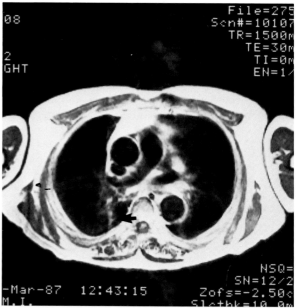

DISCUSSION: As in our reference article, we feel that the inherent contrast of lung and flowing blood offers good contrast to the adenopathy and parenchymal abnormality of our case. The parenchymal infiltrate or mass does show a slight increase in signal in the more peripheral lesions and, as suggested by the reference authors, probably represents accumulations of fluid within the obstructed portion of the tissue (arrow).

REFERENCE: Webb et al.: *Radiology* **156**:117, 1985.

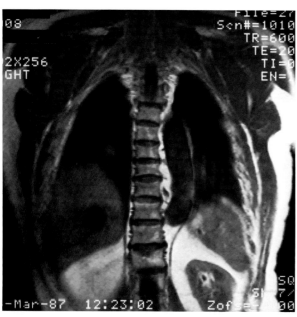

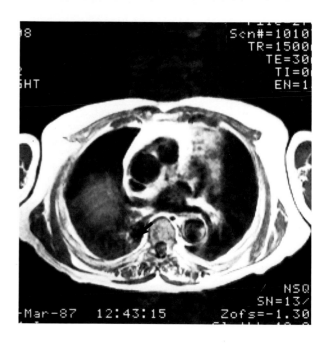

187: Superior Vena Cava Clot   (.6T)

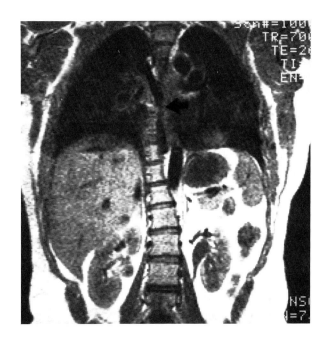

EXAM: MRI of the chest.

CLINICAL INFORMATION: A 25-year-old female with previously treated lymphoma. Rule out superior vena cava thrombus. Clinically, patient has superior vena cava syndrome.

TECHNIQUE: Coronal and axial T1-weighted views with gaiting were acquired (700/26).

FINDINGS: The coronal views show altered mediastinal fat intensity surrounding the superior vena cava with narrowing and total obstruction immediately above the right atrium. On the axial views, the lumen is identified, with an area of high signal within it representing clot. The mediastinal alteration of signal is also identified on axial and coronal views. This represents postradiation fibrosis from treatment for lymphoma.

IMPRESSION: Superior vena cava clot.

DISCUSSION: The precise location and degree of obstruction in the superior vena cava are well-demonstrated by MRI. In the reference article, the authors found the transaxial view to be the most useful. The coronal, as included here, also displays nicely the degree of stenosis and total obstruction. This can be related to the more conventional venogram orientations.

The SVC syndrome includes enlargement of the upper body veins, altered skin tone, and patient discomfort. This syndrome of vena cava obstruction is seen in postradiation patients treated for lung cancers and lymphomas.

REFERENCES: Weinreb et al.: *AJR* **146**:679, April, 1986.
Stanford et al.: *AJR* **148**:259, February, 1987.

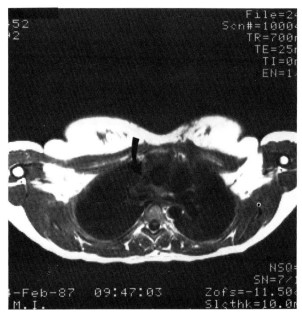

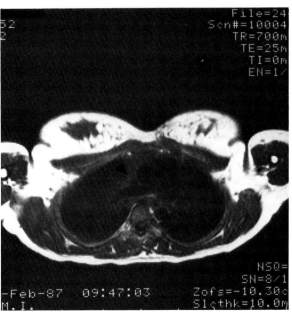

188: Hilar Mediastinal Adenopathy   (1.5T)

EXAM: MRI of the chest.

CLINICAL INFORMATION: A 43-year-old female with question of a right hilar mass on CT. Patient has a known nonpulmonary malignancy.

TECHNIQUE: Gaited scans were obtained in the axial and coronal planes (2143/30,60).

FINDINGS: Right hilar and mediastinal adenopathy are identified. These nodes are enlarged and show intermediate or low-signal intensity like that of normal mediastinal or hilar fat.

IMPRESSION: Right hilar and mediastinal adenopathy.

DISCUSSION: The side-by-side comparison of the contrast CT and MR in this case clearly shows the additional appreciation of adenopathy. Per our reference article, there is no characteristic signal from a metastatic-involved versus a benign node. Again, like CT, the most useful criteria is the enlargement of the nodes. There is, however, as demonstrated here, clear advantage to the MR, as opposed to CT alone, in differentiating between the vascular and air-containing structures for better delineation of adenopathy.

REFERENCE: Poon et al.: *Radiology* **162**:651, 1987.

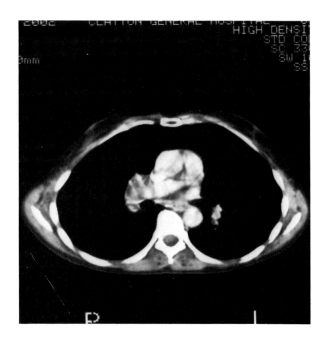

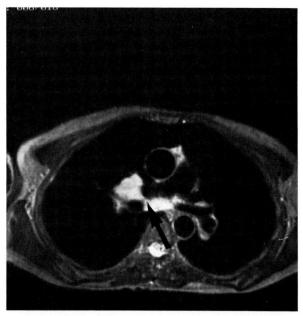

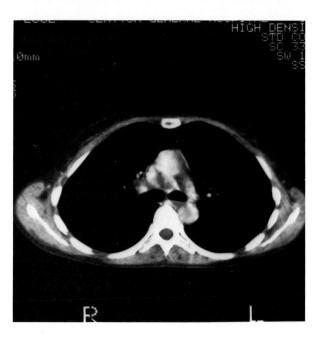

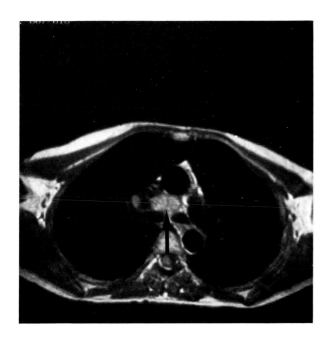

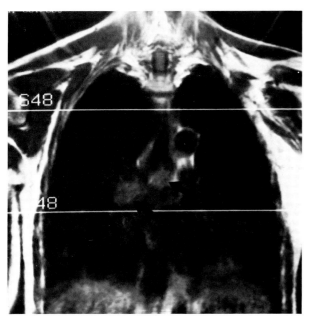

189: Apical Neoplasm (Pancoast's Tumor)   (.6T)

EXAM: MRI of the chest.

CLINICAL INFORMATION: 76-year-old with known Pancoast's tumor now being evaluated for spinal cord compression.

TECHNIQUE: Body coil coronal and axial images were used primarily to evaluate the cervical and thoracic spinal canal. There is, however, because of body coil imaging, significant information included about the lungs. The technique is predominantly T1-weighted (300/20).

FINDINGS: There is a large neoplastic mass occupying the left apical region, with extensive invasion through the pleural space, invasion into the vertebral body, as well as significant extension of tumor into the thoracic canal with total encirclement and compression of the cord at about the T3 level. This mass is isointense with that of muscle and has long irregular infiltrative edges. This also extends into the mediastinum and superior left hilar region (arrows).

IMPRESSION: The findings are most consistent with a large apical neoplasm such as a Pancoast's tumor.

REFERENCE: Musset et al.: *Radiology* **160**:607, 1986.

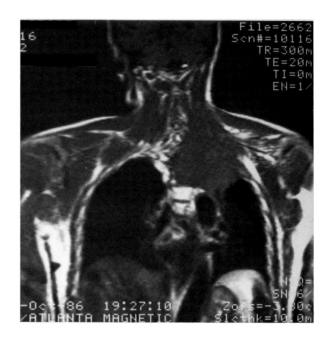

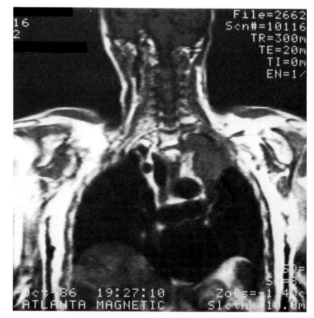

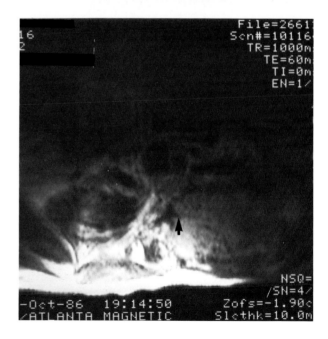

190: Ascites and Pleural Effusion (.6T)

EXAM: MRI of the chest.

CLINICAL INFORMATION: A 76-year-old being evaluated for posterior mediastinal tumor.

TECHNIQUE: Coronal and axial T1- or spin-density-weighted images were obtained with a body coil in coronal and axial planes (800/32).

FINDINGS: Large right and moderate-sized left pleural effusions are noted. There is also increased signal in the dependent portion of the lung, reflecting dependent edema and a small amount of atelectasis. This is identified as an intermediate signal that delineates the collapsed atelectatic lung (Image 3, large arrow). There is also ascitic fluid demonstrated nicely on the coronal views (long arrows). The hilar nodes are well-demarcated, as are the mediastinum paratracheal nodes (arrows). Incidental note is made of a hiatal hernia (small arrow).

IMPRESSION: Ascites, pleural effusions, and a large amount of atelectasis of the right lower lung. Cannot exclude infiltrate or even small mass. Multiple enlarged nodes in the hilar and mediastinal regions.

DISCUSSION: In our reference article, the authors studied 20 patients and felt that the detection of nodes was better accomplished with MR. They quickly added that the MR also had a higher false-positive rate. The false-positive nodes were all enlarged and did contain inflammatory, rather than neoplastic, change. The CT scan was felt to offer the optimal spatial resolution; however, the negatives include the need for intravenous contrast and radiation exposure. MR with an intrinsic contrast resolution detected more easily the nodes surrounded by the high-signal fat in the hilar mediastinal regiona. Nodes in the more peripheral hila were also easily evaluated with MR because of the presence of low signal in blood flowing through vessels.

It is felt by these authors that MR does not clearly visualize the smaller nodules within the parenchyma (3–5 mm). However, at 1.5 mm, both MR and CT were insufficient for visualization of nodules.

REFERENCE: Heelan et al.: *Radiology* **156**:111, 1985.

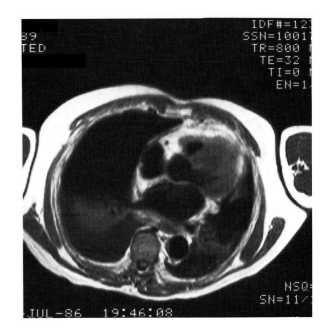

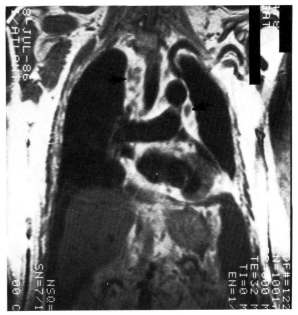

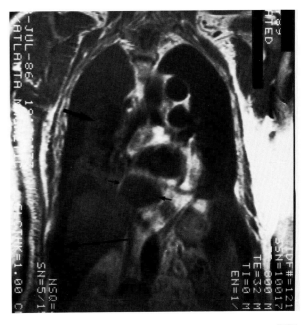

191: Adenopathy (Sarcoidosis) (1.5T)

EXAM: MRI of the chest.

CLINICAL INFORMATION: Patient with abnormal chest x-ray and known sarcoidosis.

TECHNIQUE: Body coil T1-weighted images were acquired with cardiac gaiting.

FINDINGS: Large bilateral hilar mediastinal nodes are noted. These encircle the pulmonary artery, trachea, and bronchi (arrows). Patient refused any further imaging, and there is a profound wraparound artifact from selection of a small on the coronal acquisition.

IMPRESSION: Large mediastinal hilar nodes. With history of known sarcoidosis, findings are certainly consistent with sarcoid.

DISCUSSION: The delineation of adenopathy is well-demonstrated. The T1 and T2 characteristics by investigators in the pulmonary area have found much overlap between benign and pathologic states, and MR at this time is not felt to represent an absolute modality for exclusion of malignant change. The symmetry of the clinical presentation and bilateral nature of the findings here certainly help with the confirmed diagnosis of sarcoidosis.

REFERENCES: Johnson et al.: *Canadian Medical Association Journal* **132**:765, 1985. de Gee et al.: *European Journal of Radiology* **6**:145, 1986.

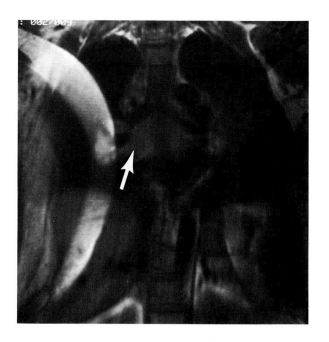
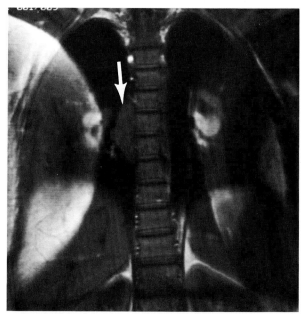
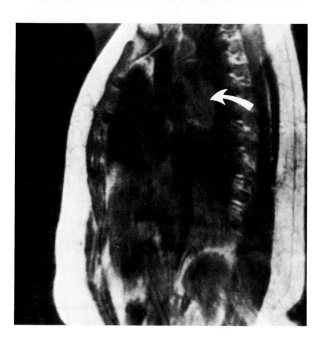

192: Metastases (Changes of Tuberculosis) (.6T)

EXAM: MRI of the chest.

CLINICAL INFORMATION: A 50-year-old male, status postradicle neck dissection on right. Now with abnormal chest x-ray.

TECHNIQUE: Coronal and axial images were acquired with spin density or T1-weighted parameters (700/32).

FINDINGS: There are numerous areas of intermittent signal, seen predominantly in the upper portion of the lung fields. No significant hilar or mediastinal adenopathy is identified. There is, in the apical regions, bilaterally significant scarring consistent with history of prior tuberculosis. The pulmonary nodules are most consistent, in light of the history, with metastatic deposits.

IMPRESSION: (1) Evidence for old tuberculosis in the apices and (2) multiple parenchymal nodules, probably metastatic.

DISCUSSION: CT remains the imaging modality of choice when the clinical concern is for detection of pulmonary nodules. MR can, however, be successful in imaging even smaller nodules. Our reference article has compared CT and MR and found that nodules less than 1.5 mm in diameter were missed by both. The CT scanning, because of the short imaging time used (3–4 s), certainly offers better spacial resolution and higher detection of nodules. MR may be of value in augmenting the study by demonstrating nodules which are adjacent to vascular structures and may be missed by CT exam.

REFERENCE: Müller et al.: *Radiology* 155:687, 1985.

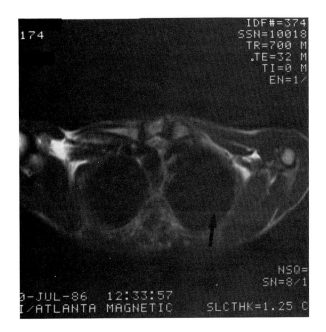

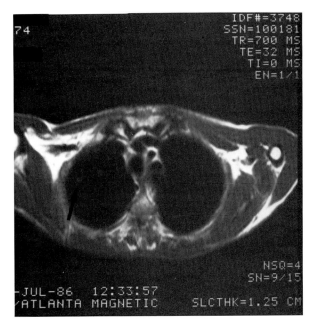

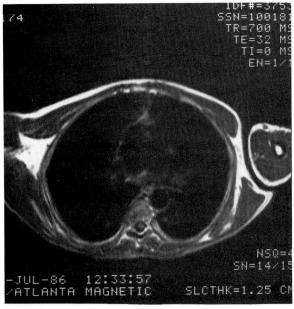

193: Apical Scarring   (.6T)

EXAM: MRI of the chest.

CLINICAL INFORMATION: Patient with known tuberculosis.

TECHNIQUE: Spin echo axial and coronal cuts were obtained (700/32).

FINDINGS: There is diffuse scarring and intermediate signal seen in both apices. There is slightly more intermediate signal or soft tissue mass in the left apical region. This is primarily based within the parenchymal, but also abuts the pleural surface. This finding is nonspecific. In light of history of prior tuberculosis, this is most consistent with a large amount of scar tissue or cicatrization of the parenchymal apical tissue. A scar carcinoma cannot be excluded, particularly in reference to the most superior axial cut.

IMPRESSION: (1) Changes in the apical region most consistent with tuberculosis. However, the scarring and proliferation of inflammatory soft tissue make exclusion of a scar carcinoma arising from this area impossible.

DISCUSSION: MR, like CT, is quite nonspecific in histology of most parenchymal changes within the lung. The diagnosis again rests on location, morphology, and clinical history. Of interest, however, is the utility of the coronal and axial images in giving a better overall appreciation of the amount of soft tissue change seen in the apex. This may be of further value in the future in establishing a baseline in patients with chronic inflammatory change to exclude any subtle change in the amount of soft tissue and better assess early detection of possible carcinomatous change.

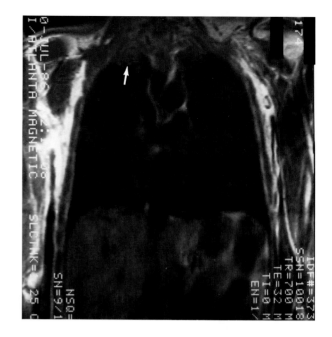

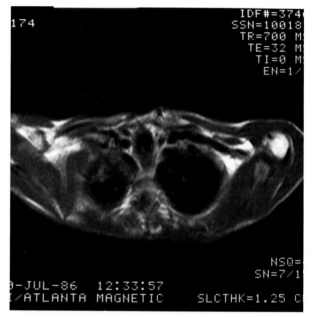

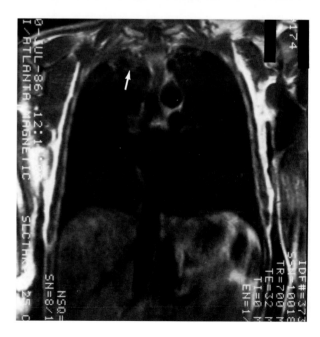

194: Recurrent Adenocarcinoma (.6T)

EXAM: MRI of the lungs.

CLINICAL INFORMATION: A 64-year-old male, with lobectomy approximately 13 months earlier. CT scan shows a definite area of abnormality near the hilum. Unable to differentiate between scar and tumor.

TECHNIQUE: Coronal and axial T1- and T2-weighted images were acquired (2200/45, 850/32).

FINDINGS: There is an ill-defined right lower lobe mass which has an infiltrative characteristic involving the hilar structures and extending out into the periphery of the right lower lobe. The longer T2-weighted images show an increase in signal in this area of abnormality, suggesting the presence of soft tissue as well as possible accumulation of secretions and fluids. Simple pulmonary scarring should remain fairly low signal intensity throughout the different T1- and T2-weighted images.

IMPRESSION: Gaited MR exam suggests that this is most consistent with recurrent lung cancer, rather than simple scarring in the area of prior resection.

DISCUSSION: As demonstrated above, the signal characteristics of certain areas which may be confused on plain film and CT can be reevaluated with the gaited MR technique. The good definition of involvement into the hilar region and the inherent contrast provided by the air and moving blood separate the tumor from the normal hilar structures.

CONFIRMATION: Recurrent tumor was removed at surgery.

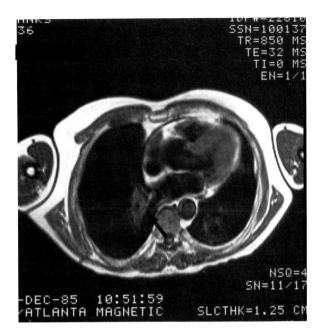

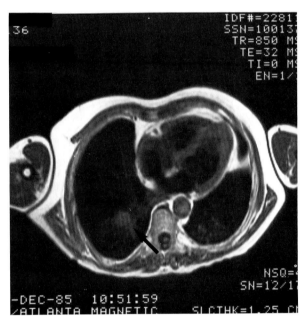

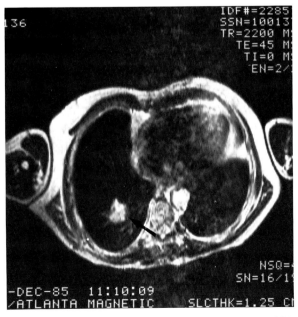

195: Mediastinal Adenopathy
(Small Cell CA)   (.35T)

EXAM: MRI of the chest.

CLINICAL INFORMATION: A 50-year-old male with biopsy-proven small cell carcinoma.

TECHNIQUE: Nongaited coronal images through the chest were obtained for evaluation of hilar mediastinal adenopathy (500/30).

FINDINGS: Large conglomerate of hilar and mediastinal adenopathy is identified. All represent secondary metastatic disease from a small cell carcinoma as proven by needle biopsy.

IMPRESSION: Large hilar mediastinal nodes from small cell cancer.

REFERENCE: Ross et al.: *Radiology* **160**:839, 1986.

Case courtesy of Dr. Walter Bednartz, Williamsport Magnetic Imaging.

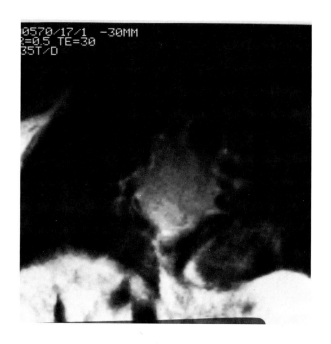

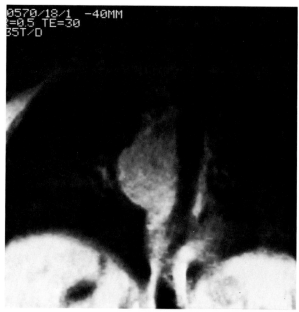

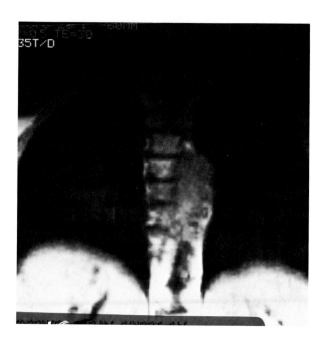

196: Adenobronchial Lesion with Distal Atelectasis   (.35T)

EXAM: MRI of the chest.

CLINICAL INFORMATION: Follow-up study of known metastases in the left chest from primary elsewhere.

TECHNIQUE: Gaited technique was employed with a TE of 40. Five-millimeter slices were obtained through the entire thoracic cavity.

FINDINGS: An indistinct 2-cm area of increased signal on the study is noted in the left upper lung. This just touches the more distal aspects of the hilar structures from the left side. No associated mediastinal adenopathy is seen.

IMPRESSION: Parenchymal lesion consistent with an endobronchial lesion and distal obstructive atelectasis or retained secretions versus a totally metastatic lung tumor.

DISCUSSION: CT remains the preferred investigative tool for small parenchymal nodules secondary to lack of good resolution of the lung tissue because of minimal amount of signal with MRI. The MR does, however, offer an excellent second investigation of the hilum and mediastinum and has been shown by various authors to detect more adenopathy than does CT.

REFERENCE: Weinstein et al.: *Diagnostic Imaging*: 58, August, 1984.
Case courtesy of R. S. Aurora, Pasadena Magnetic Imaging.

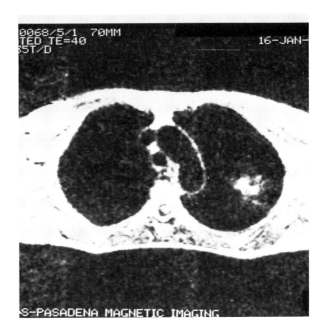

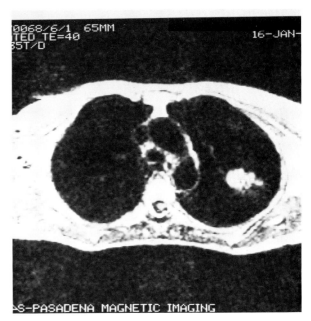

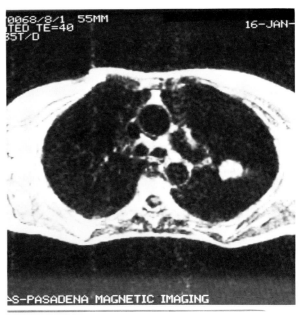

197: Apical Mediastinal Mass (.6T)

EXAM: MRI of the chest.

TECHNIQUE: Axial, coronal, and sagittal images were acquired with T1- and T2-weighted images (500/34, 1400/40-80).

FINDINGS: There is a large intermediate signal mass occupying the medial right apical region. This is within the lung parenchyma and abuts but does not invade or cross the pleural space. Location and appearance are most consistent with that of a primary lung carcinoma. Location in the apex raises the possibility that this is a Pancoast tumor.

IMPRESSION: A right apical mediastinal mass most consistent with that of a primary lung carcinoma that sits in posterior mediastinum and may involve T1-T3 roots as they exit the neuroforaminal canal.

REFERENCE: Webb et al.: *Radiology* **153**:729, 1984.

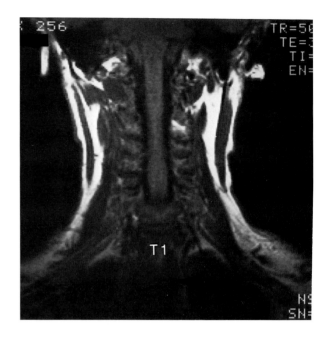

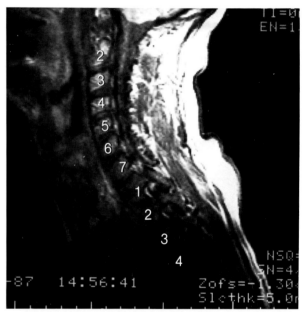

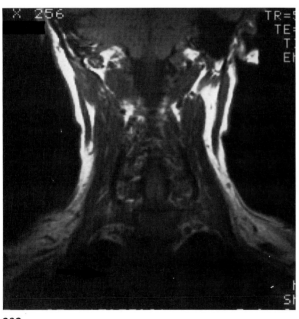

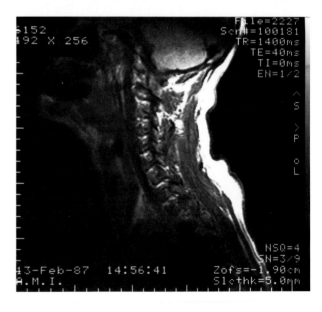

198: Right Upper Lobe Malignancy (.6T)

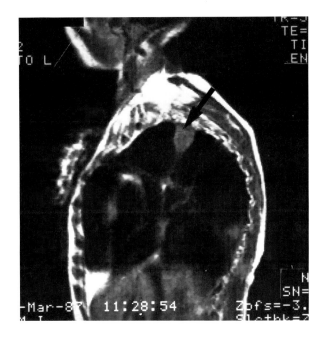

EXAM: MRI of the chest.

CLINICAL INFORMATION: Rule out metastatic disease in 58-year-old female with low back pain presenting with a known upper lobe density and proven malignancy from pericutaneous needle biopsy.

TECHNIQUE: Body coil images were employed to include as large a portion of the vertebral column as possible in the sagittal orientation. T1-weighted images were used (500/26).

FINDINGS: There is metastatic involvement of the T5 and T6 bodies. These do not appear to intrude into or obstruct the canal (arrows). The cord appears to pass by this area without obstruction.

On the sagittal, more lateral, views, there is incidental note made of a triangular area of intermediate signal which contrasts sharply to the very low signal of the normal lung. The triangular appearance suggests that this is probably a distal collapse of lung secondary to endobronchial lesion (arrow).

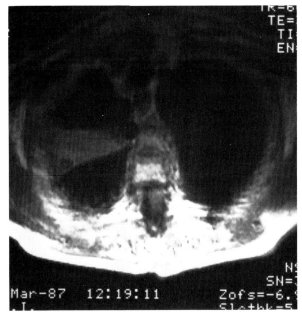

IMPRESSION: Metastatic vertebral body disease without evidence for canal compression, and demonstration of a right apical mass which has the appearance of an endobronchial lesion with distal infiltrate in a subsegmental distribution.

This demonstrates nicely the advantage of MR in being able, in one imaging sequence, to both evaluate the neurologic anatomy and elegantly demonstrate the primary cause of the metastatic deposits on the sagittal in an incidental fashion as demonstrated above (arrows).

REFERENCE: Mayr et al.: *JCAT* **11**:43, January/February, 1987.

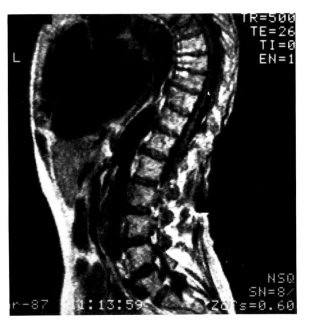

199: Normal Inferior Vena Cava (1.5T)

EXAM: MRI of the abdomen.

CLINICAL INFORMATION: Rule out clot within the inferior vena cava of 84-year-old male being evaluated for deep vein thrombus and possible pulmonary embolus.

TECHNIQUE: Coronal body coil images were obtained (1500/25,50).

FINDINGS: The inferior cava and iliac veins are well-demonstrated on the cuts. The renal veins are easily identified. The low signal seen in the lumen is good evidence against the presence of any clot. The renal veins are also well-demonstrated. Note also incidental demonstration of the hepatic venous structures (arrowhead).

DISCUSSION: The coronals nicely depict the inferior vena cava, as well as the renal, veins. In cases where deep vein thrombus has been demonstrated, this can allow for identification of clot within the inferior vena cava. The renal veins can also be identified, and they assist the vascular surgeon in placement.

REFERENCE: *Radiology* **156**:415, 1985.

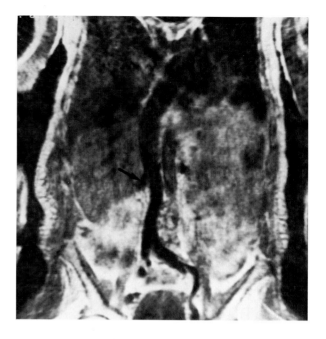

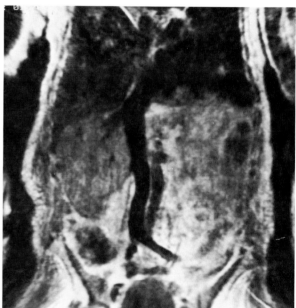

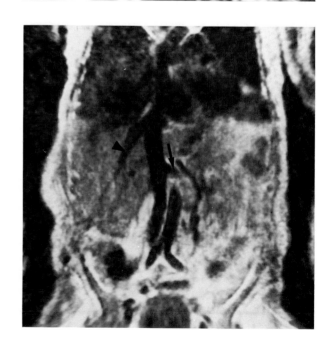

200: Extensive Clot with Inferior Vena Cava   (1.5T)

EXAM: MRI of the abdomen.

CLINICAL INFORMATION: This is a 59-year-old male with severe DVT and prior pulmonary emboli. Question patent IVC.

TECHNIQUE: Coronal and axial T1- and T2-weighted images were acquired through the abdomen with special attention to the abdomen and the inferior vena cava. (2200/5/25,50; 1000/25).

FINDINGS: High-signal intensity is seen in two separate areas of the mid- and lower IVC. This correlates with the placement of two Greenfield filters. The lack of visualization of the lumen within the IVC is consistent with thrombus throughout it. High-signal focus is seen in the lumen of the IVC. This may represent clot; however, it is difficult to differentiate from the presence of metallic filter apparatus (arrow, Image 3).

IMPRESSION: Extensive clot involving the entire inferior vena cava. Two areas of metal-type artifacts are consistent with placement of two filters.

DISCUSSION: The well-demonstrated presence of blood flow through the IVC has immediate application. The increase in signal with clotted blood is easily demonstrated on both the axial and coronal images as evidenced by our case and demonstrated in the reference article.

REFERENCE: Hricak et al.: *Radiology* **156**:415, 1985.

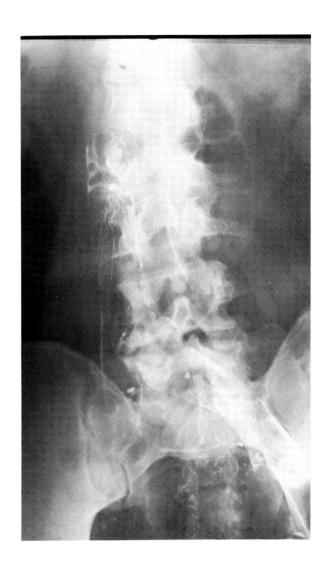

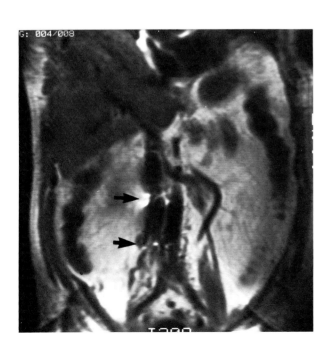

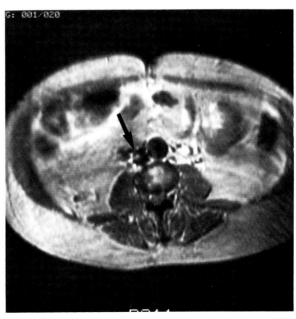

201: Fatty Normal Pancreas (1.5T)

EXAM: MRI of the abdomen.

CLINICAL INFORMATION: Rule out Pancreatic Neoplasm.

TECHNIQUE: Body coil axial images were obtained through the upper abdomen (2000/25/50).

FINDINGS: No pathology is detected. However, this allows us to show the excellent demonstration of the pancreatic tissue of this somewhat fatty replaced pancreas.

IMPRESSION: Normal fatty replaced pancreas.

DISCUSSION: The investigating authors indicated in this early article that MR can be successful in detecting pancreatic pathology. We suspect that as further opportunity for the incidental observation of the pancreas with MR presents itself, more and more pathologic states will be demonstrated. Perhaps the unique abilities of this procedure will present incidences in which it would be preferable to image with MR rather than with CT or ultrasound.

Arrows demonstrate the somewhat fatty replaced pancreatic tissue. Note that the caudate lobe circles posterior to the superior mesenteric vein (arrow). Note also, on Images 2 and 3, the body and tail as they sit upon the splenic vein and course over the celiac artery.

REFERENCE: Smith et al.: *Radiology* 142:677, March, 1982.

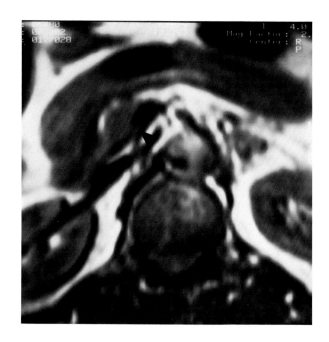

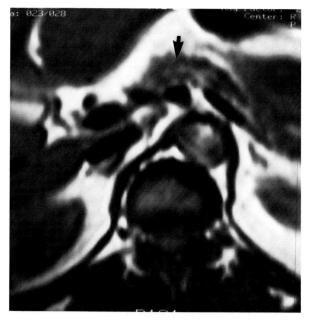

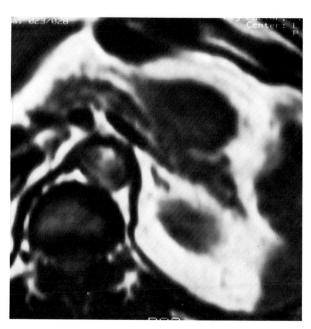

202: Hepatoma   (1.5T)

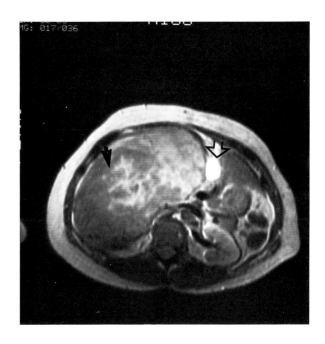

EXAM: MRI of the abdomen.

CLINICAL INFORMATION: A 56-year-old female with recent weight loss and enlarged liver. Rule out tumor.

TECHNIQUE: Axial and coronal T1- and T2-weighted images were acquired with body coil images (2000/40,80).

FINDINGS: There is diffuse enlargement and irregularity of signal seen throughout the right hepatic lobe. The T1-weighted images show lowered signal intensity through the area of abnormality when compared with the remaining normal tissue of the left hepatic lobe. (arrow, Image 1 with T2-weighting). The signal differences are further dramatically illustrated with the central portion of the tumor showing an increase in signal intensity. These correlate well with abnormality detected on CT scan through the same area (Image 3). No displacement of the normal gallbladder (open arrow).

IMPRESSION: Large amount of tumor. Differential is hepatoma and large metastatic disease.

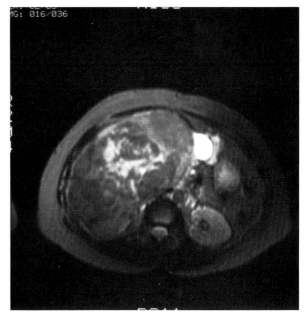

DISCUSSION: Despite the excellent delineation of the tumor on this sequence we have followed the tendency, as did our reference authors, to favor shorter TR's in 300-ms range. This allows for improved resolution and suppresses the motion artifact from respiration.

CONFIRMATION: Open biopsy confirmed hepatocellular carcinoma.

REFERENCE: Stark et al.: *Radiology* **159**:365, 1986.

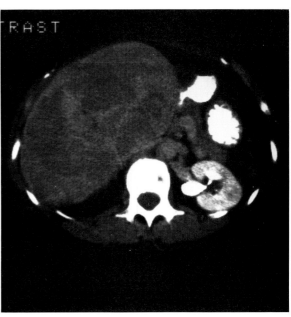

203: Cavernous Hemangioma   (1.5T)

EXAM: MRI of the abdomen.

CLINICAL INFORMATION: Well-circumscribed 6-cm mass was identified on CT scan in 47-year-old female with question of pancreatic carcinoma. Concern for metastatic involvement of the liver was raised.

TECHNIQUE: Body coil axial and coronal T1- and T2-weighted images were obtained (2000/40/80).

FINDINGS: A focal well-circumscribed area of isosignal intensity on the T1-weighted images was observed to show dramatic increase in signal on the more T2-weighted images. Findings are most consistent with a benign cavernous hemangioma, although, by MR criteria alone, a large hepatic cyst cannot be totally excluded.

IMPRESSION: Most likely a benign cavernous hemangioma, although large hepatic cyst cannot be totally excluded.

DISCUSSION: Detection of abnormality within the liver parenchyma is good on MR and CT. The added advantage of specificity particularly when a questionably focal metastatic mass is raised is well-demonstrated here. Although there are exceptions to the rule, hemangiomas seem to have pathopneumonic high-signal signature on the more T2-weighted images.

REFERENCE: Moss et al.: *Radiology* **150**:141, 1984.

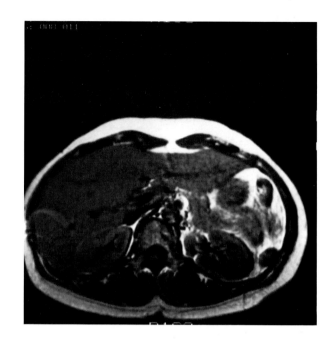

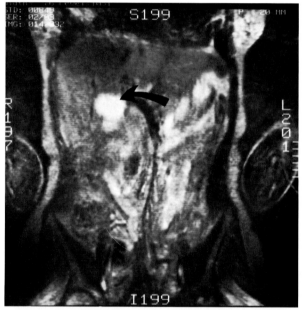

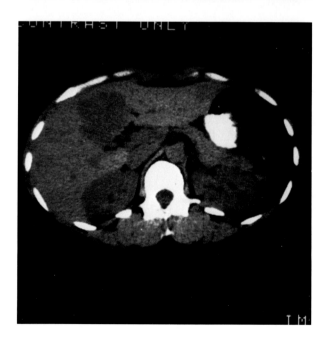

204: Simple Renal Cyst (.6T)

EXAM: MRI of the abdomen.

CLINICAL INFORMATION: An 82-year-old female, with skin cancer recently removed. Cyst demonstrated on ultrasound in kidneys. Rule out possible cystic neoplasm.

TECHNIQUE: Axial and coronal body scans were obtained with T1- and T2-weighted images (3000/32,64).

FINDINGS: The superior pole of the left kidney shows a cystic formation. The signal intensity is low on the more spin-density-weighted image and increases on the T2-weighted image. The relaxation characteristics are most consistent with a fluid-filled structure such as a simple renal cyst. There is no evidence for any asymmetric wall thickening. In addition, the venous structures are well-demonstrated, as is the IVC, and there is no evidence of a high-signal focus within the lumen to suggest thrombus. The remainder of the retroperitoneum shows no evidence of adenopathy.

IMPRESSION: Simple renal cyst.

DISCUSSION: MR shows a similar, if not higher, rate of detection of renal cell CA when compared to CT. Our reference article points out several distinct advantages, including the demonstration of vascular patency, detection of perihilar lymph nodes, and evaluation of any direct tumor extension into adjacent organs in the upper abdomen. We believe, as do the authors of this article, that MR will become an important modality in staging of renal cell CA.

CONFIRMATION: Ultrasound demonstrated renal cyst.

REFERENCE: Hricak et al.: *Radiology* 154:709, 1985.

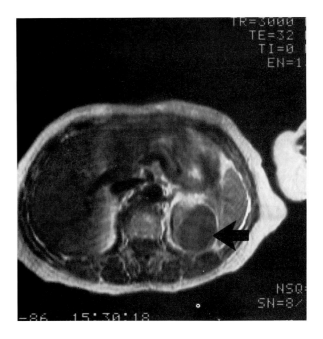

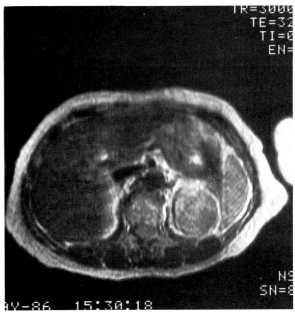

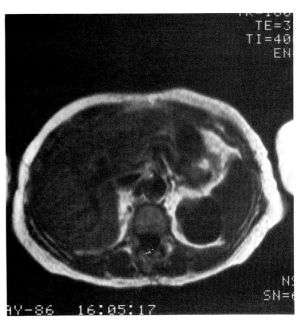

205: Gallstones (.6T)

EXAM: MRI of the abdomen.

CLINICAL INFORMATION: Unrelated to findings.

TECHNIQUE: Axial T1- and T2-weighted images were acquired with the body coil (3000/60,120).

FINDINGS: Circular low-signal intensity objects are identified in the fundus of the gallbladder. They show no increase with the more T2-weighted images. The findings are most consistent with gallstones.

IMPRESSION: Gallstones.

DISCUSSION: In severe inflammatory diseases of the gallbladder, the bile shows an altered or increased water content and remains of low-signal intensity despite the change in the T1- and T2-weighted images. With incidental observation of gallstones and appropriate clinical findings, diagnosis of cholecystitis may also be rendered.

REFERENCE: McCarthy et al.: *Radiology* **158**:333, 1986.

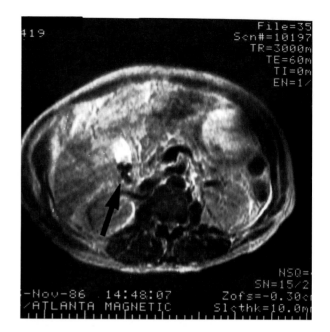

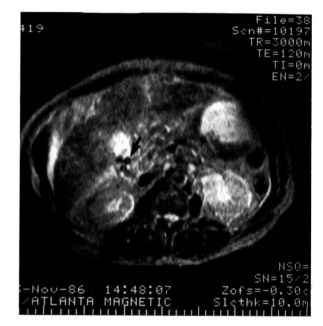

206: Metastatic Disease   (.6T)

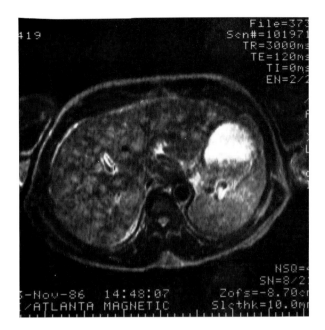

EXAM: MRI of the abdomen.

CLINICAL INFORMATION: RUQ mass in a 65-year-old.

TECHNIQUE: Coronal and body coil images were obtained with T1- and T2-weighting (3000/30/120).

FINDINGS: There are numerous areas of increased signal intensity diffusely involving the liver. The signal intensity is somewhat suppressed on the more T2-weighted images (see Image 1). Comparison with the CT scan obtained at the same time shows diffuse involvement on the latter. However, the liver is totally studded with multiple areas of abnormality.

IMPRESSION: Extensive abnormal signal involving the entire liver parenchyma is consistent with metastatic disease.

DISCUSSION: In general, our review articles indicate an increase in signal with the metastatic lesions to the liver. There is some overlap with the hemangiomas, but the benign hemangiomatous lesion normally shows a much more significant increase in signal intensity, whereas our metastases show somewhat of a less dramatic increase of signal with the T2-weighted images. The shorter TR's of 300 and the TE of 20 have been shown in recent articles to offer both a shortened scanning sequence and an increase in sensitivity to detection of liver metastases.

REFERENCE: Reinig et al.: *Radiology* **162**:43, 1987.

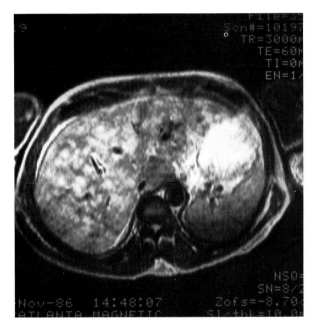

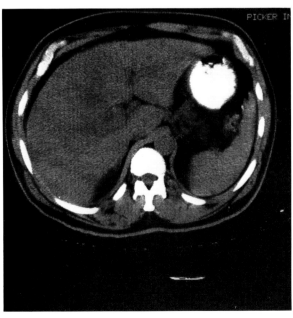

207: Benign Prostatic Hypertrophy (.6T)

EXAM: MRI of the pelvis.

CLINICAL INFORMATION: A 67-year-old male with urinary outlet syndrome.

TECHNIQUE: Coronal, sagittal, and axial T1- and T2-weighted images were obtained using the body coil (2000/30/60, 500/30).

FINDINGS: The prostatic gland is symmetric and enlarged. No altered signal or eccentric nodules are identified. The capsule is intact (Image 1, arrows). The levator ani shows no significant displacement (Image 2, arrows). No evidence of pelvic adenopathy or mass is revealed.

IMPRESSION: Benign prostatic hypertrophy.

DISCUSSION: In our review article, the inherent contrast sensitivity and multiplaner imaging is felt to be a distinct advantage over CT in stating pathologies because of the fat and high-signal intensity of the fascia surrounding the prostate, carcinomatous extension from the prostatic capsule and lymphadenopathy are well-demonstrated on MR.

REFERENCE: Lee & Rholl: *AJR* **147**:732, October, 1986.

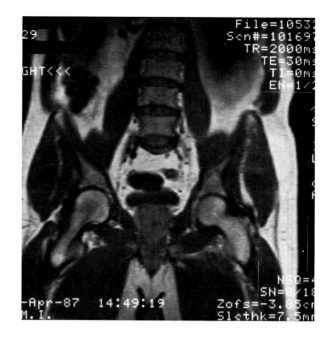

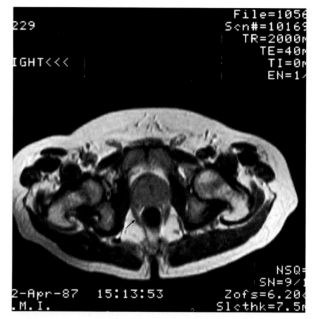

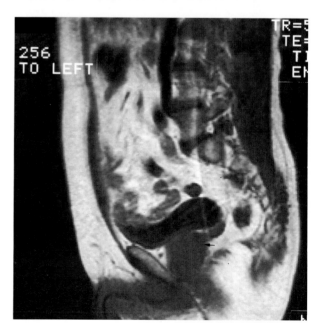

208: Retroperitoneal Adenopathy   (.35T)

EXAM: MRI of the retroperitoneum.

TECHNIQUE: Axial and coronal images were obtained with T1-weighting (500/30).

FINDINGS: Large metastatic nodes are seen surrounding the aorta and displacing superiorly the venous and arterial structures. The absence of signal within the vessel suggests the absence of any tumor thrombus. The appearance of numerous enlarged nodes is consistent with metastatic adenopathy, although the differential between lymphoma is not possible.

IMPRESSION: Marked retroperitoneal adenopathy.

DISCUSSION: MR, like CT, identifies abnormal nodes on the basis of their enlarged size and morphologic characteristics rather than by any distinctive signal differentiating benign and metastatic lymph node tissue. Our reference article states that both MR and CT are equal in their detection of lymphadenopathy. We suspect, with the ability to do coronal and sagittal views the actual sensitivity of MR should eventually exceed that of the CT scanning. The well-defined vascular structures and demonstration of patent lumens, particularly with renal neoplasms, should be of more marked value.

REFERENCE: Lee et al.: *Radiology* **153**:181, 1984.
Courtesy of Dr. Bednartz, Williamsport Imaging.

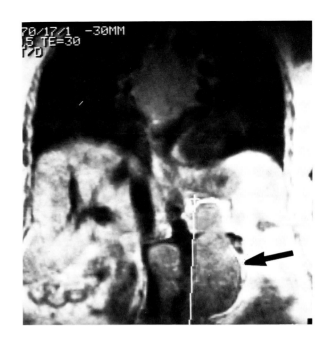

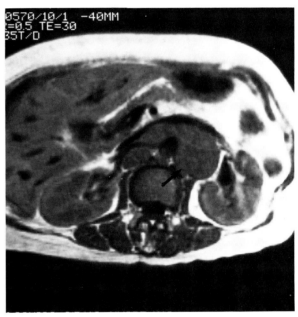

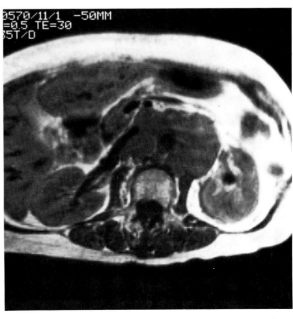

209: Metastases (Melanoma)   (.6T)

EXAM: MRI of the abdomen.

CLINICAL INFORMATION: Female patient with known metastatic melanoma.

TECHNIQUE: Sagittal and axial double-echo spin echo technique used (3000/30,60).

FINDINGS: Immediately deep to the right of the rectus muscle is a large intermediate signal intensity mass which is fixed to the muscle and consistent with a metastatic deposit. Note also is made of increased signal intensity and vertebral body destruction in an apparently metastatic lesion involving the T9 vertebral body.

IMPRESSION: Abdominal metastatic deposit and T9 vertebral body metastases presumably all related to known diagnosis of melanoma.

DISCUSSION: The sagittal and axial views offer a uniquely informative exam of the anterior wall, particularly for investigation of hernias and metastatic deposits.

REFERENCE: Glazer et al.: *Radiology* **155**:417, 1985.

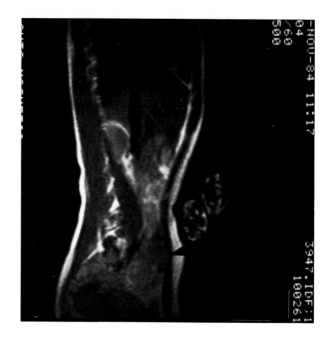

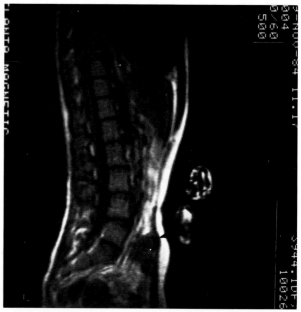

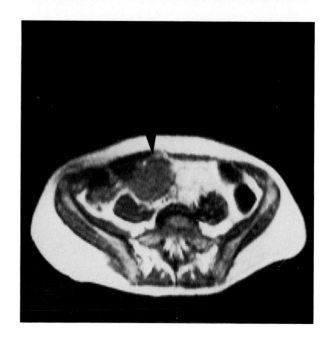

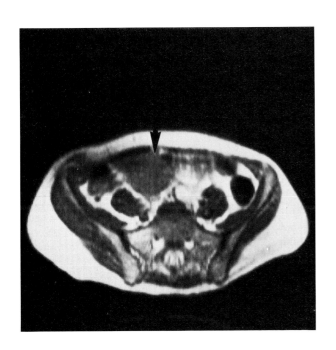

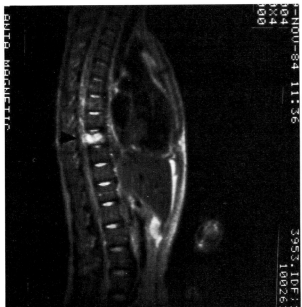

210: Hemangioma (.6T)

EXAM: MRI of the liver.

CLINICAL INFORMATION: A 26-year-old female, with incidental mass detected on ultrasound.

TECHNIQUE: Axial and coronal T1- and T2-weighted images were acquired with respiratory gaiting (2000/25/80).

FINDINGS: On a separate T1 sequence, acquired but not shown, there is little or no evidence of any mass other than an ill-defined area of low-signal intensity. With the spin echo sequence, there is now profound enhancement of a circular area within the right hepatic lobe (arrows). This correlates exactly with an area of marked echogenecity on the ultrasound and with an area of ring enhancement on the dynamic bolus scan through this region. The feature of very bright enhancement on MR is considered a fairly characteristic sign of hemangioma. The only differential would be the exclusion of hepatic cysts with this signal behavior.

IMPRESSION: Hemangioma of the liver.

REFERENCE: Glazer et al.: *Radiology* **155**:417, 1985.

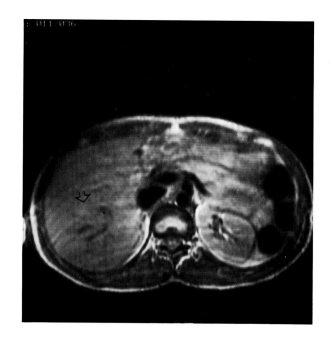

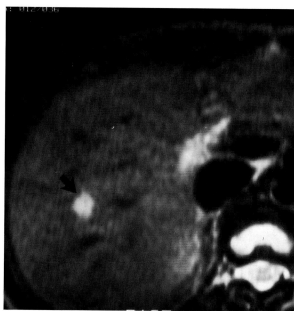

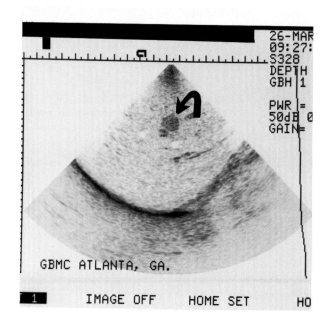

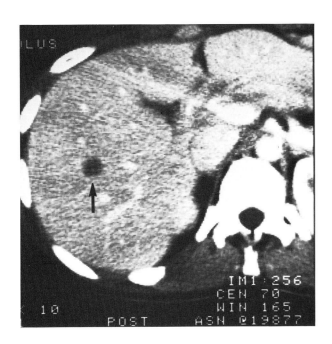

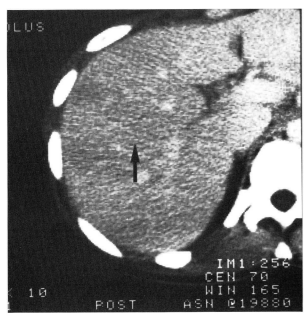

211: Metastases (.6T)

EXAM: MRI of the abdomen.

CLINICAL INFORMATION: A 75-year-old with mass revealed on routine chest x-ray. MR done to evaluate right lower lobe mass.

TECHNIQUE: Gaited coronal and axial scans were obtained through the chest. This included a greater portion of the liver.

FINDINGS: Fairly well-circumscribed lesion is identified in the posterior hepatic lobe. With T2-weighting, this increases in signal but to a lesser extent than that seen with hemangioma. A similar small lesion is identified in the left hepatic lobe.

IMPRESSION: Hepatic metastases.

DISCUSSION: The signal behavior of hepatic metastases can change slightly with the various TR and TE combinations employed. However, the lesions are usually detected when using the spin echo or double-echo technique. Although the authors of our reference article do not advocate MR at present as the modality of choice, more recent articles have indicated that MR is the more sensitive modality, particularly when employing a short TR, TE sequence.

REFERENCES: Heiken et al.: *Radiology* **156**:423, 1985. Stark et al.: *AJR* **145**:213, 1985.

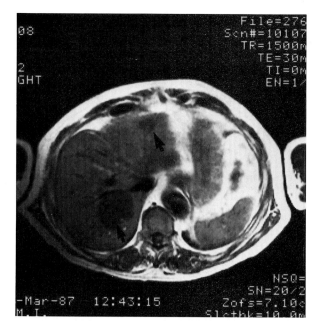

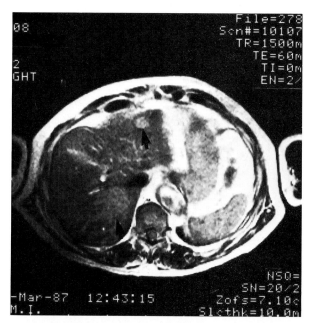

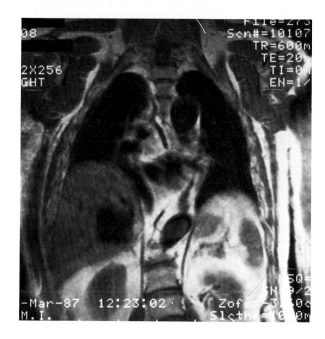

212: Reidel's Lobe   (.6T)

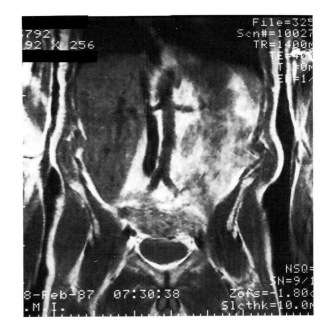

EXAM: MRI of the abdomen.

CLINICAL INFORMATION: Patient with prior colectomy for carcinoma of colon. Rising CEA. Question of metastases.

FINDINGS: The elongated liver is a normal anatomic variant. The axial films not shown demonstrated only one small peripheral lesion which was compatible with metastatic disease.

IMPRESSION: Small focus of metastatic disease is not shown on this example. Incidental note is made of Reidel's lobe and nice demonstration of the retroperitoneal vascular structures with particular reference to the renal arteries and inferior vena cava.

DISCUSSION: The detection of an incidental anatomic variant is fun, but usually of no clinical significance. Of more important note on this particular sequence is the nice demonstration in the coronal plane of both the aorta and inferior vena cava. With preoperative planning for aneurysm repair, the location and appearance of renal arteries are of key importance to the vascular surgeons, and, in other studies, we will demonstrate the utility of MR in evaluating the aneurysm of the abdominal aorta and its relation to renal arteries. Also of note is the delineation here of the inferior vena cava.

213: Ascites, Renal Atrophy (.6T)

EXAM: MRI of the thoracic spine.

CLINICAL INFORMATION: This is a 67-year-old male with no history of prior trauma with severe back pain into the right shoulder. Transported from local I.C.U. with nurse and monitoring devices.

FINDINGS: The thoracic spine portion of the study was unremarkable for metastases or disc disease. There is, however, incidental note made of free interperitoneal fluid consistent with patient's recent dialysis treatment (arrow). Also note generally atrophic appearance of the kidney (arrow). Note made of superior mesenteric arteries, originating from the celiac trunk.

IMPRESSION: Thoracic spine, negative for degenerative changes or metastases. Incidentals noted above.

DISCUSSION: Early in our experience, the body coil images were very useful for defining the abdominal anatomy, and, on more than one occasion, the chance for intraabdominal pathology imaging has presented itself. In this case, the patient with renal failure demonstrates the MRI's capacity to be a multiorgan imager. The very thin wasted kidney and the dialysis fluid were not relevant to this case but show the ability of MR to demonstrate both types of pathology.

REFERENCE: Stark et al.: *AJR* **145**:213, 1985.

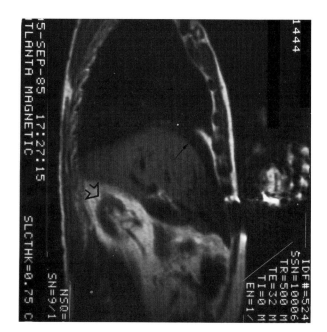

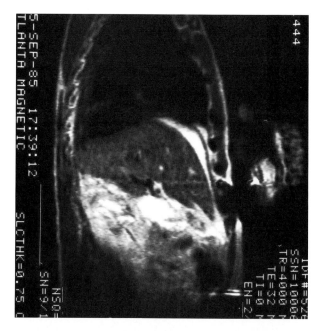

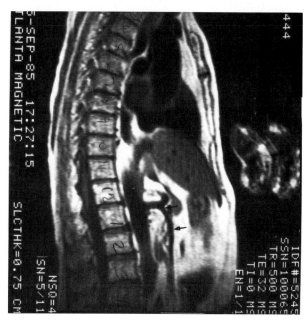

214: Abdominal Aneurysm   (1.5T)

EXAM: MRI of the abdomen.

CLINICAL INFORMATION: A 71-year-old male with palpable mass. Evaluate for abdominal aneurysm.

TECHNIQUE: Sagittal and coronal body coil images were obtained with a spin-density-weighted image (800/25).

FINDINGS: There is a large 5.6 × 5.7 cm aneurysmal enlargement of the aorta. The coronal images demonstrate relatively normal renal arteries which originate above the aneursym (arrows). There is also poor visualization of any central patent lumen in the midportion of the aorta. There is a tapered aspect and inferior portion of the lumen in the aneurysm's upper or more superior extent (arrow). There is, however, low signal seen in the iliac, suggesting that some antegrade flow does exist.

IMPRESSION: Abdominal aneurysm as described.

DISCUSSION: Coronal view nicely demonstrates the ability to visualize the renal arteries. There is difficulty in observing much in the way of a patent lumen through the midportion of the aneurysm. The relation to the renal arteries and the presence or absence of lumen in reference to intraluminal clot and the overall size of the aneurysm are all nicely displayed. In addition, the inferior vena cava is well-displayed, and the detection of clot is obvious.

REFERENCE: Amparo et al.: *Radiology* **154**:451, 1985.

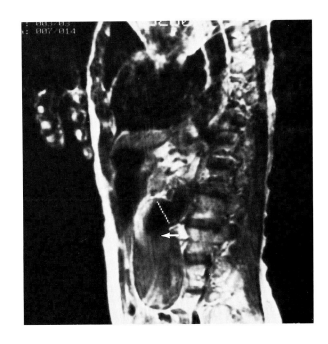

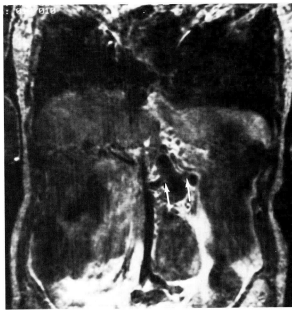

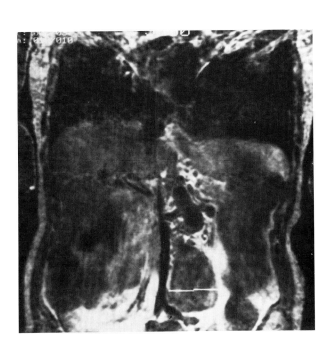

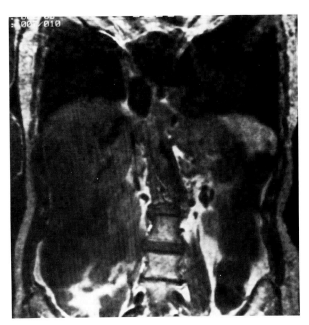

215: Abdominal Aneurysm (1.5T)

EXAM: MRI of the abdomen.

CLINICAL INFORMATION: This is for evaluation of an abdominal aneurysm in a 78-year-old female.

TECHNIQUE: Body coil coronal, sagittal, and axial T1-weighted images were acquired (500/25).

FINDINGS: There is a long fusiform aneurysm, 8 to 10 cm in length, arising approximately 1 cm inferior to the origin of the renal arteries (arrows). There is a 3-cm lumen with circumferential clot, and the total outer wall measurement of the aneurysm is 5 cm.

IMPRESSION: Abdominal aneurysm.

DISCUSSION: There is good anatomic correlation with the available angiography and CT.

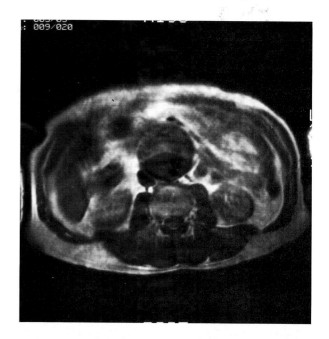

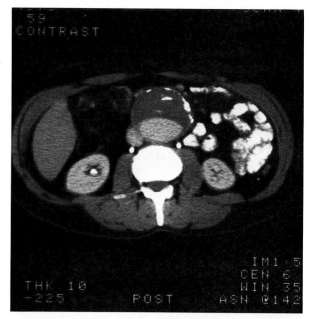

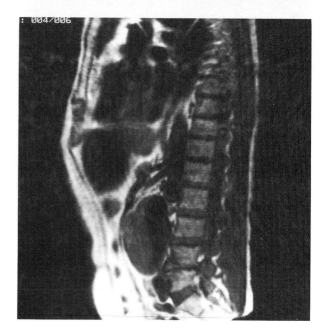

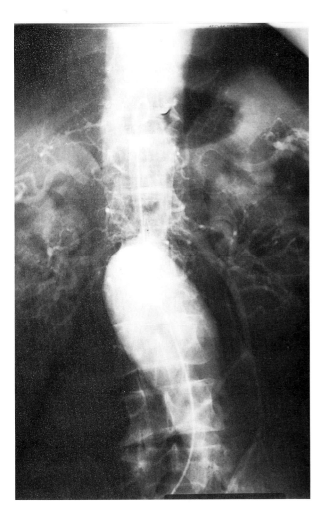

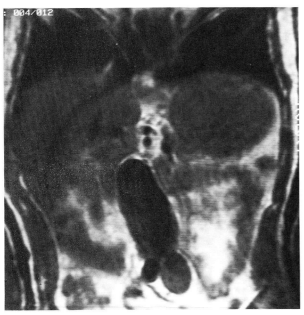

253

216: Abdominal Aneurysm with Clot (1.5T)

EXAM: Abdominal MRI.

CLINICAL INFORMATION: This is an evaluation of an aneurysm in a 59-year-old male with bilateral claudication and palpable abdominal mass.

TECHNIQUE: Respiratory gaited spin density imaging was obtained (1500/25, 1000/25).

FINDINGS: These views demonstrate an 11 × 7 × 7 cm (length × width × side to side) abdominal aneurysm. The renal artery origin is superior to the totuous neck of the aneurysm. There is also aneurysmal dilatation and involvement of the iliacs (Image 2).

In addition, along the anterior wall there is a large amount of clot which markedly narrows the aneurysmal lumen to approximately half that of the total aneurysm size from the anterior to posterior dimension.

IMPRESSION: Large abdominal aneurysm with large amount of intraluminal clot and extension into the iliac arteries.

DISCUSSION: Good correlation between MR angiography and CT is demonstrated here, suggesting the eventual replacement of the aortagram simply with MR. This would reduce significantly the total contrast load in preoperative evaluation of aneurysms. Perhaps, in the near future, the entire preoperative evaluation of aneurysms could consist solely of MR exam, gaited and angiography for runoff below the iliac bifurcation to the ankles.

REFERENCE: Amparo et al.: *Radiology* **154**:451, 1985.

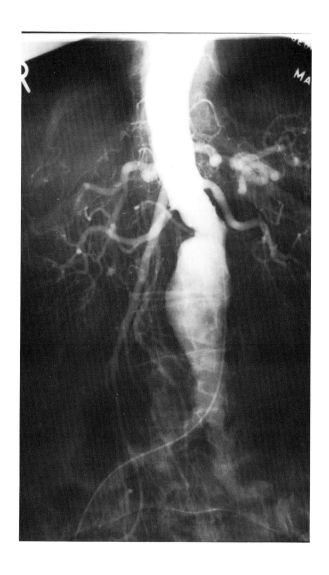

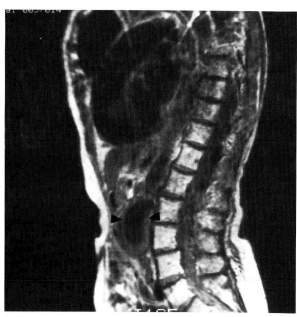

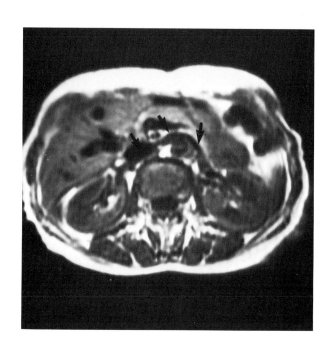

217: Renal Cyst   (.6T)

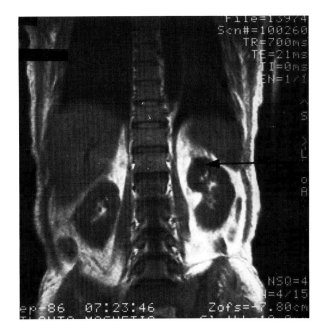

EXAM: MRI of the upper abdomen and kidneys.

CLINICAL INFORMATION: A 63-year-old with weight loss over past 8 months. Rule out occult carcinoma.

TECHNIQUE: Axial and coronal T1- and T2-weighted images were acquired (400/24).

FINDINGS: On the coronal and axial imaging, a discrete well-circumscribed low-signal-intensity lesion is identified in the upper pole of the left kidney. On the T2-weighted images (not shown), there is an increase in signal intensity in this region. Because of the sharp margins and signal characteristics, this is most consistent with a small incidental renal cyst.

IMPRESSION: Small renal cyst, left upper pole.

DISCUSSION: Recent advances in software packages of MR scanning have allowed for significant shortening of sequences. With this shortening, MR through the abdomen will improve in resolution because of the marked suppression of respiratory motion artifact.

This case demonstrates the features of a simple renal cyst. The use of the usual radiographic criteria, as well as the additional information yielded by the behavior on T1- and T2-weighted images, allows for an even more sensitive way to evaluate for renal masses.

REFERENCE: Marotti et al.: *Radiology* 162:679, 1987.

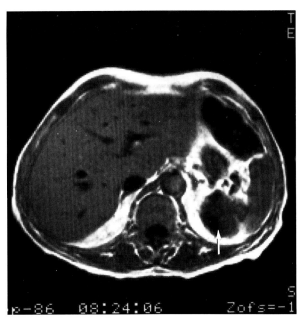

218: Normal Upper Abdomen (.6T)

EXAM: MRI of the upper abdomen.

CLINICAL INFORMATION: A 63-year-old with weight loss of 35 lb over past 8 months. Rule out occult carcinoma.

TECHNIQUE: Coronal and axial T1- and T2-weighted images were acquired (400/24).

FINDINGS: The upper abdomen, liver, and kidneys are normal with good delineation of the hepatic vascularity, as well as retroperitoneal structures. Kidneys, pancreatic region, and adrenal areas are all normal.

IMPRESSION: Normal upper abdominal MRI.

DISCUSSION: The well-delineated abdominal vascular and retroperitoneal structures are easily identified by the inherent property of flowing blood. The renal and hepatic cortex is also nicely demonstrated. Fat gives a high signal, and even sparse amounts of it are usually sufficient to outline and separate the important abdominal structures.

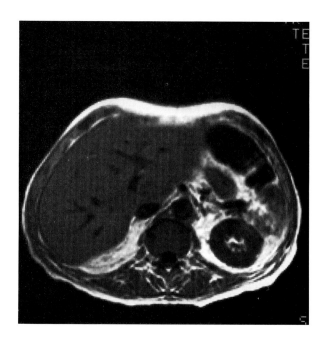

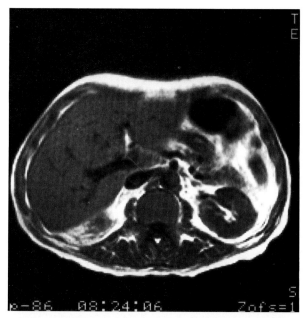

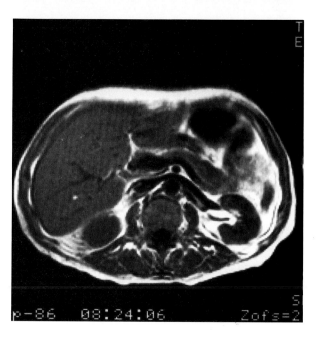

219: Abdominal Aneurysm   (.6T)

EXAM: MRI of the lumbar sacral spine.

CLINICAL INFORMATION: A 48-year-old female with low back pain for 3 years that is gradually increasing in severity.

TECHNIQUE: Sagittal and axial T1- and T2-weighted images were acquired (1500/40/80).

FINDINGS: The vertebral canal is well-aligned with normal discs. The central canal shows no evidence of intrusion from disc bulge or herniation. Incidentally noted is an aneurysmal enlargement of the distal abdominal aorta.

IMPRESSION: Abdominal aortic aneurysm.

DISCUSSION: MR can differentiate beautifully the normal aorta and also define nicely the aneurysmally enlarged aorta. In addition, the wall and intramural clot can be easily identified. The inherent property of flowing blood in yielding little or no signal also usually allows for good estimation of the total patent lumen present.

REFERENCE: Amparo et al.: *Radiology* **154**: 451, 1985.

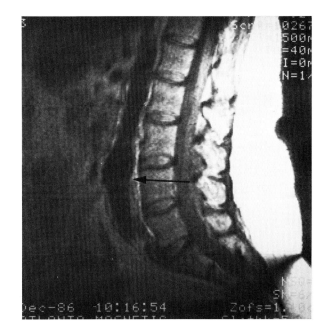

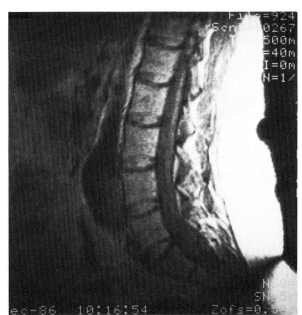

220: Coiled Pancreatic Tail Simulating Metastatic Adenopathy (.6T)

EXAM: MRI of the adrenal glands.

CLINICAL INFORMATION: Female with bladder cancer and mass in left adrenal region as detected on CT.

TECHNIQUE: Axial and coronal T1- and T2-weighted images were acquired.

FINDINGS: Aside from what appears to be an adenoma superior to the kidney, there is a mass anterior to the upper pole of the kidney. On T1, this demonstrates a low signal and on the T2-weighted images the low signal is maintained in the larger portion of this mass. There is, however, a high-signal-intensity center. Because of this heterogeneous signal, concern for a metastatic adenopathy is raised.

IMPRESSION: Question of metastatic adenopathy in lymph nodes anterior to left kidney.

DISCUSSION: This case represents one of the pitfalls of adrenal imaging. The mass is clearly seen (arrows), and there is slightly increased signal focus in the central portion. Concern at the time for adenopathy was raised. In the area superior to this, the adrenal gland and an adenoma was correctly detected. This second mass was considerably more difficult to diagnose. Our review article demonstrated 28 patients with adrenal gland abnormalities which were correctly diagnosed given the signal characteristics listed. These, however, did not include the pitfall that we encountered. At surgery, the tail of the pancreas was found to be coiled and located in the area of concern on the MR scan.

FOLLOW-UP: Pancreatic tail coiled upon itself at surgery.

REFERENCE: Glazer et al.: *Radiology* **158**:73, 1986.

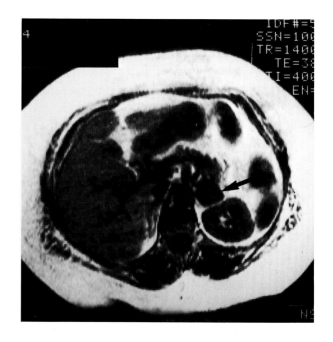

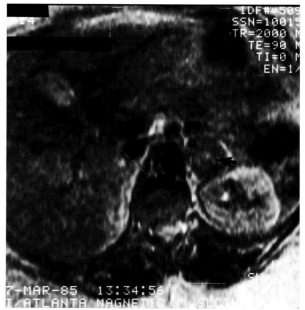

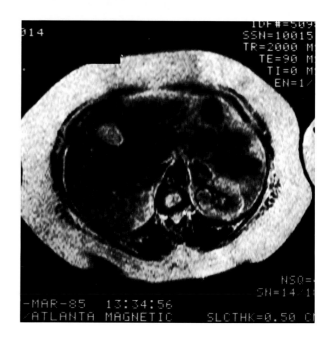

221: Adrenal Adenoma   (.6T)

EXAM: MRI of the adrenal glands.

CLINICAL INFORMATION: Female with cancer of the bladder. Mass detected in the left adrenal gland.

TECHNIQUE: Axial and coronal T1- and T2-weighted images were acquired through the adrenal glands (1400/38, 2000/90).

FINDINGS: There are what appears to be two large masses arising in the arms of the left adrenal gland. The more superior mass (arrows) shows a low intermediate signal on both T1- and T2-weighted images through this region. This is most consistent with a nonfunctioning adrenal adenoma.

IMPRESSION: Adrenal adenoma.

DISCUSSION: The nonfunctioning adenomas show little signal change and can be compared to the signal from the adjacent liver. This is a sharp contrast to the appearance of metastatic and pheochromocytoma masses within the adrenal glands which show increased signal on the more T2-weighted images. The nonfunctional adenomas are the most common adrenal masses and are encountered in approximately 60 percent of autopsy specimens. Metastatic involvement of the adrenal gland is the second most common involvement and, in the recent articles which we have reviewed, they usually display increased signal intensity on T2-weighted images. There is some overlap; however, neoplastic and metastatic involvement of the adrenal gland with low T2 signal is uncommon.

REFERENCE: Reinig et al.: *Radiology* **158**:81, 1986.

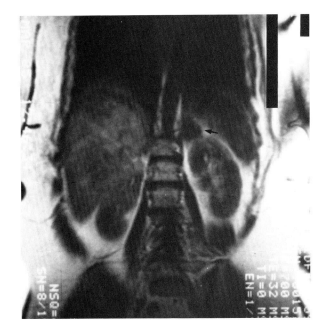

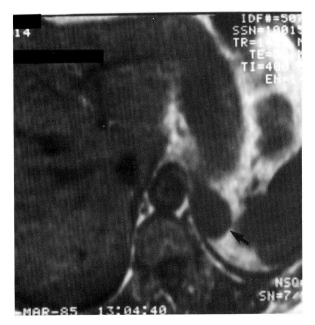

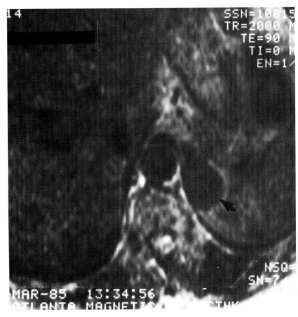

222: Hemochromatosis (1.5T)

EXAM: MRI of the abdomen.

FINDINGS: The liver is of normal size. However, there is markedly decreased signal when compared to the surrounding viscera, such as the kidneys and spleen. Such diffuse low signal raises the possibility of hemochromatosis. Our case demonstrates a characteristic low-signal intensity observed with increased hepatic iron.

IMPRESSION: Consistent with hemochromatosis.

DISCUSSION: Our reference article indicates that idiopathic dietary and transfusional hemochromatosis cannot be distinguished on the basis of distribution, but all have characteristic low-signal intensity within the liver. Our case and another patient's CT scan illustrate the fairly classic appearance of hemochromatosis on CT (Image 3) and the typical appearance on MRI (Images 1 & 2).

REFERENCE: Stark et al.: *Radiology* **154**:137, 1985.

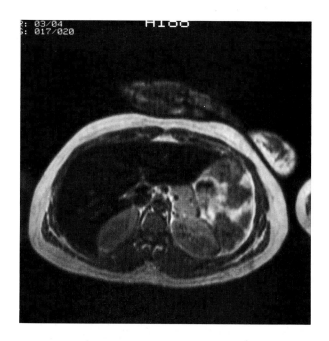

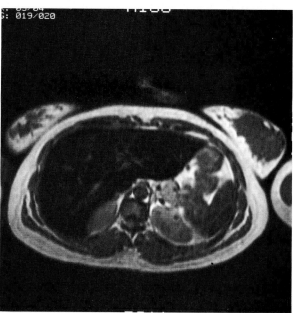

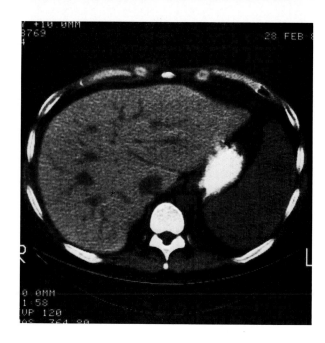

223: Ascites with Thrombus in the Inferior Vena Cava (.6T)

EXAM: MRI of the abdomen.

CLINICAL INFORMATION: Rule out Chiari syndrome in a 76-year-old male.

TECHNIQUE: Body coil T1- and spin-density-weighted images were obtained (1200/32/40; 800/32).

FINDINGS: Free interperitoneal fluid is identified. In addition, high signal persists in the right atrium extending up into it from the left renal vein. This is consistent with thrombus. No increased signal is identified within the hepatic veins themselves.

IMPRESSION: Ascites and thrombus in the inferior vena cava extending from the left renal vein to the right atrium.

DISCUSSION: Flowing blood leaves a signal or black void within the lumen of vascular structures. Here, the increased signal is consistent with clot. This can be substantiated by checking the axial slices above and below this level showing the normal signal characteristics. Care should be taken that interpretation of thrombus is not made on the first or last axial cut in a sequence where paradoxical blood movement may, in fact, increase signal intensity. When the question of thrombus or vascular occlusion is raised, inspecting both T1- and T2-weighted images, as well as imaging in two planes or using gaited methods, can exclude false intraluminal enhancement from true intracanal thrombus.

REFERENCE: Stark: *AJR* **146**:1141, June, 1986.

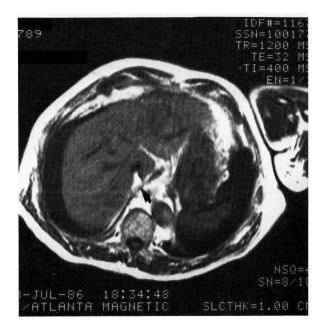

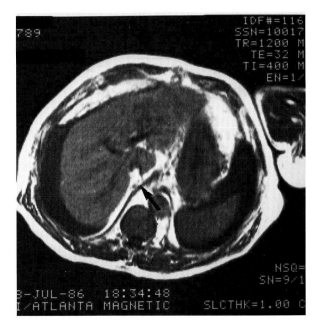

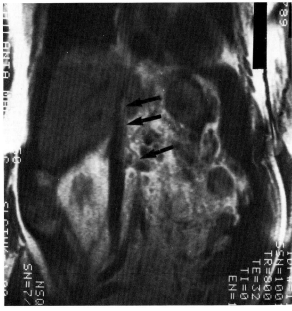

224: Abdominal Wall
Metastases   (.35T)

EXAM: MRI of the abdomen.

CLINICAL INFORMATION: Patient with a right abdominal wall palpable mass and known primary. Rule out adenopathy.

TECHNIQUE: Body coil T1- and T2-weighted images were acquired (1000/30; 2000/60).

FINDINGS: Metastatic mass is identified arising from the lateral aspect of the rectus muscle on the right. In addition, along the iliac bone large metastatic nodes are identified. There is also a large amount of parapsoas adenopathy or metastatic disease which appears to be invading the right psoas muscle (Image 2).

IMPRESSION: Evidence for multiple areas of metastatic involvement, including the right anterior wall, right pelvis, and right psoas muscle.

DISCUSSION: Dramatic metastatic masses can be easily displayed. Nodes within the peritoneum may be confused with bowel loops. In addition, iron-fortified vitamins, such as Geritol, given as an oral contrast agent in diluted amounts, can enhance the intestinal lumen and help to differentiate bowel loop from a node or metastatic mass.

REFERENCE: Stark et al.: *AJR* **145**:213, 1985.

Courtesy of H. C. Ibarra, M.D., Pasadena Magnetic Imaging.

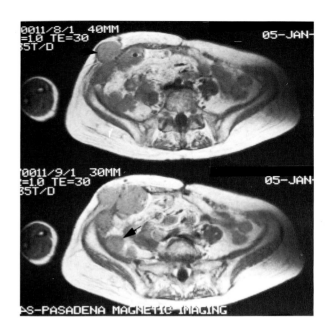

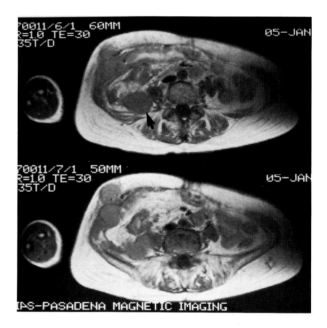

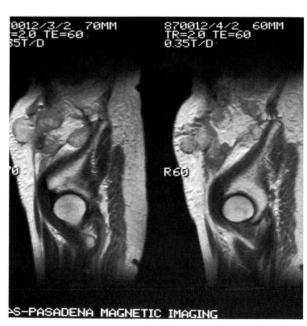

225: Enlarged Pancreatic Uncinate Process (.35T)

EXAM: MRI of the abdomen.

CLINICAL INFORMATION: A 65-year-old male; question of a possible pancreatic mass.

TECHNIQUE: Body coil T1- and T2-weighted images were obtained (500/40; 2000/40).

FINDINGS: There is a prominent or increased uncinate process. This is isointense with that of the remainder of the pancreas on the more T1-weighted image. On the T2-weighted image, there is a slight increase in signal intensity in this region. Note is also made on the more T2-weighted images of a small cyst in the pancreatic tail (Image 3).

IMPRESSION: Enlarged uncinate process raises the possibility of a neoplastic mass.

DISCUSSION: Through our limited experience with the pancreas, we too agree with the conclusions of the authors of our reference article that MR functions best at present as a complementary or confirmatory test following CT. However, secondary to the marked improvement in software and multislice one breathhold features which are soon to be made available, MR may replace CT as the initial screening modality.

REFERENCE: Tscholakoff et al.: *AJR* **148**:703, April, 1987.
Courtesy of S. Fein, M.D., Pasadena Magnetic Imaging.

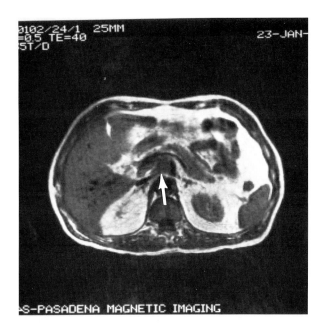

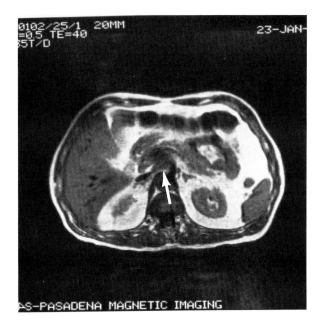

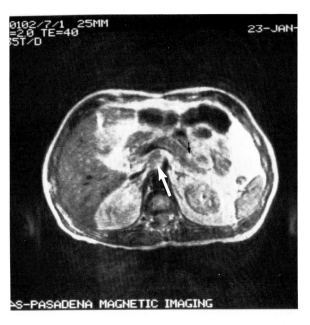

226: Metastases to the Liver   (.35T)

EXAM: MRI of the abdomen.

CLINICAL INFORMATION: Rule out metastatic involvement in the liver.

TECHNIQUE: T1- and T2-weighted images were obtained (2000/30,60).

FINDINGS: Numerous areas of low-signal intensity which are fairly well-circumscribed throughout the right hepatic lobe are identified on the more T1-weighted images (Image 1). These show slight increase in signal intensity on the more T2-weighted images. This increase in signal is heterogeneous, and the findings are most consistent with metastatic disease.

IMPRESSION: Metastatic disease to the liver.

DISCUSSION: Image 1 suggests that there may be some edema surrounding the metastatic disease (arrows). On the spin density images, the lesions or abnormalities are nearly invisible. On the more T2-weighted images, increased signal is identified; however, compared to hemangiomas, this is less intense and is heterogeneous rather than homogeneous. Additionally, inspection of other areas of the liver show altered signal also consistent with metastatic disease (small arrows).

REFERENCE: Henkelman et al.: *Radiology* **161**:727, 1986.

Courtesy of M. T. Smolkin, M.D., Pasadena Magnetic Imaging.

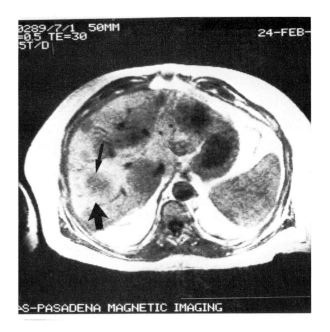

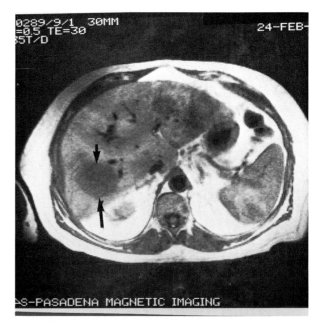

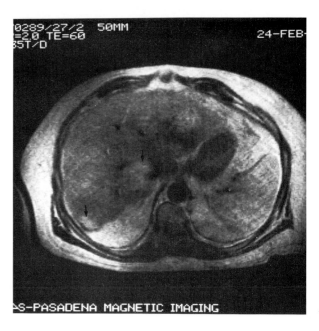

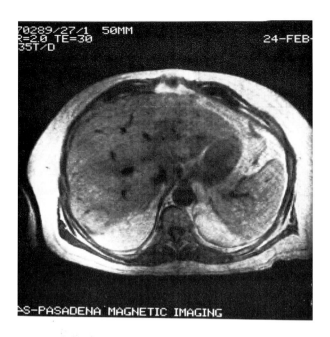

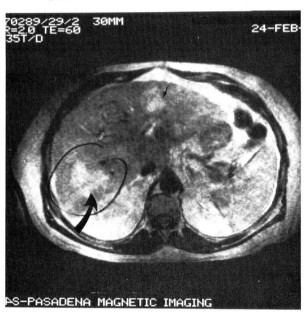

227: Hydronephrosis   (.35T)

EXAM: MRI of the abdomen.

CLINICAL INFORMATION: Patient with known primary lung carcinoma.

TECHNIQUE: Body coil T1- and T2-weighted images were obtained (500/30,2000/30).

FINDINGS: There is hydronephrotic dilatation of the pelvis and collecting system on the left. No evidence of associated retroperitoneal adenopathy is identified. The retroperitoneal vascular structures are free of any evidence of deviation or invasion. No retroperitoneal adenopathy is identified.

IMPRESSION: Left-sided marked hydronephrosis.

REFERENCE: Hircak et al.: *Radiology* **159**:435, 1986.

Courtesy of R. S. Aurora, M.D., Pasadena Magnetic Imaging.

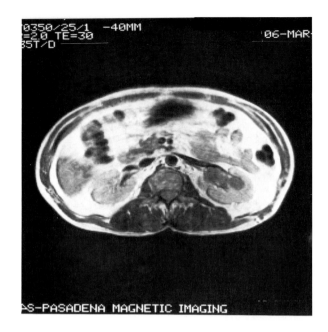

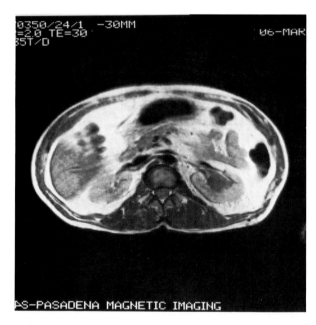

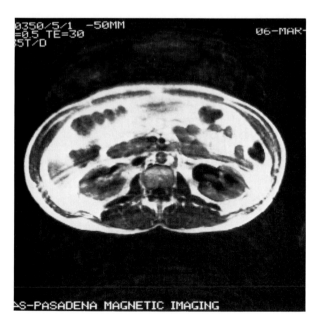

228: Renal Neoplasm (.35T)

EXAM: MRI of the abdomen.

CLINICAL INFORMATION: A 76-year-old male. Rule out renal neoplasm.

TECHNIQUE: Axial T1- and T2-weighted images were acquired (500/30; 2000/30,60).

FINDINGS: A medial right-upper-pole renal neoplasm is identified. This shows increased signal intensity on the more T2-weighted images. The renal vein on the right is draped over this mass, but the low signal suggests that this remains patent and contradicts any suggestion of renal vein thrombosus. The mass appears to be contained within the renal capsule, and no extension beyond the paranephric fat is identified. No retroperitoneal nodes can be seen.

IMPRESSION: Findings are consistent with an upper-pole renal neoplasm. The vascular structures, including the right renal vein and inferior vena cava, show no evidence of renal vein tumor thrombus.

DISCUSSION: The most promising application of MR for the evaluation of renal tumor staging is its excellent delineation of the tumor thrombus involvement of the inferior vena cava. It can, also demonstrate the same morphology and extension through the capsule, as seen with CT.

REFERENCE: Fein et al.: *AJR* **148**:749, April, 1987.

Courtesy of Paul Hicks, M.D., Pasadena Magnetic Imaging.

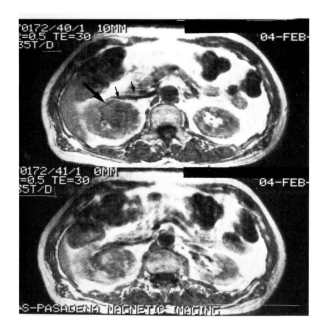

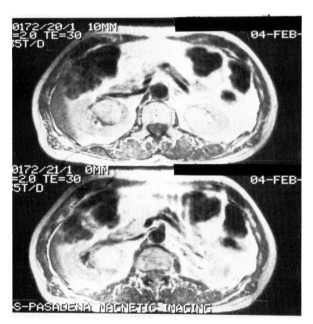

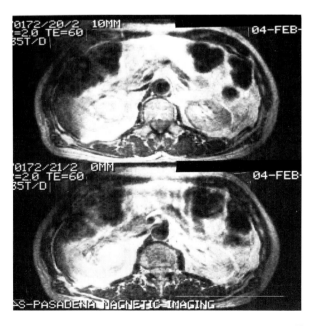

229: Renal Neoplasm with Venous Tumor Thrombus (.35T)

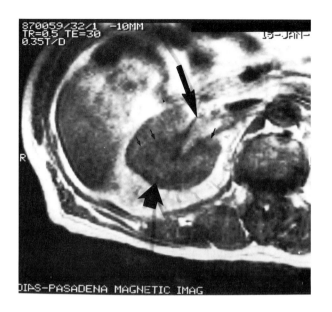

EXAM: MRI of the abdomen.

CLINICAL INFORMATION: This is a 63-year-old male. Rule out renal neoplasm.

TECHNIQUE: T1- and T2-weighted axial images were obtained. The T1 images are shown (500/30).

FINDINGS: A right-upper-pole renal neoplasm is noted with intermediate-to-high signal intensity within the renal vein lumen. The findings are consistent with a renal neoplasm which shows evidence of tumor thrombus within the renal vein.

DISCUSSION: The renal mass is identified (Image 1, large arrow). The separation of normal renal tissue from the renal neoplastic tissue is suggested by the small arrows. In addition, there is good evidence (large arrow, long stem) for the alteration of the normal low-signal intensity in the renal vein consistent with tumor thrombus.

Courtesy of M. Quraishi, Pasadena Magnetic Imaging.

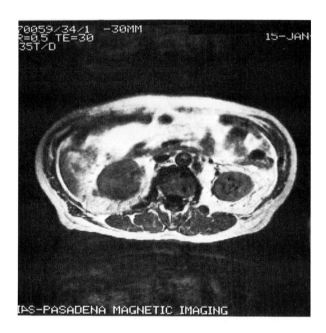

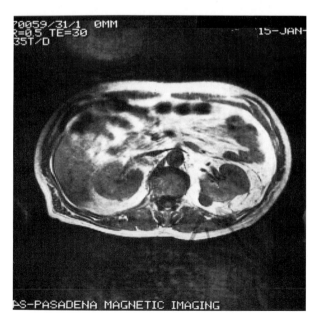

230: Left Renal Cyst   (.35T)

EXAM: MRI of the abdomen.

CLINICAL INFORMATION: Rule out neoplastic mass in the kidneys.

TECHNIQUE: Axial and coronal T1- and T2-weighted images were obtained (500/30; 2000/30,60).

FINDINGS: A well-rounded mass in the left renal cortex is identified. This shows very low signal intensity on the more T2-weighted images and increased signal intensity on the T2-weighted images.

This is consistent with the behavior of fluid. The edges or margins of the mass are quite smooth and well-rounded. Findings are consistent with a simple renal cyst.

DISCUSSION: Although the same features on CT that differentiate a cyst from a mass in the kidney can be used in MR interpretation, analysis of the T1- and T2-weighted portions of the study can yield additional information about the contents of these apparently cystic structures. Blood within the cysts shows a definite increase in signal. In addition, renal neoplasms which simulate a cyst can be separated from the real cysts by their behavior in the obtained double-echo sequences. The ability to separate simple cysts containing fluid which behaves in a manner like urine in the bladder from those which may have higher protein or blood content allows for increased proof of simple renal cyst benignity and attention to the hemorrhagic cyst which may harbor renal neoplasm.

IMPRESSION: Left renal cyst.

REFERENCE: Marotti et al.: *Radiology* **162**:679, 1987.

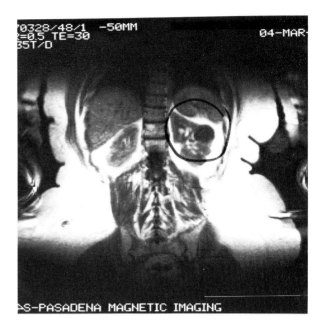

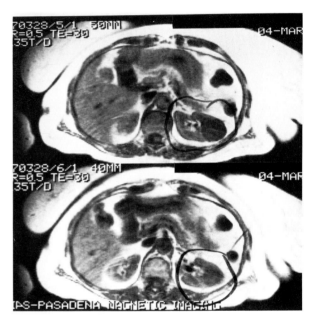

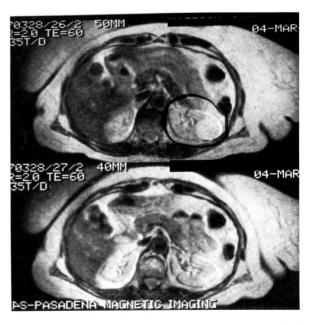

231: Sacral Histiocytoma   (.6T)

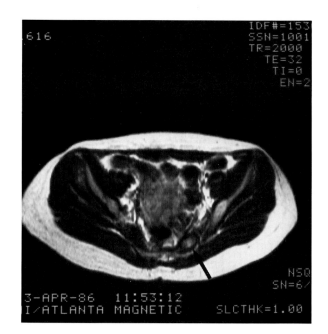

EXAM: MRI of the pelvis.

CLINICAL INFORMATION: Rule out sacral bone malignancy in 40-year-old female.

TECHNIQUE: Axial, coronal, and sagittal T1-weighted images were obtained (T1- and T2-weighting) (2000/32,64; 500/32).

FINDINGS: At approximately the third sacral level within the bone and extending into the sacral ala of the third sacral body, there is an intermediate signal which contrasts to the bright or increased signal intensity of the normal bone marrow fat. There is a degree of bony expansion and remodeling. A portion of this mass extends outside the confines of the bone. On the more T2-weighted images, this area of abnormality is shown to increase slightly in its signal intensity. This is consistent with a metastatic or primary bone tumor. There has been, prior to this study, a biopsy diagnosis of histiocytoma.

IMPRESSION: Sacral lesion, left side, consistent with histiocytoma.

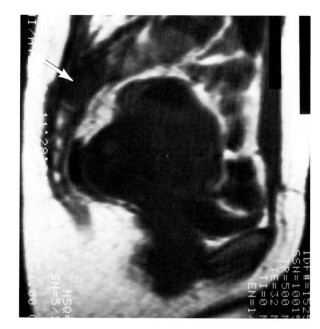

DISCUSSION: Although the signal characteristics of benign and malignant bone tumors can overlap, the value of imaging in the three different planes lies in its full assessment of the lesions.

REFERENCE: Resenthal et al.: *AJR* **145**:143, 1985.

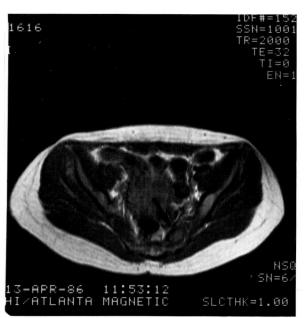

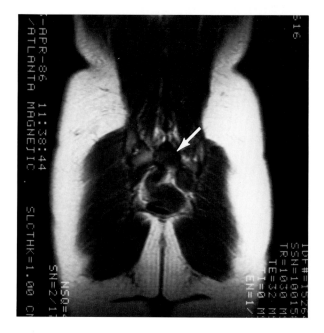

232: Fibroids   (.6T)

EXAM: MRI of the pelvis.

CLINICAL INFORMATION: Known sacral histiocytoma in 40-year-old female.

TECHNIQUE: Body coil axial, sagittal, and coronal scans were obtained (2000/32,64; 500/30).

FINDINGS: An enlarged abnormal uterus is identified with several variously sized areas of low-signal intensity within the uterine fundus. These are well-circumscribed and do not extend beyond the uterine myometrium. The overall uterine size is grossly enlarged. The findings are consistent with numerous uterine leiomyomas.

IMPRESSION: Uterine fibroids.

DISCUSSION: In the reference authors' evaluation, more leiomyomas were detected with MR than with ultrasound. The size in relationship to these masses could be easily appreciated. Their particular investigation was evaluation of pregnant patients. They do, however, point out that low-signal leiomyomas were found to be without degeneration. The more high-signal-intensity leiomyomas were correlated histologically with degeneration of the leiomyoma.

REFERENCE: Weinreb et al.: *Radiology* **159**:717, 1986.

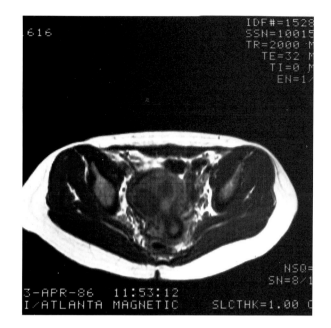

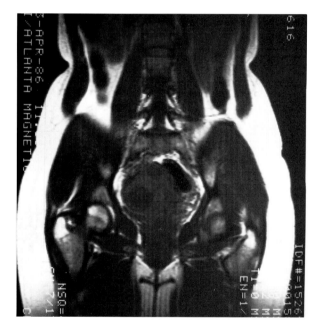

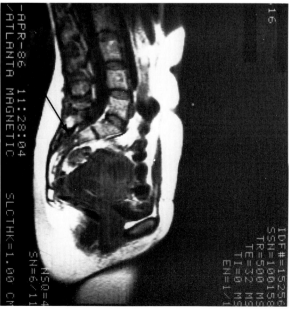

233: Normal Uterus   (.6T)

EXAM: MRI of the pelvis.

CLINICAL INFORMATION: Evaluation for leg pain following MVA.

TECHNIQUE: Coronal views were obtained using spin echo technique (1600/40,80).

FINDINGS: This study is essentially normal. There is good delineation of two myometrial layers with a bright endometrial signal intensity. No masses in the pelvis are detected.

IMPRESSION: Study is normal. The prominent uterine lumen and myometrial layers are consistent with active menstruation.

DISCUSSION: Myometrial and endometrial areas increase slightly in size during menstruation. This can be followed with MRI and, as done in our reference article, was followed in six healthy patients. The importance of this to investigators is in the recognition of the normal slight change in size of the uterus, endometrial layer, and myometrium.

REFERENCE: Haynor et al.: *Radiology* **161**:459, 1986.

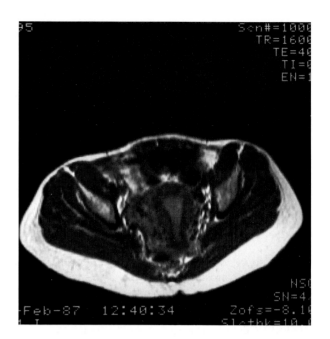

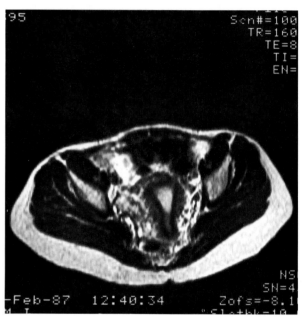

234: Prostate Calcification (.6T)

EXAM: MRI of the pelvis.

CLINICAL INFORMATION: Patient evaluated for avascular necrosis.

TECHNIQUE: Axial and coronal images were obtained (1500/30).

FINDINGS: The hip exam was normal. There is, however, note of a low-signal-intensity void seen included in the prostate parenchyma. These areas of low-signal intensity represent calcification.

IMPRESSION: Prostate calcification. Remainder of the exam is normal.

DISCUSSION: We feel that MRI offers a superior modality for investigation of prostate abnormality as evidenced by the good anatomic delineation of the prostate and the incidental calcifications in this case.

REFERENCE: Bryan et al.: *AJR* **146**:543, March, 1986.

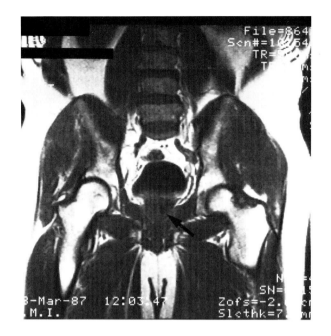

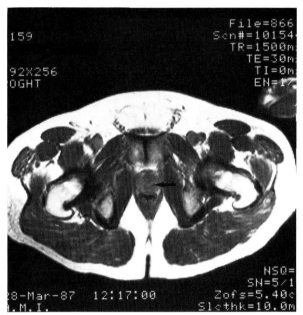

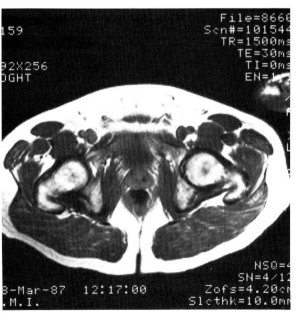

235: Bladder Carcinoma   (.6T)

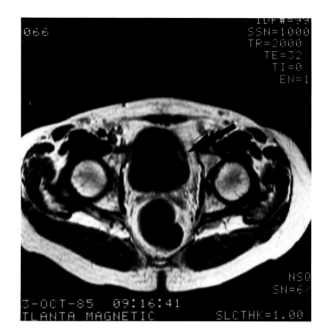

EXAM: MRI of the pelvis.

CLINICAL INFORMATION: A 67-year-old with urinary bleeding on blood thinner for recent stroke. Cystoscopy revealed bladder CA.

TECHNIQUE: Coronal and axial scanning with double-echo technique was obtained (2000/32,64).

FINDINGS: The focal thickening is identified in the left bladder wall. No associated adenopathy is seen. The parapelvic fat planes remain well-preserved.

IMPRESSION: Focal bladder wall thickening is consistent with bladder CA.

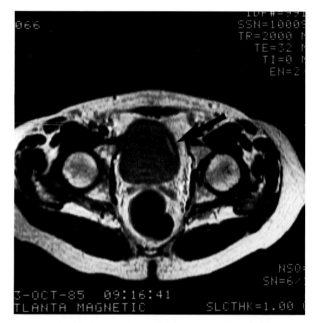

DISCUSSION: As per our reference article, we too feel that the T1-weighted images are optimal for depicting focal bladder wall thickening, and the ability to scan in several orientations allows for good evaluation of the wall. The lack of any enlarged nodes makes exclusion of any metastatic adenopathy to the nonenlarged nodes similar to that of CT. However, the elegant demonstration of the bladder wall and focal thickening, as seen with involvement of carcinoma, represents an imaging modality superior even to that of the excellent CT scan evaluation.

REFERENCE: Bryan et al.: *JCAT* **11**:96, January/February, 1987.

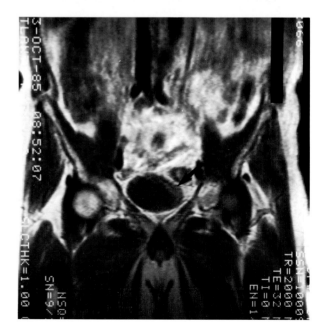

236: Normal Pelvis/Testes   (.6T)

EXAM: MRI of the pelvis.

CLINICAL INFORMATION: This is a 44-year-old male being evaluated for orthopedic reasons.

TECHNIQUE: Coronal T1-weighted images were acquired (500/20).

FINDINGS: The testicles and epididymis are normal and symmetric.

IMPRESSION: Normal.

DISCUSSION: This particular case shows no abnormality. However, the well-displayed anatomy in both our incidental examination of the testes (usually during hip evaluation) and in the authors' reference articles points to the future utility of MR in evaluating the testes. Although ultrasound offers an excellent scanning modality, this is highly dependent upon the expertise of the operator observer.

REFERENCES: Baker et al.: *Radiology* **163**:89, 1987.
Bretan et al.: *Radiology* **162**:867, 1987.

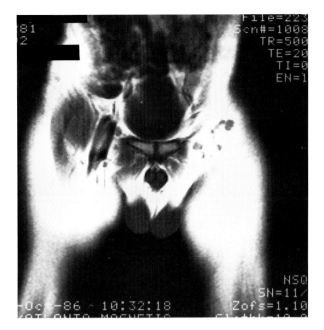

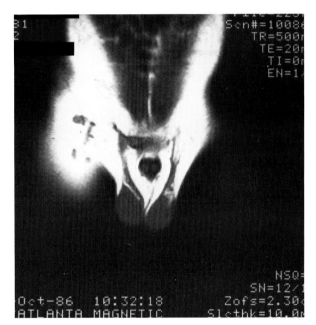

237: Enlarged Prostate (Status Post-TURP for Adenocarcinoma) (.6T)

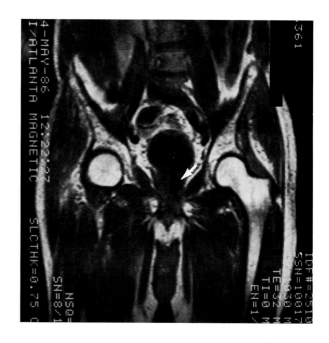

EXAM: MRI of the pelvis.

CLINICAL INFORMATION: Adenocarcinoma of the prostate.

TECHNIQUE: Axial, sagittal, and coronal views were obtained (1000/30,60; 550/32).

FINDINGS: Enlarged prostate is seen with an eccentric defect seen through the midportion of the prostate. This is consistent with the patient's previous transurethral prostatectomy (TURP). The prostatic capsule is intact. No evidence of inguinal adenopathy is seen.

IMPRESSION: Moderate prostatic enlargement. Defect in glandular tissue is consistent with recent TURP.

DISCUSSION: The defect from the transurethral prostatectomy is identified. This demonstrates the ability of MRI to define what portion of the prostate has been removed and may explain any complications, such as excessive bleeding, following the procedure. Note the eccentricity of the defect; it is not a symmetric paraurethral defect. Note also the well-delineated prostatic capsule, seminal vesicles, and the pelvic fat which outline associated prostate adenopathy.

REFERENCE: Fisher et al.: *Radiology* **157**:467, 1985.

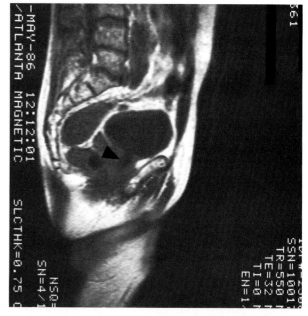

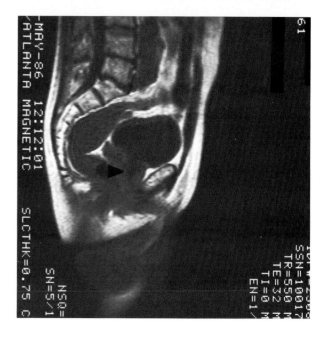

238: Ovarian Cyst   (1.5T)

EXAM: MRI of the abdomen.

CLINICAL INFORMATION: A 30-year-old female with postgravid state, being evaluated for unrelated renal problems.

TECHNIQUE: Coronal body coil images were obtained through the kidneys for purposes of evaluating the anatomy of the renal arteries.

FINDINGS: The uterus is enlarged and shows a right cystic structure in the region of the adnexa, probably representing a simple ovarian cyst instead of a cystic degenerating fibroid within the right uterine fundus.

REFERENCE: Hricak et al.: *Radiology* **158**:385, 1986.

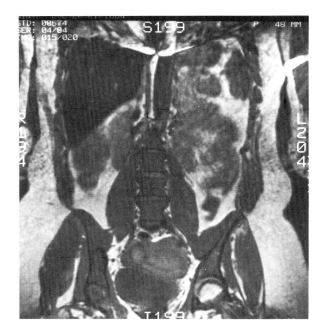

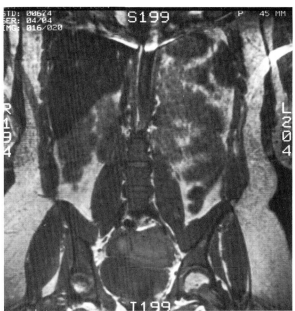

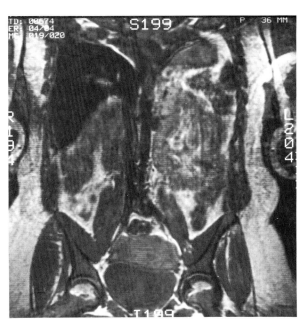

239: Bilateral Cyst (Ovarian) (.6T)

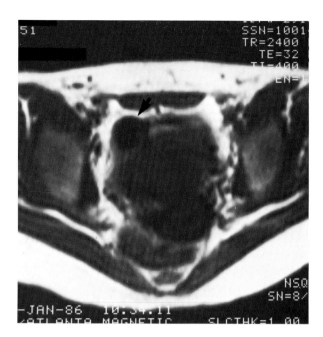

EXAM: MRI of the pelvis.

CLINICAL INFORMATION: A 27-year-old female with laparoscopy in the past, revealing a cyst in the left ovary. Now recurrent left side pain.

TECHNIQUE: Coronal and axial T1- and T2-weighted images in the body coil were obtained (2150-60/120).

FINDINGS: There are bilateral cystic masses measuring approximately 2 to 3 cm on the left and 1 to 2 cm on the right. T1 images show low-signal intensity, or long T1, and the T2 images show increased signal consistent with a long T2. The signal characteristics and morphology are consistent with that of simple ovarian cysts.

IMPRESSION: Bilateral ovarian cysts. Note made of incidental fibroid extending from right uterine fundus (small arrow).

DISCUSSION: Adnexal structures can be well-evaluated with MR in patients on whom ultrasound is inconclusive or not suitable (for example, obese patients). The bilateral cystic structures are well-displayed, as are the incidental findings of a fibroid. Note also the well-demonstrated uterine lumen and the normal delineation between the endometrial and myometrial layers (small arrow).

REFERENCE: Kulkarni et al.: *RadioGraphics* 5:611, July, 1985.

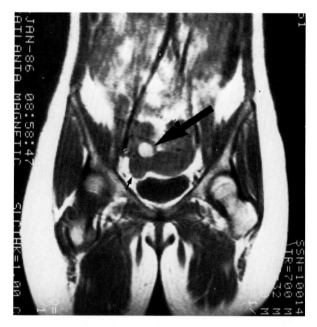

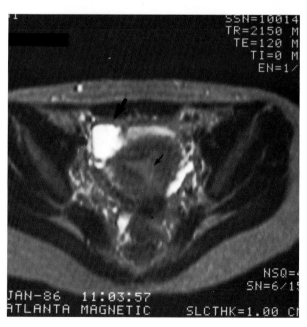

240: Status Post Hysterectomy (.6T)

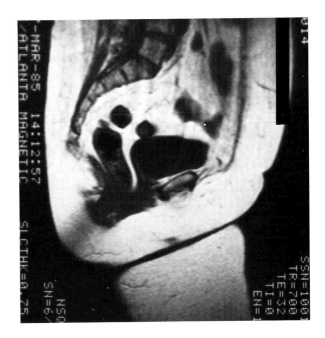

EXAM: MRI of the pelvis.

CLINICAL INFORMATION: A 55-year-old female with diagnosis of bladder cancer is now submitted for MR to rule out metastases. By history, patient has had prior hysterectomy.

TECHNIQUE: Coronal, sagittal, and axial spin density imaging was obtained with body coil (700/32).

FINDINGS: The uterus is surgically absent. No nodes are identified. The contours of the bladder wall are smooth without evidence of intraluminal defect or focal bladder-wall thickening. The rectosigmoid and mesenteric structures are well-displayed and unremarkable.

IMPRESSION: Changes consistent with prior hysterectomy.

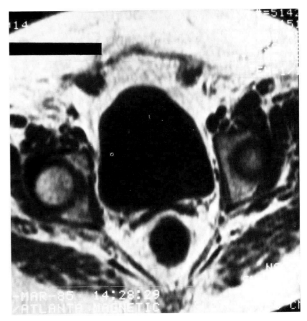

DISCUSSION: The intrinsic contrast of body fat allows for good separation of the pelvic viscera, and the contrast of the urine and the soft tissue of the bladder wall allows for a good exam for infiltrative processes. This is a typical appearance of a pelvis which has undergone total hysterectomy. Of particular note is the ease of evaluating the vaginal cuff, cul-de-sac, and bladder.

REFERENCE: Hricak: *AJR* **146**:1115, June, 1986.

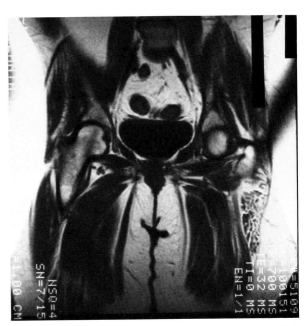

241: Pelvis   (1.5T)

EXAM: MRI of the pelvis.

CLINICAL INFORMATION: A 47-year-old male with focal ureteral stricture on retrograde pyelogram. CT shows poor delineation of the retroperitoneal vessels. Question of metastatic adenopathy or mass versus retroperitoneal fibrosis.

TECHNIQUE: Body coil T1- and T2-weighted images were acquired in the coronal and axial projection (25-50/100; 800/25).

FINDINGS: There is good delineation of a focal area of intermediate signal encasing the iliac artery and inferior vena cava.

DISCUSSION: Retroperitoneal fibrosis, may be idiopathic or related to methylsergide use. Perianeurysmal inflammation or radiation may also be a cause. Medial deviation and stricture of the ureter with hydronephrosis are the characteristic uroradiographic findings. Malignant retroperitoneal adenopathy may mimic this situation. The MR's ability to demonstrate the retroperitoneal vessels and show discrete, smooth borders, rather than the lumpy, bumpy borders of retroperitoneal adenopathy, helps in separating these two diagnoses. The nondisplacement of the aorta with retroperitoneal fibrosis versus the separation away from the vertebral body on malignant lymphomas, adenopathy, or masses is another sign which MR can demonstrate well.

CONFIRMATION: Retroperitoneal fibrosis confirmed at surgery for repair of ureteral obstruction.

REFERENCE: Degesys et al.: *AJR* **146**:57, January, 1986.

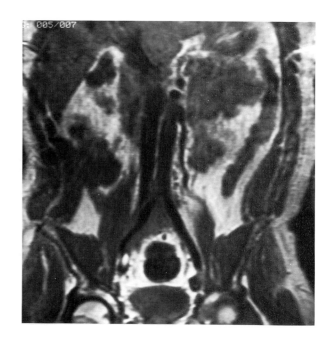

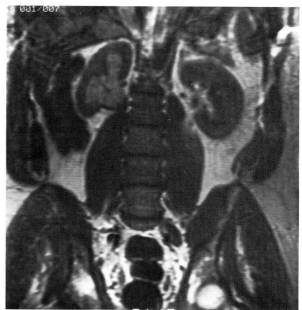

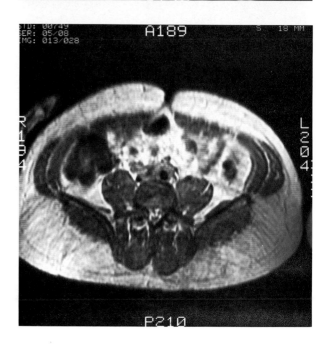

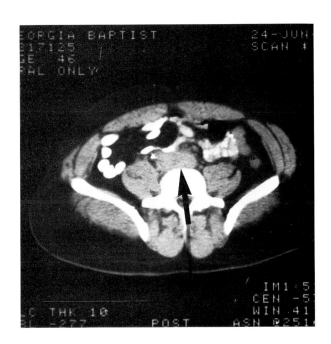

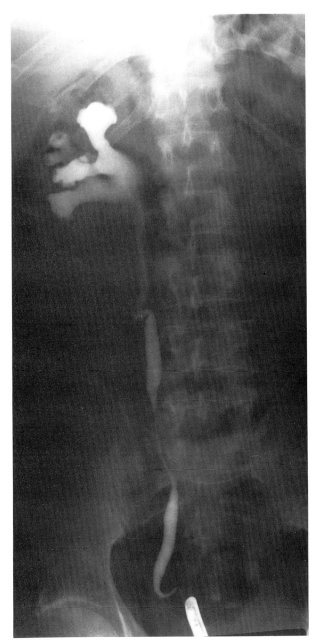

242: Retroperitoneal Fibrosis (.6T)

EXAM: MRI of the pelvis.

CLINICAL INFORMATION: A 65-year-old male with biopsy-proven prostate CA.

TECHNIQUE: Body coil T1- and T2-weighted images were acquired through the pelvic region (2000/32,64).

FINDINGS: The prostate is enlarged and extends beyond its capsule. There is metastatic invasion of the seminal vesicles. In addition, note is made of large iliac chain nodes, greater than 1 cm bilaterally. Findings are consistent with a Stage D-1 prostate CA.

IMPRESSION: Prostate CA.

DISCUSSION: For prostate CA, the evaluation of lymphadenopathy is essential in correct staging. At best, an 80% correlation using lymphangiography and CT can be obtained. MR offers an accuracy rate quoted at 83 percent in our reference article. This is due in part to multiplaner imaging capacity as well as the nodes inherent intermediate signal versus low signal of blood vessels and the lower signal of soft tissue in the pelvic region. Note the ease of detection of adenopathy (arrows, Images 1–3). The enlarged prostate is extending out of the capsule with seminal vesicle invasion.

REFERENCE: Hricak et al.: *Radiology* **162**:331, 1987.

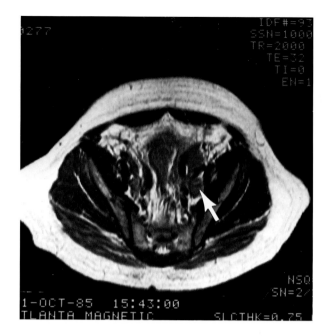

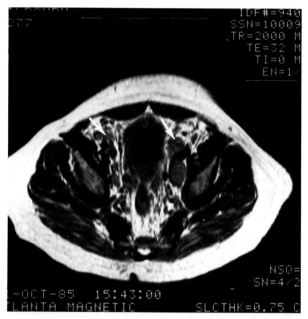

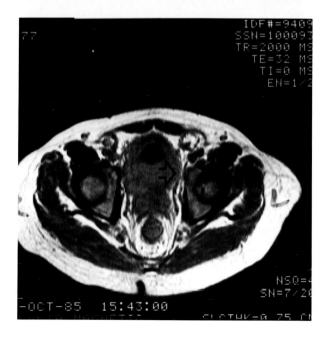

243: Prostatic Carcinoma   (.6T)

EXAM: MRI of the pelvis.

CLINICAL INFORMATION: A 60-year-old male with biopsy-proven cancer of the prostate. Exam for staging purposes.

TECHNIQUE: Axial and saggital body coil images were acquired with body coil (2000/32,64; 500/30).

FINDINGS: There is diffuse enlargement of the prostatic gland which appears to be elevated and inseparable from the posterior bladder wall and seminal vesicles. The bladder wall is thickened, particularly along its posterior and superior aspect. The seminal vesicles are also markedly enlarged, and the normal pelvic fat lying separate from the prostate is absent. In addition, there is loss of the normal fat separating the prostatic capsule from the levator ani muscle (Image 3, arrow).

IMPRESSION: Findings compatible with Stage C prostatic cancer.

DISCUSSION: In both our experience over the past 1½ years and the reference article, a higher stage of accuracy is available with MR. This is due in part to the inherent contrast available, as well as the significant added information on the sagittal and coronal views. Staging the prostate cancer is important for the urologist in his or her plan of management. Stage B includes tumor contained only within the gland. Stage C is seen when the tumor spreads into the extracapsular area. Stage D is demonstration of pelvic lymphadenopathy (Stage D-1). Bone metastases changes the classification to Stage D-2. Also, the seminal vesicles are well-defined and early metastatic involvement to them can be more fully appreciated than with CT.

REFERENCE: Steinbert et al.: *Radiology* **162**:331, 1987.

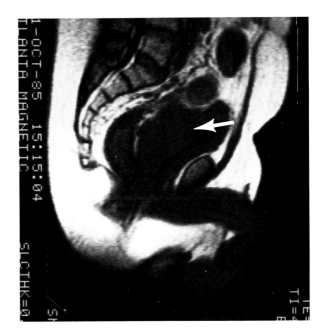

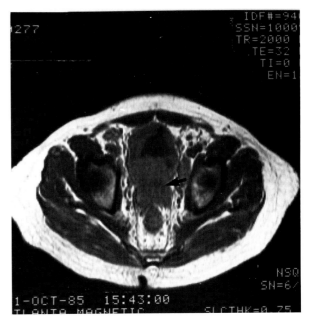

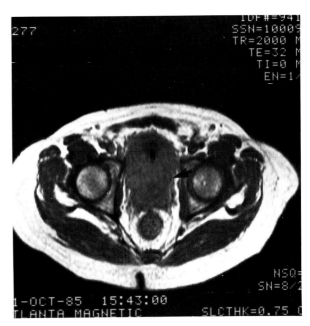

244: Ovarian Mass   (.6T)

EXAM: MRI of the pelvis.

CLINICAL INFORMATION: A 49-year-old female with radicular pain radiating into the ischium.

TECHNIQUE: Body coil axial and coronal T1- and T2-weighted images were acquired (1400/80, 160).

FINDINGS: There is a 3.8-cm mass in the right adnexa arising from the region of the right ovary. The signal intensity is greater than that of the soft tissue or muscle structures and is an intensity similar to fat on the T2-weighted images. The signal is slightly heterogeneous, suggesting that this is solid, rather than cystic, in nature. The uterus is also well-displayed and normal with normal endometrial signal. The myometrium also shows normal signal.

IMPRESSION: Right adnexal, solid ovarian mass.

DISCUSSION: Although ultrasound remains the preferred diagnostic modality, some patients, because of sheer size or complexity of lesions, require complementary studies such as CT or MR. MR, in our review article, was successful in delineating adnexal masses as well as specifying whether they represented solid or cystic masses. Simple cystic masses behaved in a similar fashion to the urine contained within the bladder. Solid masses, such as ours (arrows), show a slightly more intermediate signal than does urine on the more T1-weighted images. They also suggest their solid character by the heterogeneity of the signal (as seen above).

REFERENCE: Dooms et al.: *Radiology* **158**:639, 1986.

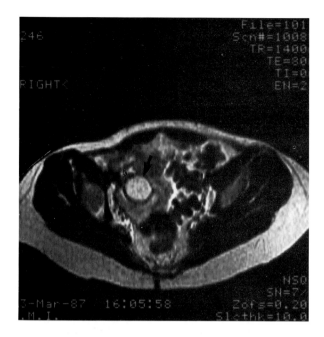

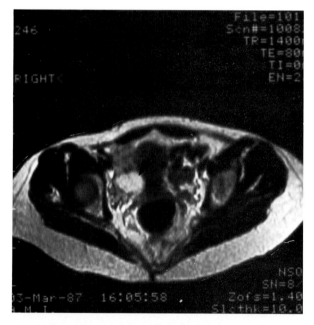

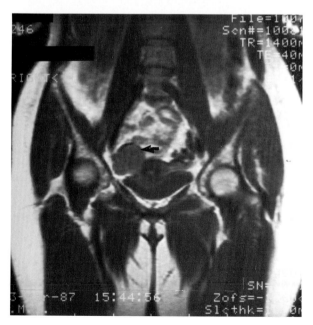

245: Nabothian Cyst of the Cervical Os   (.6T)

EXAM: MRI of the Pelvis.

CLINICAL INFORMATION: Rule out pelvic mass.

TECHNIQUE: Body coil axial and coronal images were acquired (1400/80,160).

FINDINGS: There are several small, round, discrete areas of increased or long T2-weighted characteristics on image (arrow). These are in the region of the uterine cervix and are most consistent with small nabothian cysts.

DISCUSSION: Increased signal intensity on both T1- and T2-weighted images is observed in our case and in the reference article. The nabothian cysts are simply incidental blocked glands in the region of the cervix and, in themselves, serve only to demonstrate the ability of MR to delineate the uterine structure. Note the myometrial endometrial separation of signal and the well-displayed size and nature of the uterine lumen.

REFERENCE: Lee et al.: *Radiology* **157**: 175, 1985.

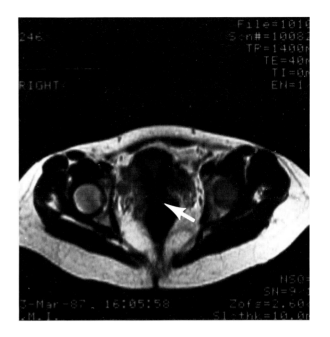

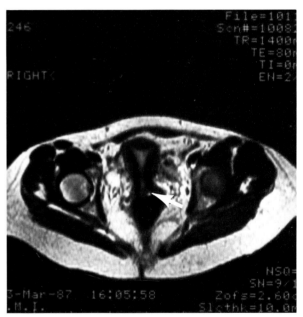

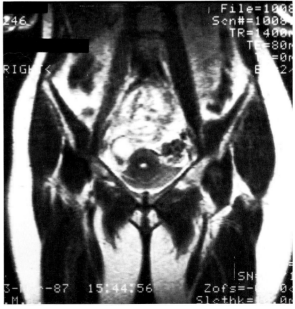

246: Ovarian Cyst (Question Hemorrhagic Content)   (.6T)

EXAM: MRI of the pelvis.

CLINICAL INFORMATION: This is a 28-year-old female with left anterior pelvic and hip pain.

TECHNIQUE: T1-weighted images were obtained in the coronal and axial plane through the hips (700/32).

FINDINGS: The study is essentially normal with the exception of a rounded, smooth cystic structure in the right adnexa with increased signal similar in intensity to fat. These are morphology and signal characteristics of simple ovarian cyst, possibly with high protein or old hemorrhage to explain the increased signal intensity on the more T1-weighted images.

IMPRESSION: Small ovarian cyst, right side. Question of high-protein or hemorrhage content.

DISCUSSION: Incidental examination of the male and female pelvic viscera is available when evaluating the hips for avascular necrosis. Numerous incidental adnexal masses have been detected, showing MR as a useful modality for study of adnexal masses. Ultrasound will remain the primary modality of choice with MR adding supplemental information.

REFERENCE: Mitchell et al.: *Radiology* **162**:319, 1987.

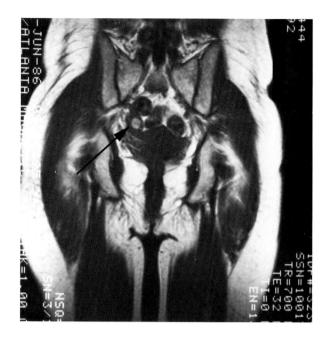

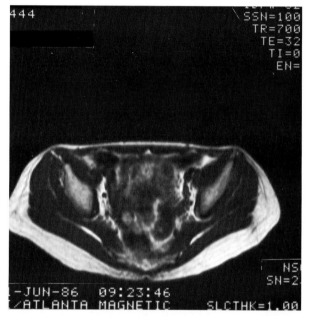

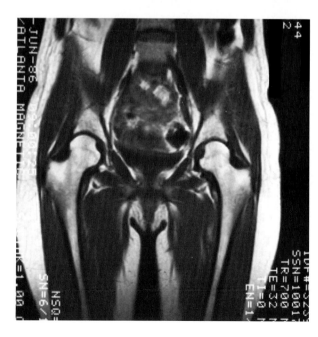

247: Bladder Carcinoma (.6T)

EXAM: MRI of the pelvis.

CLINICAL INFORMATION: This is a 72-year-old male with hematuria.

TECHNIQUE: Body coil axial and coronal scans were obtained with T1- and T2-weighting (1600/32,74; 600/32).

FINDINGS: There is a lobulated mass arising from the posterior wall of the bladder identified on both coronal and axial views. This appears to be confined to the bladder-wall musculature. No evidence of extension beyond the bladder is identified.

IMPRESSION: Bladder-wall neoplasm.

DISCUSSION: Patient's urine provides an excellent inherent contrast to the MRI's ability to image the bladder in three different planes. There is an increase in sensitivity to the detection of focal areas of thickening, which may represent transitional cell carcinomas. In addition, the inherent contrast of the fat allows for good definition of any early extension of a bladder or prostate malignancy to the adjacent pelvic viscera. The bladder wall is well-imaged, and any subtle thickening or invasion can be imaged early with MR.

REFERENCE: Rholl et al.: *Radiology* **163**:117, 1987.

Courtesy of Al Alexander, M.D., Lancaster Magnetic Imaging.

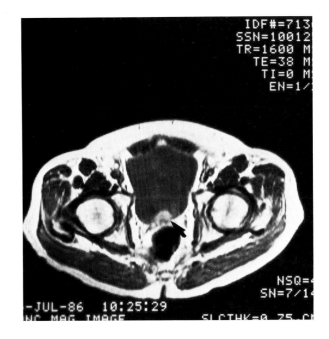

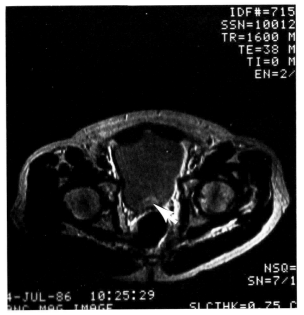

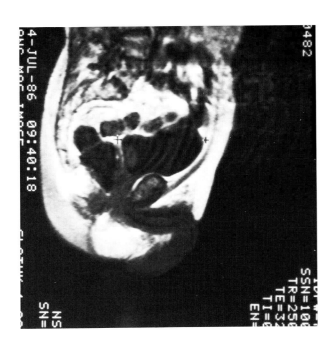

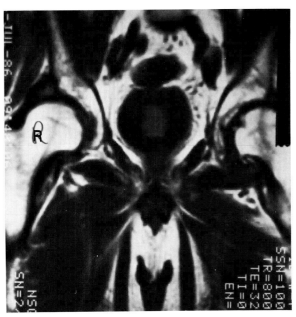

248: Recurrent Cancer of the Fallopian Tubes   (1.5T)

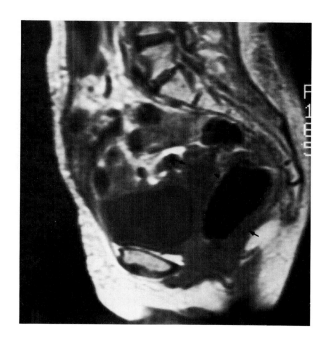

EXAM: MRI of the pelvis.

CLINICAL INFORMATION: This is a 65-year-old female with proven cancer of the fallopian tubes. Patient returns for follow-up to exclude recurrence.

TECHNIQUE: Sagittal and axial T1- and T2-weighted images were obtained (500/25; 2000/40,80).

FINDINGS: A midline pelvic mass in the cul-de-sac, measuring approximately 4 × 4 × 2 cm, is identified. This is separate and anterior from the rectosigmoid, posterior to the bladder, and felt to represent recurrence, given history of prior hysterectomy. In addition, there is increased soft tissue in the retrorectal space consistent with additional metastatic involvement. Note is also made of a medial neoplastic mass laterally displacing the left psoas muscle.

IMPRESSION: Recurrent carcinoma with a large midline pelvic mass and evidence for diffuse extension into the retrorectal space as well as metastatic implants in the retroperitoneum.

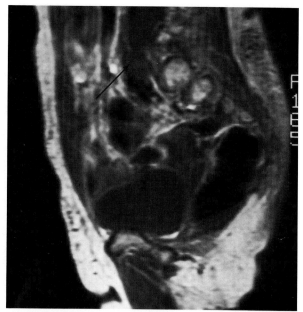

DISCUSSION: Although our case does not directly involve the rectum, the reference case demonstrates the possible application of MR in the evaluation of primary rectal lesions. The perirectal fat and the demonstration of the rectal anatomy is at least equivalent, if not superior, to CT in its delineation of pathology.

The differentiation between tumor and stool within the rectum is difficult, and, if pelvic imaging becomes advantageous, this may include the need for a limited bowel prep.

REFERENCE: Butch et al.: *AJR* **146**:1155, June, 1986.

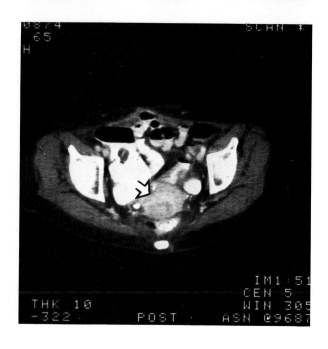

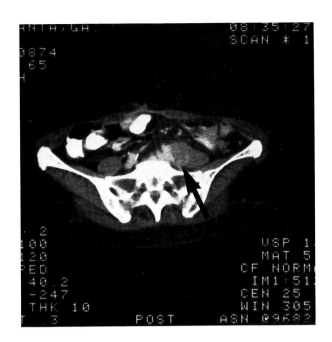

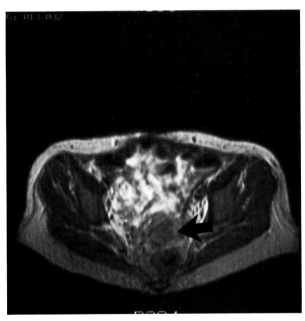

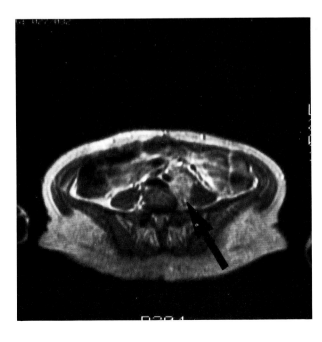

249: Postgravid Uterus   (1.5T)

EXAM: MRI of the pelvis.

CLINICAL INFORMATION: Patient is a 34-year-old female several days post delivery. Rule out pelvic vein thrombosis.

TECHNIQUE: Coronal and axial T1- and T2-weighted images were obtained (1000/20; 2000/20,90).

FINDINGS: The uterus is boggy and diffusely enlarged with some minimal increased signal intensity in the lumen representing minimal amount of fluid and blood. The remainder of the study was normal.

IMPRESSION: Postgravid uterus. No increase in signal is seen in the pelvic veins or IVC to suggest thrombus.

DISCUSSION: MRI is an excellent screen to exclude large clot in the large retroperitoneal vessels; however the incidental inclusion of the postgravid uterus also points to the use of MR in evaluating the uterus during pregnancy. As in our reference article, we agreed that the cervix and gravid uterus can be better visualized on MR. We have not yet had the chance to image a pregnant patient, but MR should be considered superlative for evaluation of any head and pelvic discrepancy, incompetent cervical os, or clot within the large vessels.

REFERENCE: McCarthy et al.: *Radiology* **154**:421, 1985.

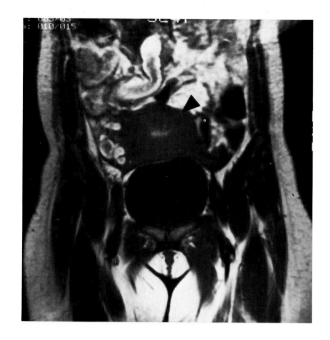

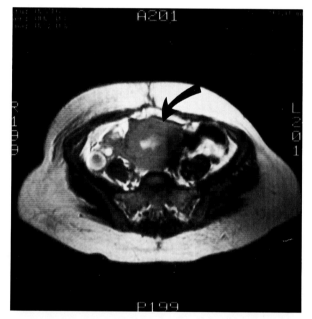

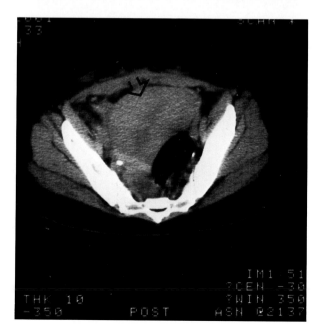

250: Recurrent Uterine Malignancy (.6T)

EXAM: MRI of the pelvis.

CLINICAL INFORMATION: Rule out recurrent malignancy following hysterectomy in proven uterine neoplasm.

TECHNIQUE: Sagittal and axial T1- and T2-weighted images were obtained (2000/32,400/32).

FINDINGS: A 5 × 3 cm lobulated mass appears to be rising from the posterior bladder wall. It extends to the right. It has fairly well-marginated edges and does not appear to invade the pelvic musculature. This has a fairly homogeneous signal, slightly more intense than that of normal pelvic musculature.

IMPRESSION: Large right-sided pelvic mass, with invasion into the posterior bladder, is consistent with local recurrence of patient's prior uterine malignancy.

DISCUSSION: The bladder-wall invasion is well-identified (Image 2, large arrows). The ability to do sagittal imaging demonstrates the invasive behavior which may not be appreciated on the axial images of CT.

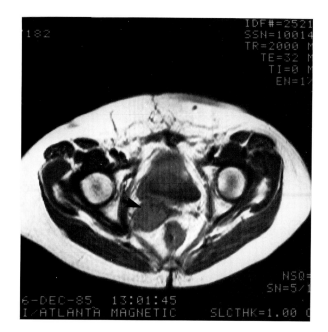

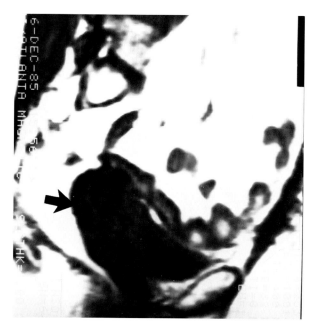

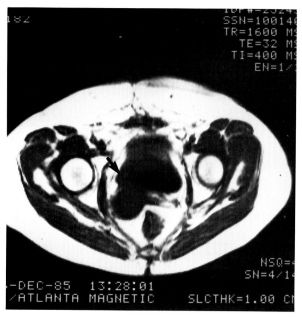

INDEX